The court and country cook : giving new and plain directions how to order all manner of entertainments, ... Together with new instructions for confectioners : ... How to prepare several sorts of liquors

François Massialot

The court and country cook : giving new and plain directions how to order all manner of entertainments, ... Together with new instructions for confectioners : ... How to prepare several sorts of liquors, ... Faithfully translated out of French into Englis
Massialot, François
ESTCID: T120659
Reproduction from British Library
Anonymous. By F. Massialot. A translation of 'Le cuisinier roial et bourgeois' and 'Nouvelle instruction pour les confitures, les liquers, et les fruits'. 'New instructions for confectioners' and 'New instructions for liquors' have separate pagination ;
London : printed by W. Onley, for A. and J. Churchill, and M. Gillyflower, 1702.
[48],276,130,20p.,plates : ill. ; 8°

neceſſary Proviſions; ſo it is no leſs requiſite, that he know how to make uſe of them to the beſt Advantage.

In this Book is alſo contain'd a very great number of common Meſſes, as of Chickens, Pigeons, and even of Butchers-meat, which may give a great deal of ſatisfaction, for indifferent Ordinaries, more eſpecially, in the Country: And in ſhort, it may be averr'd, That nothing has been omitted, which may contribute either to the Honourable Entertainment of a Perſon of Quality, or to the Aſſiſtance of the Officers employ'd in preparing it: Since without deviating from the beſt Ways, that are now in Uſe, a particular Deſcription has been always given, of every Thing, that may ſerve for all kinds of Tables, except thoſe of the meaner ſort of Country-People, on which it would be needleſs to inſiſt; becauſe the Management of them may be eaſily perform'd, when that of the others above-mention'd, is ſufficiently underſtood.

After having thus given an Account of the Deſign of this Book, and of the Uſefulneſs and Certainty of the Inſtructions contain'd in it; our *Court* and *Country Cook* does not fear the Cenſure of malevolent Carpers, unleſs it were for divulging the Secrets of his Art, to oblige the Publick; which is a very pardonable Offence, conſidering, That the Advantage of the Common-wealth ought to be preferr'd before that of private Perſons. It may happen, That in managing the Buſineſs ſeveral Ways, it may alſo be brought to good Effect, and therefore every Man is left to his liberty, to follow his own Method, which may tend to the ſame purpoſe; provided, that care be taken, to order the reſpective Meſſes, with all poſſible Neatneſs; to ſeaſon them well, and to dreſs them according to Art.

It

It was defign'd to add here, what relates to thofe Officers, whofe Bufinefs it is to look after the Deferts, that is to fay, the Fruits, Sweet-meats, Comfits, Liquors, &c. But forafmuch as the prefent Volume has already attain'd to a fufficient Bulk, we have contented our felves only to touch upon fome Articles, by the Way; *viz.* fuch as are proper for Intermeffes, and others that ferve for the garnifhing of particular Difhes; referring the reft, to be treated of at large, in another Volume hereto annex'd, which is of no lefs Importance, and equally deferves a favourable Reception. It is alfo to be hop'd, That the *Court and Country-Cook*, will be as acceptable here, in an Englifh Drefs, as in that of his native Country; where three feveral Editions of his Work have been printed and fold, in a fhort fpace of Time: To that purpofe, care has been taken to make a faithful and fignificant Tranflation of it, and for the greater benefit of the Reader, to annex a Table, explaining all the difficult Terms of Art, and French Words us'd throughout the whole Work.

A

A TABLE of the Entertainments and Instructions contain'd in this Book.

[b]

A

A

A TABLE *explaining all the Terms of Art and French Words us'd in this Treatise of Cookery.*

A.

Andouille, a fort of Chitterling made either of Hoggs or Calves-gut, the former being stuff'd with Pork, and the other with Calves-chaudron, Udder, &c

Andouillet, minc'd Veal, with Bacon and other Ingredient rolled into a Pelt. *Andouillets for birthdays*, are also made of Eels and Carps flesh chop'd small or pounded in a Mortar

B.

Barbe Robert, a particular Way of dressing Hoggs ears

Bards, thin broad slices of Bacon, with which Capons, Pullets, Pigeons and other forts of Fowl are sometimes cover'd, before they are roasted, bak'd, or otherwise dress'd.

Beatilles, certain Tid bits, such as Cocks-combs, Livers, Gizzards and other Appurtenances of Fowls, of the same nature as Goose gibblets, which are usually put into Pies, Potages, &c. There are also *Beatilles* of Fish, as Roes, Livers, &c

Becafigo, or *Fig eater*, a little Bird like a Wheat-ear, being a kind of Ortolan

Beef a la mode, see the last Article of Beef in the Body of the Book.

Bignot, minc'd Meats made of the Breasts of Partridges and fat Pullets.

Bisk, a rich kind of Potage,

made of Quails, Capons, fat Pullets, and more especially of Pigeons roasted

Biset, a fort of Stock dove, or Wood-pigeon.

Blanc manger, a kind of Jelly made of Calves feet and other Ingredients, with pounded Almonds.

Bottons, Veal slice roll'd up with thin slices of fat Bacon and Gammon.

Boutilans, little Pies made of the Breasts of roasted Capons or Pullets, minc'd small with Calves-udder, Bacon, Herbs, &c

Bourgeoise, as Veal dress'd *à la Bourgeoise*, i.e. after the Country-fashion. See the second Article of Veal in the Body of the Book, under the Letter V

Bouton, a Dish of large *Bards*, or thin Slices of Bacon cover'd with a Farce and Ragoo, and bak'd between two Fires

Braises, or Meat dress'd *à la Braise*, that is to say, either broil'd upon the live Coals, or bak'd in a Pot, Pan, or Campain oven, between two Fires, *viz.* one underneath, and the other on the top of the Lid. This last Way of dressing Meat is much in vogue, and extremely heightens its relish

Brochette, as Chickens fried and stew'd *à la Brochette*, for which particular Way, see the fifth Article of Chickens

Burjous, or *Burjoles*, Strikes of

[b 2] Veal

Veal or other Meat, laid in a Stew-pan between thin Slices of Bacon, with the usual seasoning Ingredients, and bak'd between two Fire, pouring a Ragoo or Cullis upon them before they are serv'd up to Table

Butter may be us'd in Sauces, after three several manners, that is to say, 1 Natural, or only melted without any alteration, 2 Burnt, or fried brown till it turns as it were to an Oil, 3. Refined, or clarified, by boiling, and taking off the Scum.

C.

Apitalade, a particular Way of dressing Capons, Partridges and other sorts of Fowl.

Casserole, a Stew-pan, also a Loaf stuff'd with a Hash of roasted Pullets, Chickens, or other Roast meat, and dress'd in a Stew-pan of the same bigness as the Loaf Also a kind of Soop or Potage of Rice, &c. with a Ragoo

Cervelas, or *Cervelas*, a large kind of Sausage, well season'd and eaten cold in slices.

Ciboule, a young Chibbol, a sort of little Onion

Citrull, a kind of Cucumber of a Citron colour.

Civet a particular Way of dressing Chickens, Hares, and other sorts of Venison, first frying them brown in Lard, and afterwards stewing them in Broth. See the several Articles of Civet in the Body of the Book, under the Letter C.

Civet, or *à la Civet*, another manner of dressing Chickens, for which see the seventh Article of Chickens

Compote, Fruit, or Meat stewed For a *Compote* of Pigeons, see the fourth Articles of *Pigeons*.

Court-bouillon, a particular Way of boiling Fish, in Wine, Verjuice and Vinegar, with all sorts of Spice For Carp dress'd in a *Demi-court-bouillon*. See the sixth Article of *Carp*.

Crepines, a sort of Farce wrapt up in a Veal caul, call'd *Crepine* in *French* For Capons - livers dress'd *à la Crepine*, or in a Veal-caul, see the first Article of *Livers*.

Croquets, a certain Compound made of a delicious Farce, some of the bigness of an Egg, and others of a Walnut, the former may serve for a Side-dish, and the others only for Garnishing.

Cicutade, a peculiar manner of dressing a Loin of Mutton.

Cullis, a strained Liquor, made of any sort of Meat or other things pounded in a Mortar and pass'd thro' the Hair-sieve. These Cullises are usually pour'd upon Messes, either of Flesh or Fish, and into Pies, a little before they are brought to Table.

Cutlets, are made of the short Ribs of a Neck of Mutton or Veal, and take their Name from the *French* Word *Cotelette*, signifying a small Rib

Civet, a kind of oval Dish.

D

Dame Simonne, a particular Way of farcing Cabbage-lettice *à la Dame Simonne*, for which see the Article of Lettice

Daube, a certain peculiar manner of dressing a Leg of Veal, as also several sorts of Fish and Fowl,

Fowl, to find out which, recourse may be had to the General Table of the Messes

Dauphine, as Veal sweet breads farced *à la Dauphine,* as it were for the Dauphin's Table. This Dish is explain'd in the first Article of *Veal sweet breads.*

Demi-court bouillon, see *Court-bouillon.*

Douillet, as a Pig dress'd after a particular Way, call'd *au Pere Douillet.* See the fourth Article of *Piggs.* For Pigeons so order'd, see the last Article of *Pigeons* under the Letter P.

E.

Epigramme, as a Knuckle of Veal *à l' Epigramme,* a particular manner of dressing it.

Essence de Jambon, see *Gammon-essence.*

Estoufade, a particular Way of stewing Meat or other Things in an earthen Pan For a Leg of Veal so dress'd, see the last Article of *Leggs,* in the Body of this Work, under the Letter L.

F.

Farces, are usually made of several sorts of Meat and Herbs chopt small and well season'd with Spice, in order to stuff any Joint of Meat, Fowl, or Fish. Of these Farces there is very great variety, and some are distinguish'd by particular Names, as *Godivors, Mirotons, Poupetons, Salpicons,* &c.

Feuillantins and *Fleurons,* certain small Tarts or Puffs of fine Pastry work, proper for Garnishing, fill'd with Sweet meats, they serve for the garnishing of other Pies of a larger size, and are usually set among the Intermesses.

Filets, any sort of Butchers-meat, Fowl, or Fish cut into slices and dress'd in a Ragoo.

Filets mignons, large slices of Beef, Veal, or Mutton, spread over with a rich Farce, well roll'd up, and cover'd both underneath and on the top, with *Bards* or thin slices of Bacon; in order to be bak'd in a Stew-pan, between two Fires, and serv'd up with a good Cullis or Ragoo.

Fricandoes, a sort of *Scotch* Collops, made of thin slices of Veal well larded and farced, which are afterwards to be dress'd in a Stew-pan, close cover'd, over a gentle Fire.

G.

Galantine, as a sucking Pig serv'd up in *Galantine,* which remarkable manner of dressing is explain'd at large in the third Article of *Piggs.*

Gallimawfry, a kind of Hash; see a Shoulder of Mutton so dress'd in the Article of *Gallimawfry,* under the Letter G.

Gammon essence, is made of thin slices of Gammon dress'd in a Stew-pan with a Ragoo and afterwards strain'd thro' the Hair-sieve; to be put into all sorts of Messes, in which Gammon is us'd. See the first Article of *Gammon*

Gatee of Soles, a particular Way of dressing them

Gibelote, as Chickens dress'd *à la Gibelote,* for which see the tenth Article of *Chickens.*

Godard, or *à la Godard,* a particular Way of dressing a short Rib of Beef, described in the first Article of *Beef.*

Godivoe, a kind of delicious Farce

Farce made of Veal and several other sorts of Meats, or else of Carps, Pikes and other Fish, for Days of Abstinence.

Grenade, a Dish of larded Veal-collops bak'd in a round Stew pan between two Fires, with six Pigeons and a Ragoo in the middle, and cover'd on the top and underneath with thin slices of Bacon.

Grenadin is made of a good *Godrue,* or Farce laid upon thin slices of Bacon in a Baking-pan, with a hollow Place, to receive a Fowl cut into halves and dress'd in a Ragoo. *Grenadins* may be made of fat Pullets, Chickens, Pigeons, Partridges and all other sorts of Fowl.

Grillade, Meat broiled upon the Grid-iron.

H.

Haricot, a particular Way of dressing Mutton cutlets and several sorts of Fowl and Fish in a Ragoo, with Turneps, specified in the General Table of the Messes. Also a kind of *French Beans.*

Hatlets, a Dish of Veal-sweet-breads, Capons livers and young Bacon, cut into small pieces and fried, with a little Flower, in order to be spitted on small Skewers, breaded, and broil'd or fried

Hugenote, or *a la Huguenote,* a particular Way of dressing Eggs with Gravy. See the tenth Article of *Eggs.*

I.

Jale bre, a kind of Potage, with Cheese.

Intremesses, Courses set on the Table between other Dishes

Julian, a very considerable Po-

tage made of a Leg of Mutton roasted and put into a great Pot or Kettle with a good piece of Beef, a Fillet of Veal, a fat Capon, all sorts of Roots and some Herbs Another sort of *Julian* is also prepar'd for Fish days.

Jus lie, thick Gravy of Beef or Veal.

L.

Lardoon, a small slip of Bacon proper for Larding.

M.

Marinade, pickled Meat, either of Flesh or Fish.

Matelotte, as Cucumbers dress'd *à la Matelotte,* or after the Seaman's Way, for which see the second Article of *Cucumbers.*

Mavurette, a kind of Mavis or Thrush

Mazarine, or *à la Mazarine,* a particular Way of dressing several sorts of Fowl, more especially Pigeons and Chickens, for the latter, see the third Article of *Chickens*

Menehout, or *à la Sainte Menehout,* a peculiar Manner of baking Meat cover'd with Buds or thin slices of Bacon, either in an Oven, or between two Fires For a Loin of Mutton so dress'd, see the fifth Article of *Mutton,* for Piggs petitoes, the last Article of *Piggs,* for fat Pullets, the third Article of *Pullets,* and for Pigeons, the seventh Article of *Pigeons*

Menus droits, or *Mine droit,* a certain Dish proper for Intermesses, made of different Things, among others of an Ox palate, or of Stags flesh, cut into thin slices, and fried. See the Article of *Me-*

nus-

nus drotts, under the Letter M.

Meringues, a sort of Confection made of the Whites of Eggs Whipt, fine Sugar and grated Lemmon-peel, of the bigness of a Walnut They are proper for the garnishing of several Dishes.

Miroton, a kind of Farce made of Veal, Bacon, &c. or else of Fish, and dress'd several Ways, for which see the respective Articles in the Body of the Book under the Letter M.

Miroir, as Eggs dress'd *au Miroir*, that is to say, broken into a Plate full of Gravy, over a Chafing dish, and afterwards ic'd with the red-hot Fire shovel.

Mode, as Beef *à la Mode*, a particular Way of dressing it See the last Article of *Beef*.

Morille, the smallest and most delicious kind of red Mushrooms.

Mousseron, a sort of white Mushroom.

N

Antilles, Lentils a sort of Pulse.

O.

Il, a very rich *Potage* after the *Spanish* Way, made of Buttock-beef, part of a Fillet of Veal, a piece of a Leg of Mutton, and another of raw Gammon, as also Ducks, Partridges, Pigeons, Chickens, Quails, Sausages and a Cervelas, all fried brown and afterwards boil'd with all sorts of Roots and Herbs Other kinds of *Oils* are also prepar'd for Fish-days, with Peas soop, several sorts of Fish, Roots and Pulse.

Omelet, a kind of Pancake made of Eggs

Ortolan, a delicate Fowl of an exquisite taste, about the bigness of a Lark.

Out works, Courses of Dishes set on the out side of the Table.

P.

Ains, i e. Loaves, divers Messes proper for Side-dishes so call'd as being made of Bread stuff'd with several sorts of Farces and Ragoo's· See the respective Articles in the Body of the Book.

A la Parisienne, a particular Way of making Pies, after the Mode of the City of *Paris*

Parmesan, Cheese brought from the City of *Parma* in *Italy*.

Petits choux, i e. small Coleworts, a sort of Paste for garnishing, made of fat Cheese, Flower, Eggs, Salt, &c. bak'd in a Pie-pan and iced over with fine Sugar: See the Article of *Cabbage* and *Coleworts*.

Petits patez, little Pies.

Poleacre, or *a la Poleacre*, a particular Way of dressing Chickens and other sorts of Fowl.

Poor man's Sauce, or Carrier's Sauce, a Sauce made of Shalot cut very small, with Salt, white Pepper, Vinegar and Oil of Olives.

Potage de Sante, i. e. *health potage*, a rich Potage made of the Broth of Buttock-Beef, with a knuckle of Veal and Mutton, boil'd again in a Pot with Capons, fat Pullets or other sorts of Fowl, proper for that purpose *Potage de Sante* for Fish day is likewise prepar'd, with chopt Lettice, Purslain, Sorrel, Beets, and other savoury Herbs first stew'd in an earthen Pot with Butter, and afterwards boil'd in Water.

Potpourri, a Hotch-potch, or

Dish

Difh of feveral forts of Meat, as Ducks, young Turkeys, Leverets, &c. firft larded and fried in Lard to give them a colour, and afterwards ftew'd in Broth with white Wine, Pepper, Salt, a Bunch of Herbs, &c.

Poupeton, a particular Mefs made in a Stew-pan, as it were a Pie, with thin flices of Bacon laid underneath, Pigeons, Quails, or other forts of Fowl drefs'd in a Ragoo in the middle, and a peculiar Farce call'd *Godivoe* on the top, in order to be bak'd between two gentle Fires. For Days of Abftinence, the *Poupeton* muft be prepar'd with a good Fifh-*Godivoe* and Sole-*Filets*, or others in a Ragoo, as alfo a fine Artichoke-bottom in the middle. See the Articles of *Godivoe* and *Poupeton*.

Poulets Mignons, a Difh of roafted Chickens larded and barded. See the eighteenth Article of *Chickens*.

Poupiets, are made of fomewhat long and thin flices of Bacon, cover'd with Veal flakes of the fame bignefs, as alfo with a good Farce, in order to be roll'd up, and roafted on a little Iron-Spit, wrapt up in Paper.

Profitrolles, certain fmall round Loaves farced and fet in the middle of feveral forts of Potages. See the Article of Potages

Prunes de Brignoles, Prunelloes.

R.

Ragoo, a high feafon'd Difh, after the *French* Way

Ramequins, fmall flices of Bread-crum cover'd with a Farce made of pounded Cheefe, Eggs and o-ther Ingredients, and bak'd in a Pie-pan. They may be made of a round or fquare Figure, and ferve, either for Out works, or to garnifh other Difhes

Ramolade, a particular Sauce, made of Parfley, Chibbol, Anchovies and Capers, all chopt fmall and well temper'd in a Difh, with a little Pepper, Salt, Nutmeg, Oil, and Vinegar

A la Reyne & à la Royale, certain peculiar Ways of dreffing Meat, more efpecially Beef, as it were for the King and Queen's Table. There are alfo feveral Potages fo call'd, for which fee the refpective Articles.

Riffoles, a fort of minced Pie made of Capons-breafts, Calves-udder, Marrow, Bacon, fine Herbs, &c and fried in Lard to give it a fine colour. *Riffoles* may be alfo prepar'd, for Days of Abftinence, with a delicious Fifh farce, or even with white Mufhrooms and Spinage.

Robert fauce, a Sauce made of Onions, Muftard, Butter, Pepper, Salt and Vinegar

Rocambole, a kind of fmall Garlick of the bignefs of a Shalot

Roulades, Veal flakes, thin flices of Bacon and other flices of a Calves or a Sheep's Tongue, all cover'd with a particular Farce, roll'd up together, and boil'd in a Pot.

S.

Saingaraz, as Rabbets drefs'd à la *Saingaraz*, that is to fay, larded, roafted and put into a Ragoo of Gammon. Fat Pullets, Pigeons and Chickens may alfo be drefs'd in the fame manner. See the Article of *Rabbets.* S4

Salmigund, a kind of Hotch-potch, or Ragoo of several sorts of cold Meats cut into pieces and stewed on a Chafing-dish, with Wine, Verjuice, Vinegar, &c.

Salpicon, a kind of Ragoo or Farce made of Gammon, Capons-livers, fat Pullets, Mushrooms, *Truffles*, &c. proper for large roasted Joints of Beef, Veal, or Mutton, more especially Leggs, making a Hole in them, taking away the Meat, and substituting this Ragoo in its room. See the Article of *Salpicon*, in the Body of the Book, under the Letter S.

Sauce, see *White Sauce*.

Souse, a certain compound Souse or Jelly made of Hoggs-Ears and Feet, boil'd in Water, and afterwards being cut into small pieces, stew'd in Vinegar and Sugar

Spatula, a Spatule or Slice to stir Liquors or any sort of Butter

Sur tout, as Pigeons dress'd in *Sur tout*, that is to say, farced, tied up, and every one cover'd on the Breast with a larded Veal collop, in order to be roasted, wrapt up in Paper, and serv'd up in a Ragoo or Cullis Partridges, Wood cocks and other sorts of Fowl may also be dress'd in this manner. See the eighth Article of *Pigeons*.

T

Tartre, or *a la Tartre*, a particular Way of dressing

Chickens, after they have been breaded and cut upon the Grid-iron

Terrine, a very considerable Mess made of a Breast of Mutton cut into pieces, with Quails, Pigeons and Chickens all stew'd in an earthen Pan call'd *Terrine* in French, cover'd with slices of Bacon on the bottom and set between two certain Fires.

Tourte, a Pie bak'd in a Pan of which there are several sorts See the Article of *Tourte*, under the Letter T, in the Body of the Book.

Truffles, a kind of Mushroom, or Puff, cover'd with a blackish Skin, without either Stalk or Root, which grows within the Ground, especially after great Rains.

V.

Vermicelli, i.e. *little Worms*, a sort of Italian Dish made of very small thin slips of Paste, season'd with white Pepper, Salt and *Milan* Cheese, all grated and put into Potage or Soop, with some other Ingredients.

W.

White Sauce, a Sauce made of blanched Almonds and the Breast of a Capon, pounded together, adding Cinnamon, Cloves, Ginger Rose-water and

A General TABLE of the Messes, the particular manner of preparing which, is described at large in this Work.

[c 2]   CHIT-

Filets

[d 2] With

SE a·

THE

THE
PREFACE
TO THE
READER.

SInce this Work is not the firſt that has been ſet
forth on the ſame Subject, there is no neceſſity
of juſtifying the Deſign of it againſt the Cavils
of malevolent and cenſorious Carpers, who are
no leſs ready to debar Mankind of the Uſe of theſe
ſorts of Dainties, than of that of Ragoo's and high-
ſeaſon'd Meats, a juſt Vindication of which is in-
ſcrib'd in the Preface to the *Court and Country-Cook*,
equally oppoſing their erroneous Opinion, That theſe
Dainties tend only to the impairing of the Health and
the ſhortening of Humane Life: And indeed, nothing
is more natural than ſuch an Apology, in this Caſe;
not to make mention of Fruits, againſt the uſe of
which, without doubt, no Objection can be made, as
being the moſt innocent Productions of Nature. As
for the reſt of theſe Varieties, when us'd with due
moderation (which is always to be preſuppos'd) do
they not afford almoſt innumerable Delights and Ad-
vantages; to deny which to the Exigencies of Mankind would be a ſignal Piece of Injuſtice, more eſpecially in regard that they are of ſo great energy in the
comforting as well of healthful Perſons, as of thoſe
that are ſick, or indiſpos'd?

[a a]   This

THIS is a Truth fo well known, that the Ufe of Sweet-meats, is allow'd even in the moft retired Families, and befides the peculiar Trade of Confectioners, there are many Perfons of Quality, and accomplifh'd Ladies, who fometimes divert themfelves with making feveral forts of Comfits. Therefore perhaps it may be objected, That there is no need of any new Inftructions in a Matter that is fo obvious, but if other Arts are daily improv'd, is there not ground to believe, that this may alfo be brought to farther Perfection? Which will be more plainly made manifeft by means of this Treatife, wherein are contain'd feveral Methods of Preferving Fruits and other particular Circumftances, that are altogether new, and quite different from the common Practice, as alfo from what has been before written on this Subject by any Authors: For it may be fufpected, That in laying down fuch imperfect Rules and Directions, (not to mention the unprofitable Repetitions us'd by them, on purpofe to augment the Bulk of their Volumes) they had no other Defign but to abufe the Publick; being fully refolv'd before hand, not to difcover the Secrets of their Art.

Indeed, it is certain, That fuch a Difcovery (as it ought to be expected here) cannot be really made by any Perfon, without doing himfelf a confiderable Injury, in regard, that by reafon of the eafinefs of making all forts of wet and dry Sweet-meats, according to the Inftructions that are given, the meaneft Houfe-keepers, or Chamber-maids might afterwards fet up for Confectioners and Butlers, and perform the greateft Part of the Functions of thofe Officers: Hence it comes to pafs, that fo great a Number of Noble Families ufually difpenfe with fuch Officers; and how many other Artifts of the firft Rank would be likewife difregarded, if the Oeconomy of that Northern Prince were in requeft, who having once caus'd his Defert

to

to be dreſs'd, orders it to be carefully lock'd up in his Preſence, in the Appartment, where he takes his Royal Repaſt, every time that it is ſerv'd up to his Table, which is as long as it laſts, and always keeps the Key in his Pocket?

Foraſmuch as the Officers of the Mouth are employ'd to ſomewhat better purpoſe, in theſe Parts, it is here deſign'd to do them a Pleaſure, by cauſing them to be inſtructed in every Thing that is moſt modern, generally receiv'd, and moſt curious, relating to the principal Part of their Employment, that is to ſay, the Art of Preſerving Sweet-meats, treating of it as methodically, and with as much Perſpicuity, as is poſſible. It is acknowledg'd, That if any Perſons be deſirous to attain to Perfection in this Art, and to comprehend all its abſtruſe Myſteries, with greater Facility, 'tis requiſite, that they work for ſome time, under thoſe that are Maſters of it; ſo that by the means of frequent Practice, they'll ſoon underſtand, at a caſt of the Eye, ſeveral Preparations, which cannot otherwiſe be well explain'd: Among theſe, the particular Way of making Sugar-plums, is more eſpecially remarkable, as abſolutely depending upon an habitual Exerciſe, and this Reflection affords Matter of Conſolation, to Maſter-Confectioners and other Officers, who have laid out Money and ſpent a conſiderable time in acquiring their Skill, and who may perhaps take it ill, that the Grounds of their Art are ſo freely communicated to Perſons, that may make uſe of it to their Prejudice.

However, if the Advantage, in this Particular redounds to the Publick, they themſelves may alſo receive ſome Benefit, from the aſſiſtance of theſe Inſtructions, which may ſerve, as it were a Manual, for the refreſhing of their Memories, ſo that it will be an eaſy matter for them to take notice in every Seaſon, what is moſt proper to be Preſerv'd and brought to

Table,

Table, according to the Entertainments which are requifite upon feveral Occafions, and the particular Cuftoms of Noble-mens Houfes, in which they are entertain'd. If their Methods are not altogether conformable, in certain Articles, to that which is here exprefs'd, neverthelefs let them not reject it, till they have made a Tryal; and if after fuch an Experiment, they ftill have an Inclination to follow their accuftomed Practice, they may be at liberty to continue it: Altho' it may be averr'd, That nothing is here deliver'd, but what has been confirm'd by Experience, with refpect to the feveral Ways of Preferving the richeft and moft delicious forts of Sweet-meats and Comfits.

The whole Work is concluded with different Models for Deferts, or entire Banquets of Sweet-meats, and a fhort Treatife of Liquors, the ordering of which, belongs likewife to certain peculiar Officers: But no notice is here taken of fome other Circumftances relating to their domeftick Concerns; fuch as the diftribution of Bread and Wine, the care that ought to be taken of the Plate in their Cuftody, the particular manner of laying the Cloth, furnifhing the Table, &c. Becaufe the management of Affairs of the like nature is never committed to Novices, or Perfons who are fo ignorant, as to ftand in need of any other Inftructions in thefe Matters, than what their own Difcretion, or their Mafters Orders may readily fuggeft to them.

The

The Contents of the New Instructions for Confectioners.

Chap.

The

The Contents of the New Instructions for Liquors.

A TABLE

A TABLE *explaining certain Terms of Art and* French *Words us'd in these Instructions for Confectioners.*

B.

Bigarrade, a kind of great Orange.

Biscotin, a sort of Confection made of fine Flower, the Whites of Eggs, Powder-sugar, Marmelade, &c.

Blanquet, a sort of Pear.

C.

Caramel, the sixth and last Degree of Boiling Sugar : Also, a curious Sugar-work so call'd.

Cedre, a kind of Citron, or Lemmon.

Certoe, a sort of *French* Pear.

Compote, stewed Fruit, more especially Apples, Pears, Plums, &c.

D.

Dauphine, as a *Compote a la Dauphine,* a particular Way of stewing Apples; as it were, for the Dauphin's Table.

Desert, a Banquet of Sweetmeats.

F.

Feuillantins, certain small Tarts of the breadth of the Palm of a Man's Hand, fill'd with Sweetmeats.

I.

Indigo, a Stone brought out of *Turkey,* commonly us'd by Dyers to die blew; as also by Confectioners, to give their Jellies, Pastes, Sugar-works, &c. a blew Tincture.

M.

Mazarines, a sort of small Tarts fill'd with Sweetmeats.

Mirabolans, certain Plums, which are cold in the first Degree and dry in the second; serving to strengthen, purge and bind at the same time.

N.

Nompareil, a kind of small Sugar-plum.

O.

Orangeade, a cooling Liquor made of the Juice of Oranges and Lemmons, with Water and Sugar.

P.

Parmesan, a sort of Cheese made at *Parma,* a City of *Italy.*

Pastille, a kind of odoriferous Sugar-paste, of which there are several sorts specified under that Article, in the Body of the Book

Petit-choux, a kind of Paste, proper for garnishing and other uses made of Cheese, Flower, Eggs, Salt, &c. bak'd in a Pie-pan and ic'd over with fine Sugar.

R.

R.

RAtafiaz, a delicious Liquor made of Cherries, or Apricocks and other Fruits with their Kernels bruis'd, infus'd in Brandy, adding Sugar, Cinnamon, white Pepper, Nutmeg, Cloves, Mace, Ginger and some other Ingredients.

Rousselet, a kind of Russet-pear.

A la Royale, a particular Way of preserving Cherries as it were, after the Royal Manner.

S.

SIamoise, as *Amandes a la Siamoise,* a particular Way of preserving Almonds, explain'd under the first Article of that Fruit, Chap 7.

Sultane, a kind of Sugar-work, made of Eggs, Powder-sugar and fine Flower.

Sur-tout, as Pistachoes in *Surtout,* that is to say, cover'd with Sugar and order'd after the same manner, as Almond-sugar-plum: See the last Article of Almonds, Pag. 26.

T.

TAmbour, a kind of fine Sieve call'd a Drum, proper for the sifting of Sugar, &c.

Turning, a particular Way of paring Oranges and Lemmons This Term of Art signifies to pare off the superficial Rind, or Peel, on the out-side very thin and narrow, with a little Knife, proper for that purpose, turning it round about the Lemmon or Orange, so as the Peel may be extended to a very great length, without Breaking.

Z

ZEsts, certain Chips of Orange, or Lemmon-peel, cut long-wise, from top to bottom, as thin, as it can possibly be done. See the second Article of *Lemmons.*

[bb]   A

A General TABLE of the Sweet-meats, Comfits, Sugar-works, Fruits and other Matters contain'd in this Treatise of the Confectionary Art.

A **Table** *of the Waters, Syrups, Juices, and other Matters contain'd in the Instructions for Liquors.*

N E W.

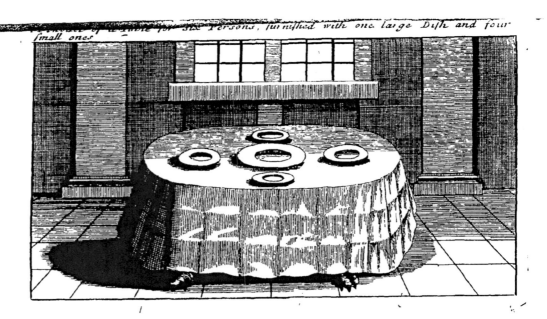

...... of a Table for six Persons, furnished with one large Dish and four small ones

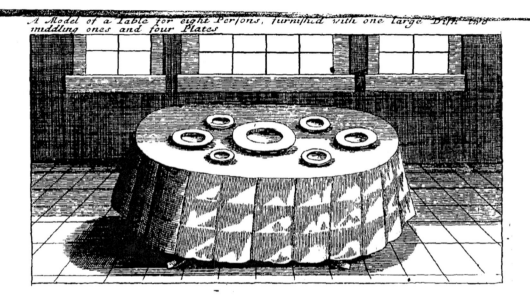

A Model of a Table for eight Persons, furnished with one large Dish two middling ones and four Plates

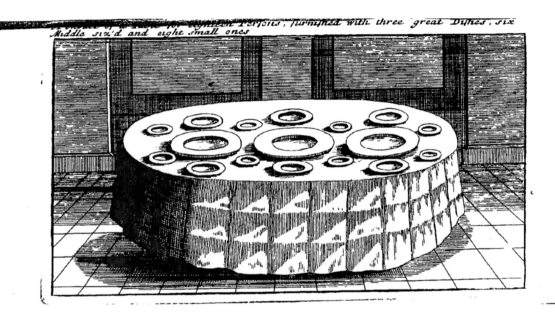

A Frame of a Table for eighteen Persons, furnished with three great Dishes, six Middle siz'd and eight small ones

A Model of a Table for fourteen or fifteen Persons furnished with one large Dish two middling ones six small ones and four Plates

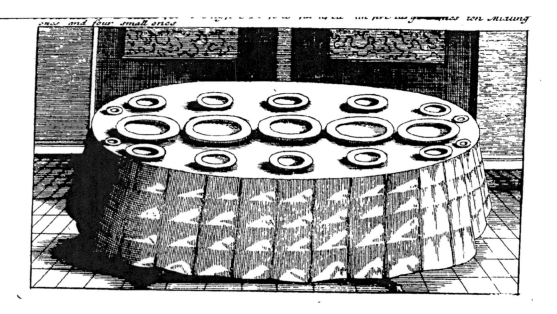

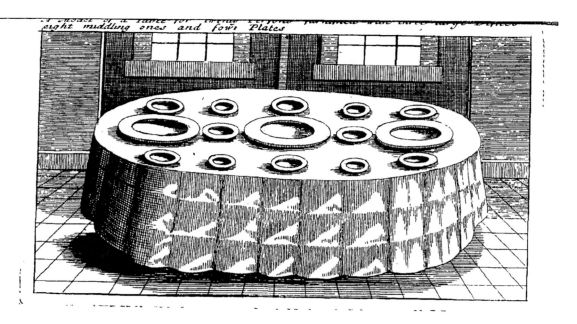

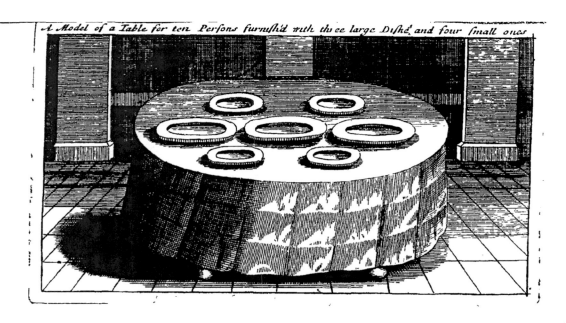

A Model of a Table for ten Persons furnish'd with three large Dishes and four small ones

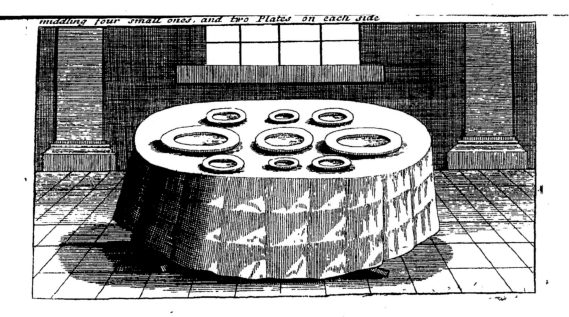

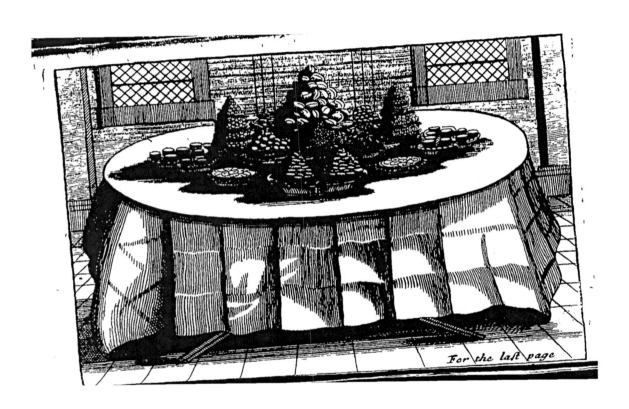

For the laſt page

THE

Court and Country Cook:

DIRECTING

How to Order all manner of ENTER-
TAINMENTS and the beſt ſort of the
moſt exquiſite *a-la-mode* RAGOO's.

The Entertainment which may be made in the Month of
January.

SUppoſe a Table were to be furniſhed for twelve Perſons,
one large Diſh in the middle, four leſſer Diſhes, and four
Out-works may ſerve for each Courſe: For Example,

The Firſt Courſe.

Potages and Side-diſhes.

Two Potages, one middling Diſh of a *Biſk* of Pigeons, and
the other of Capon with Roots

Two other middling Diſhes for Side-diſhes; *viz.* one a Partridge pye hot.

The other of a large fat Pullet and *Truffles* garniſh'd with
Fricandoe's.

The great Diſh in the middle

This ſhall conſiſt of two Pieces of roaſt Beef, garniſh'd with
Cutlets of marinated Veal fried, with good Sauce.

B   *For*

For the Out-works.

A *Poupeton* of Pigeons.
A Dish of Quails broil'd upon the Coals.
One of farced Pullets, with Cullises or strained Liquor of Mushrooms.
One of Partridges, with Spanish Sauce.

The Second Course.

The Roast-meat.

This shall consist of two middling Dishes, *viz*
One of a young Turkey garnish'd with Partridges, Chickens, Wood-cocks and *Mauviettes*
And the other of a Quarter of Lamb garnish'd after the same manner.

For the Intermesses.

A Cream-tart for the great Dish in the middle, garnished with Puffs, *Feuillantins, Fleurons*, and Milk-*bignets* or Fritters.
The two other smaller Dishes, one of them of *Pain au Jambon*, garnish'd with small Toasts of Bread and Lemmon.
And the other of Gammon of Bacon and other Salt-meats.

The Out-works

One of these shall consist of a *Blanc-manger*.
Another of the Livers of Capons
The third of Asparagus in a Sallet.
And the fourth of *Truffles* in a *Court-bouillon*.

The Third Course.

This is to consist of Fruits and Confits, of which we shall say nothing in this place, that being the particular Business of another Officer and not of the Cook.

Such an Entertainment as this above-mentioned was made *Feb.* 15, 1691, by the Duke of *Chartres* for Mademoiselle his Sister.

Instead of what was served up for Roast-meat, two Dishes may be prepared, *viz* one consisting of two fat and large young Hens, four Barn-door Pullets, and six wild Pigeons:

The other of Water-fowl, four Partridges, four Wood-cocks, and a douzen of Snipes.   The

The Particulars hereafter fpecified may ferve inftead of the reft for the Side-difhes and Intermeffes as well as for the following Entertainments *See* Page 7

According to this firft Entertainment you may eafily regulate the Ordering and Difpofition of the reft, which you would have made greater, by increafing the Number or Largenefs of the Difhes in proportion to the Number of the Guefts and Tables.

An Entertainment for the Months of February *and* March

The First Courfe.

Side-difhes

FOr the firft Courfe, An hot Pye of young Rabbets and Partridges, in which may be put, during the time of ferving, fome good Cullife of Partridge or other Ragoo's

A *Poupeton* farced with twenty or thirty young Pigeons, according to the number of Guefts entertained, with all forts of Garnitures

A Difh of *Brufelles*, broiled upon the Coals, with a Cullife pour'd upon it

A Difh of farced Sweet breads of Veal, broiled upon the Coals, with a Ragoo

A *Marinade* of fryed Chickens.

A large fat Pullet roafted after the Englifh Way, with a Ragoo put thereupon in ferving it up

A Difh of *Filets* cut in flices, with Gammon

A Difh of *Croquets*

One of *Filets* of a young fat Hen with Cucumbers.

One of farced *Fricandoe's* in a Ragoo

The Second Courfe

The Roaft-meat

Let there be three great Difhes of all forts of wild Fowl that are in feafon, and four Sallets in the Corners, proportionably to the Courfes that are ferved up, and the Guefts that fit at Table

For the Intermeffes

Twelve Difhes, viz. One of Gammon, garnifh'd with dry'd Tongues, and *Bolonia*-faufages

B 2   A

A Cream-pye garnifh'd with little Tarts.

A *Blanc-manger* of Gellies of divers Colours.

A Difh of Afparagus in Cream

One of *Morilles* in Cream

One of Sweet-breads of Veal and Cocks-combs farced in a Ragoo.

One of marinated Sweet-breads of Veal fryed.

One of Capons-livers *à la Crêpine,* broil'd upon the Grid-iron.

One of the Kidneys of Capons.

One *Pain au Jambon*

A Difh of *Truffles* in a *Court-bouillon*

A Ragoo of the Sweet-breads of Veal, white Mufhrooms and *Morilles.*

Monfieur *Langlois* caus'd fuch a Supper as this to be made, *March* 28, 1690, for the Duke of *Orleans* There was for the Duke himfelf *Potage de Sante* prepared of a fat Pullet with Eggs in her, and of a Capon

For this Entertainment they roafted fat and large Hens, Chickens and Partridges, that were ufed only in making of the farced Meats; particularly a Farce of *Croquets* For this purpofe, they took the Breafts and Legs of thefe Fowls, and left fome *Filets* for the Side-difhes. This fort of farc'd Meat was made with parboil'd Bacon, Calves-udder boil'd, Sweet-breads of Veal parboil'd, *Truffles* and minc'd Mufhrooms, fome Marrow, Crums of Bread fteeped in Milk, all forts of fine Herbs, a little Cream-cheefe, and fome Milk cream: The whole being well minced and feafoned, four or five Yolks of Eggs were put thereto, and the Whites of one or two: And this Farce was made ufe of for the *Fricandoe's, Croquets,* and *Filets Mignons.* The *Croquets* are made round, of the bignefs of an Egg; they are to be breaded at the fame time, and left in a Difh, to be fryed with Lard and ferved up hot.

The Carcaffes of Fowls may ferve to make different forts of Cullifes for the diverfifying of the Ragoo's, Strainings may alfo be made of Bread, Partridge, young Hens, Pullets, *Effence de Jambon,* Beef and Veal-gravy The Ragoo's of Side-difhes and Intermeffes are drefs'd apart into different Stew-pans with a Faggot of fweet Herbs always put thereto

Thofe that have Cream put to them, ought to be tofs'd up with good Butter, and a little Flower muft be put to each Ragoo; which being ready, the Cream is to be poured on them, and

in

in ſerving up the ſame they are thickned with ſome Yolks of Eggs.

You may hereafter obſerve the Method of managing the reſt we have taken notice of, as well for Side-diſhes as Intermeſſes, when we have run through the other Months of the Year, and ſeen what is proper, to be ſerved up every Seaſon, as we have already begun to do.

An Entertainment for the ſame Month of March.

The Firſt Courſe.

Potages.

A Potage of Capons, with Culliſes of Lambs-livers, may be uſed.

One of Lambs-heads in green Peaſe-potage, garniſh'd with their Feet

And a large fat Pullet in a *Bisk.*

Great Side-diſhes.

A great Piece of Beef

A Breaſt of Veal farced in a Ragoo.

A Fricaſſy of Chickens, garniſh'd with a *Marinade* of Chickens.

The ſmall Side-diſhes.

One of Cutlets of Mutton broiled upon a Grid-iron.

And the other of ſmall *Bouillans* made of the Breaſts of Capons.

The Second Courſe.

For the Roaſt.

A Diſh of a roaſted Capon, breaded and garniſh'd with three Pigeons and three Chickens.

A Leg of Mutton, breaded and garniſh'd with the ſame.

A Loin of Veal garniſh'd with a *Marinade* of Veal round a-bout.

A Diſh of two roaſted Ducks with Sauce.

One of two Rabbets.

And for the ſmaller Diſhes, ſome large and fat Pullets breaded.

The

The Intermesses.

Shall be of a Ragoo of Artichokes

A Dish of *Truffles* and Capons-livers in a Ragoo

A Cream tart and a *Blanc-manger*.

A Dish of breaded Mushrooms baked

One of new-laid Eggs, *à la Huguenotte*.

One of *Pain au Jambon*

Apple-fritters

And two Plates of Salt-meat

This was the Duke of *Orleans*'s Dinner, *March* 26, 1690, being Easter-day

---

For Supper.

Potages

A *Potage de Santé* with a Capon

A Bisk of Capons, or of Pigeons

And a Potage of a young Hen with Eggs in her, nothing but good Gravy to be put into it

The Side-dishes

The Sweet-breads of Veal larded and roasted, with good Sauce.

Two large fat Pullets roasted with a Ragoo underneath

And a Dish of stewed Pigeons

The Roast.

A Loin of Veal garnished with three Pigeons and three Chickens, one half larded and the other barded

A Leg of Mutton breaded and garnish'd after the same manner

A Dish of two larded Rabbets

And one of six roasted Pigeons

This is the ordinary Supper of the Duke of *Orleans*, all the difference is, that the Potages and Intermesses vary according to the Season of the Year

The Dutchess's Table is usually served with a large Potage, a great Dish of Roast-meat, a Dish of Intermesses, and two small Dishes at each Service.

A List of what may serve, during the Months of January, February *and* March, *besides the forementioned Dishes.*

Potages.

A Potage of Larks according to the English Mode.
A Potage of Quails with a *Bouillon-brun*
A Potage of boned Capon with Cardons and Cheese.
Potage of a Sucking-pig
Potage of a Chine of Pork with strained Pease
Potage of Pheasants with a *Pot-pourri*, or Hotch-potch.
Potage of Cheese, or *Jacobine*
Potage of a Leg of Veal farced.
Potage of a young fat Hen, with *Milan*-cabbage.
Potage of young Rabbets according to the Italian Mode.
Potage of *Mauviettes* with a *Bouill-n-brun*
Potage of a fat Goose with Turneps.
Potage of Partridges with Mushrooms
Potage of Partridges, *a la Reine* and *à la Royale*, (as they call it)
Potage of young Pigeons crammed
Potage of Turkey according to the German Mode.
Potage of farced Pullets
Potage of Wood-pigeons with green Cole-worts
Potage of Rice.
Potage of Teals with strained Turneps.

Side-dishes

Lamb in a Ragoo
Larks in a Ragoo, according to the English Mode
A short Rib of Beef, after the English Manner
Andouilles, or Chitterlings of Hoggs-guts
Andouillets according to the Spanish Way
Puddings
A Sucking-pig *au Blanc*
Legs of Mutton prepared divers ways
A Shoulder of Mutton in a Ragoo
A Leg of Veal stewed.
A Turkey broiled and served up cold.
An Hash of Partridge-breasts.
A Leveret or young Hare, according to the Swiss Mode
A Partridge in a Ragoo.

Young

Young Pigeons according to the Italian Mode.
A Turkey in a *Pot-pourri.*
Pullets according to the Spanish Way.
A *Pot-pourri* of Green-geese
A Loin of Mutton according to the Swiss Mode.
Sausages.
Beef with Vinegar and Pepper.

They also make use of hot Pies of several sorts, which may be hereafter specified, when we have done with that which belongs to every Season, together with cold Pies and Tarts, which may serve for Intermesses; because they hold out almost the whole Year

There are also several other sorts of Intermesses, of which a general Supplement may be made, tho' there are very many in the Entertainments that are set down for the ensuing Months

As for Rost-meats, the following Fowls may be used:

Larks,	Wood-hens,
Wood-cocks,	Rabbets,
Snipes,	Leverets,
Bitterns,	Fat Geese,
Stock-doves,	*Mauviettes,*
Quails,	Plovers,
Ducks,	Turkies,
Fat Capons,	Capons or Wood-pigeons,
Barn-door Capons, or Pullets,	Young fat Hens,
Partridges,	Teals,
Wild Pigeons,	Lapwings.
Pheasants,	

These sorts of Meats are also in their Season for the Months of *October,* *November* and *December,* and some of the following Months, may be added; which will be remarked hereafter in due Place.

Enter-

Entertainments for the Month of April.

The First Courfe.

Potages

TWo forts of Potages, *viz.* A *Bisk* of Pigeons, and a *Potage de Santé*, with a young fat Hen.

The Side-difhes.

A Quarter of Mutton farced.
A large fat Pullet in a Ragoo.
A Breaft of Veal farced.
Pigeons with fweet Bafil in their Bodies, together with a fmall Farce ; and a large Piece of Beef in the middle.

The Second Courfe.

For the Roaft.

A great Difh of Roaft-meat, confifting of feveral Fowls, according to their Seafon, and two Sallets.

The Intermeffes.

A Difh of *Pain au Jambon.*
Boil'd Cream.
A Ragoo of Sweet-breads of Veal and Capons-livers.
A Difh of Afparagus with Sauce of *Jus lié,* or thick Gravy.
And fo there may be feven Difhes for each Courfe.

The Marquefs *d'Arci,* formerly the French King's Ambaffadour at *Turin,* and fince Tutour to the Duke of *Chartres,* gave fuch an Entertainment at his Houfe on the 10th Day of *April,* 1690.

Another

Another Dinner for the same time.

The First Course.

Potages

TWo Potages, one of farced Pullets with Asparagus, and the other *Potage de Santé*, with a young fat Hen garnish'd with Roots.

For the Side-dishes

A *Poupeton* farced, with six Pigeons in a Ragoo
Pullets or Chickens with Gammon.
Calves-tongues farced and ragoo'd.
One or two young fat Hens in a Ragoo with *Truffles*
A large Breast of Veal, garnished with farced Cutlets of Mutton.

The Second Course.

The Roast

A great Dish of Roast-meat, consisting of divers Fowls and two Sallets.

The Intermesses

The Sweet-breads of Veal in a Ragoo with Mushrooms and *Truffles*, besides good Cullises put into it.
Asparagus with Sauce of *Jus lié*.
A Marrow-pye.
A *Blanc-manger*.

The Out-works.

A Dish of the Bottoms of Artichokes with Cream
One of Salt-meat in Slices.

This Dinner was prepared at the Marquess *d'Arci*'s, as also that which follows, for the Duke *de Chartres* and Mademoiselle his Sister, *April* 18, 1690.

Another

Another Dinner for the Month of April.

The First Course.

Potages.

TWo *Potages de Sante* with two young fat Hens, garnished with Aſparagus-tops
One of farc'd Pullets, garniſh'd with farc'd Lettices.
A *Bisk* of Pigeons.
A Potage of Partridges, with Cullifes *à la Reine.*

The Side-diſhes of the Table.

For the grand Side-diſh, you are to have a Quarter of Veal, garniſh'd with fried Bread and Cutlets of fried Veal, larded with *Hatlets,* and a *Salpicon* put upon the Leg
The others are a *Poupeton* farc'd with ſix young Pigeons
A *Miroton*
Sweet-breads of Veal, larded and farced in a Ragoo
A Diſh of *Filets* of large fat Hens with Oiſters
And a Rabbet-pye

The Second Courſe.

For the Roaſt.

Two great Diſhes of Roaſt-meat, and two little ones conſiſting of ſeveral Fowls, with two Sallers

The Intermeſſes

A Diſh of Gammon, garniſh'd with Sauſages and dryed Tongues
A Tart of Almond-paſte farced with Marmelade of Apricocks
A *Blanc-manger*
A Diſh of Aſparagus, with ordinary Sauce.
One of *Morilles* in Cream.
One of *Mouſſerons,* or white Muſhrooms in a Ragoo with the red.
One of Capons-livers in a Ragoo.

The

The great Entertainment for the Month of May.

The First Course.

Potages.

FOur Bisks of Pigeons.

Four Potages of farced Pullets, garnished with farced Lettices.

Three Potages of Geese with green Pease, garnish'd with Asparagus-tops.

Three young Turkies with white Succory.

Two *Oils* served up in *Cuvets.*

The Side-dishes of the Table.

Four great Side-dishes and twelve middling ones.

Two of two Rumps of Veal, *de riviere,* garnish'd with Cutlets and larded with *Hatlets,* the Veal being half larded, and a *Salpicon* pour'd upon the Leg.

Two Dishes of Roast-meat, one of Beef, the other of Mutton, garnish'd with fried Bread, and *Marinade* of Mutton-cutlets.

For the twelve lesser Dishes.

Two Pies of young Rabbets.

Two Pigeon-pies.

Two hot Pies of young Turkies.

Two Pieces of powder'd Beef, with a Hash of Gammon thereupon

Two farced *Poupetons.*

Two *Mirotons.*

The Out-works.

Thirty two Dishes in number, *viz.*

Two of Pigeons with sweet Basil.

Two of Pullets with Gammon

Two of roasted Partridges with Spanish Sauce.

Two of *Filets Mignons,* with a Ragoo apart.

Two *Filets* of Beef with Cucumbers

Two Fricassies of Chickens with Cream.

Two of young Rabbets roasted, cut into two Parts, with Gammon-sauce.

Two of Mutton-*filets* in a Ragoo with *Morilles.*

Two

Two of farced Pullets in a Ragoo.
Two of farced Pullets broiled on the Coals with a Ragoo.
Two of farc'd *Fricandoe's*.
Two of Sweet breads of Veal and farced Gammon.
Two of farced Lettices, *à la Dame Simonne*
Two of Sweet-breads of Veal larded on the Spit, and when basted a good Ragoo put upon 'em
Two of *Fricandoe's* without being farced.
Two of *Pains au Veau*.

The Second Course.

For the Roast.

Sixteen Dishes of Roast-meat, and as many Potages, consisting of all sorts of Poultry, wild Fowl, young Boars, sucking Pigs, &c.
Ten small Sallets.

The Intermesses.

Two great Gammon-pies
Two others of young fat Hens and Mutton.
Ten lesser Dishes, viz.
Two of *Blanc-manger*.
Two of Salt-meats.
Two of Calves ears farc'd.
Two of *Galantine*
Two of Asparagus.

The Out-works.

Twenty two Out-works, which, with the ten Sallets, make up the same Number as in the first Course, *viz.*
Two of *Mine-droit*.
Two of Pigs-pettitoes, *à la Sainte Menehout*
Two of *Hatlets* broiled upon a Grid-iron and breaded.
Two of the Bottoms of Artichokes with Gammon-sauce.
Two of *Pain au Jambon*
Two of farced *Morilles* and *Mousserons* in a Ragoo.
Two of Cocks-combs farced and of Capons livers in a Ragoo.
Two Pies of the Breasts of Capons.
Two of small Pease in Cream
Two of *Rissoles*, made of the Breasts of Capons
Two of boil'd Cream.

For

For a like Entertainment, Provifion muft be made the Evening before, and at Night three or four great Kettles are to be hang'd over the Fire with ftore of Meat therein, Faggots of fine Herbs and whole Onions   You muft at the fame time boil a great many Pullets and fat Hens, and roaft fome Partridges, which, with parboil'd Bacon and Fat, fhall ferve for the farced Meats that are to be made for the next Day's Entertainment, and the *Bouillons* will ferve to make Beef and Veal-gravy, Soops, Cullifes, and *Effence de Jambon*

As for the Potages, the Gravies and ftrained Liquors are to be made apart, as alfo for the Side-difhes and Intermeffes You muft moreover have good ftore of *Chibbols* and chopped Parfly, and feveral Bunches of fine Herbs to be put into the Ragoo's Great quantities of Cullifes of Partridges, Pigeons and Pullets are likewife to be made, all by themfelves.

The Marquefs *de Seignelay* made fuch a fort of Entertainment at *Seaux* for the *Dauphin*, the Duke and Dutchefs of *Orleans*, the Duke of *Chartres* and Mademoifelle his Sifter, and the whole Retinue of the Court, *May* 14, 1690

The Kitchen-tackling ufed there, confifted in fixty fmall Hand-Stew-pans, twenty round ones, as well great as fmall, twenty Kettles or Pots of all forts, thirty Spits, and, to prepare this Entertainment, thirty fix Officers were employ'd , as well Mafter-Cooks as Affiftants, *&c*

Another Entertainment for the fame Month of May.

The Firft Courfe.

Potages

THree *Bisks* of Pigeons
    Three Potages of green Geefe with Peafe or Afparagus
Three of farced Pullets with green Peafe-foop.
Three *Julians* with young fat Hens.

The *Julians*, were garnifh'd with Cucumbers , the Geefe, with flices of young ftreaked Bacon , the Peafe-potage, with farced Lettices and Afparagus-tops , and the *Bisks*, with Lemmon

Side

The Side-dishes of the Table.

Two Pigeon-pies

Two Side-dishes of Beef somewhat corned.

Two of *Filets* of Beef with Cucumbers.

Two of the Fricassies of Chickens with Cream.

Two of young fat Pullets broiled upon the Coals.

Two *Mirotons*.

The Out-works

Two of Pies according to the Spanish Mode.

Two of Cutlets of Veal broiled upon the Grid-iron.

Two of young Rabbets, *à la Saingaraz*.

Two of Pigeons with sweet Basil.

Two *Grenadins* of a large fat Pullet.

The Second Course.

For Roast-meat.

Two Dishes of young wild Boars.

 Eight lesser Dishes, viz

Two with four young Turkies in each Dish.

Two of Chickens, garnish'd with young Pigeons.

Two of young Rabbets.

Two of Pheasants.

And eight small Sallets.

The Intermesses.

Two great Dishes of Gammon-pye.

Two dried Neats-tongues and Sausages

 Twelve lesser Dishes, viz.

Two of common Pease with Cream

Two of Artichokes *à l'Estoufade*.

Two of Mushrooms and Capons-livers

Two of *Pain au Jambon*.

Two of Asparagus in Cream.

Two of the Sweet-breads of Veal and Cocks-combs.

The Out-works

 Eight in number, viz

Two of *Blanc-manger*.

Two of Fritters

Two

Two of Calves-feet, *à la Sainte Menehout.*
Two Pies of the Breasts of Capons.
This Entertainment was made, *May* 18, 1690.

An Entertainment for the Month of June.

The First Course.

Potages

A Potage of young wild Ducks or Chickens with Pease, garnished with Cucumbers.
A *Bisk* of Pigeons.
A Potage of Turneps with a Duck.
A Potage of Cole-worts with a Partridge.
A *Potage de Sante* with a Capon.
A Potage of a *Casserole* with Parmesan.
A Potage of young Stock-doves
And another of Quails with Roots.

The Side-dishes of the Table.

The Leg of a Fawn with the Rump to it, half larded and half breaded, garnished with small Pies, and Sauce of Pepper and Vinegar.
A Piece of Beef somewhat corned and broil'd upon the Coals.
And for the great Side-dish, a Piece of roast Beef, garnish'd with a *Marinade* and Cutlets of fried Veal
Having taken off the Potages, the following Dishes were serv'd up:

The Out-works.

Sheeps-trotters farced, after the same manner as the *Croquets.*
A *Filet* of a young fat Hen with Oisters.
Sheeps-tongues broiled, with a *Ramolade* for Sauce
A Fricassy of Chickens with a Pike
A Turkey-powt farced with fine Herbs.

The Second Course.

The Roast-meat

Consists of a great Dish of all sorts of wild Fowl, with four Sallets.   T*he*

The Intermesses.

An Almond-pye.
A Dish of Artichokes, *à la Saingaraz,* garnish'd with fryed Artichokes
A Ragoo of Capons-livers Mushrooms and Gammon.
Pease in Cream, garnish'd with Cheese-*Ramequins.*

The Out-works.

Four in number, viz
One of Fritters made with Water.
One of *Rissoles*
One of Mushrooms in Cream
One of Eggs with the Juice of Oranges.

These are the ordinary Courses serv'd up at the French King's Table, and here follows the Model of an Entertainment made at Court for Monsieur *de Livri,* Principal Steward to his Majesty, *A. D.* 1690.

Another Entertainment for the Month of June.

A Table furnished for Twelve Persons.

The First Course.

A Great Potage, and six Side dishes The Potage is an *Oil* serv'd up in a *Cuvet* of Silver gilt, or another in a large Dish.

For the Side-dishes.

A Leveret-pye, hot.
A Side-dish of Pigeons, with Fennel.
A *Filet* of a young fat Hen, with Cucumbers.
A Side-dish of Veal-sweet-breads, *à la Dauphine.*
One of Loins of Mutton, *à la Sainte Menehout.*
One of farced *Fricandoe's*
The Dishes garnish'd with fryed Bread, *Croquets, Marinades* and *Pain aux Perdrix.*

C   *The*

The Second Course.

The Roast.

Four Dishes of all sorts of Fowl roasted, according to the Season; and a Piece of Roast-beef between others, garnish'd with *Hatlets* and two Sallets.

The Intermesses.

Stewed Artichokes, garnish'd with fried Artichokes; for the great Dish.

An Almond-pye, garnish'd with Apple-fritters.

Pease in Cream, garnish'd with Cheese-*Ramequins.*

A Dish of Gammon.

And one of *Rissoles.*

Another Entertainment for the Month of June.

The First Course.

Potages.

FOur in number, viz
  A *Bisk* of Pigeons.
A *Potage de Santé*, with a large fat Pullet
A Potage of farc'd Chickens, with green Pease-soop,
A Potage of Quails, after the manner of an *Oil.*

Side-dishes.

A great Side-dish, of a Loin of Veal, half larded and a *Salpicon* thereupon; garnish'd with Cutlets of Marinated Veal.

  Two *middling* Side-dishes, viz.

One of a Rabbet-pye, and the other of farc'd Cabbage or Cole-worts, garnish'd with farc'd *Fricandoe's.*

  Two *small* Side-dishes, viz.

One a white Fricaffy of Chickens, garnish'd with *Marinade,*
And the other of young Rabbets *à la Saingaraz.*

The Out-works.

A Dish of a young fat Pullet farced, in Cream.
One of Chickens *à la Polacre,* with a *Ramolade.*

One

One of *Pain de Perdrix*.

And one of a Loin of Mutton *a la Sainte Menehout*.

After having taken off the four Potages, four other Out-works were set on the Table, *viz.*

One of *Pain de Veau*

One of Pigeons with sweet Basil in their Bodies.

One of *Hatlets*.

And a *Grenade*.

There were also two other Out-works, consisting of Sturgeons prepared, as for Flesh-days, two different ways, *viz.*

One after the manner of larded *Fricandoe's*

And the other, *à la Sante Menehout* in thick Slices.

The Second Course.

The Roast-meats and Intermesses are of the Nature of the Preceding

Such a sort of Entertainment was made *June* 20, 1690, in the Presence of the Cardinal *d' Estrees* and the Ambassadours, at the Table of the Grand Chamberlain and Purveyor to the French King.

As for the Potages served up in the Second Service, recourse may be had to those that have been already set down for the three first Months of the Year Let us now observe what may be added, as well to the Side-dishes, as with respect to the Roast-meats.

A List of what may be served up, besides the abovementioned Dishes, during the Months of April, May *and* June.

POtage of Lamb, with Roman Lettice.
Potage of Quails, with a natural *Blanc-manger*.
Potage of boned Capon, with Mushrooms
Potage of Kids, with white Broth
Potage of white Cabbage farced
Potage of small Citrulls, farc'd after the Spanish Mode.
Potage of Artichoke-bottoms, Cucumbers and Lettice.
Potage of young Turkies, with farced *Morilles* and white Cabbage
Potage of young Rabbets, with small Turneps

Po-

Potage of green Geese, with Asparagus
Potage of farced Bread with farced Lettice.
Potage of Partridges with brown Broth.
Potage of a farced Breast of Veal
Potage of Chickens with farced Cucumbers,
Potage of Chickens in a Ragoo.
Potage of a *Poupeton* in form of a Triangle.
Potage of Calves-feet and Chaldrons.
Potage of Lambs-heads
Potage of Calves-heads *à deux Faces.*
Potage after the Italian Mode.

Side-dishes.

Andouilles of Veal.
A Quarter of Mutton roasted.
Calve's-livers
A Calve's Chaldron fried.
A Leg of Veal larded small, in a *Daube.*
Collops of Veal broiled, with Parsley-sauce.
Young Rabbets, with white and brown Sauce,
A Loin of Veal in a Ragoo
Green Geese in a Ragoo
Young Geese, in a *Daube.*
Calves-feet larded, with white Sauce
Young Pigeons marinated, in a Fricassy.
A Breast of Veal marinated.
Boned Chickens.
Stew'd Chickens.
Chickens in a Fricassy, with Cream
Young Turkies after the Swiss Mode, fried with Cucumbers.
Little Chickens with Cherry-sauce
A *Poupeton* farced with young Pigeons.
A Cow's Udder, with sweet Sauce.

For the Roast.

This is the Season for Lambs, Kids, sucking Piggs, young Turkies a Year old, Pheasants, young Rabbets, *January*-Leverets, green Geese, young wild Boars, Partridges, young Pigeons, Chickens, and young Ring-doves, or Wood-pigeons.

A

A great Entertainment for the Months of July *and* August.

The First Course.

Potages.

TWo *Bisks* of Pigeons
Two *Julian*-potages with large fat Pullets.
Two of Quails with sweet Basil.
Two of Pease with a Duck.
Two Potages of farced Cucumbers with a Capon.
Two of *Oils,*
Two of *Casseroles.*
Two of Roots, with young Ring-doves
Two of Turneps, with farced Chickens
Two of Leaks, with Geese
Two of Succory, with young Turkies

The Side-dishes

Two Pigeon-pies
Two Rabbet-pies
Two Legs of Mutton, *à la Royale*
Two Side-dishes of Partridge fried on the Coals.
Two of young fat Hens, *à la Saingaraz.*
Two of large Pullets, farced in Cream.
Two *Mirotons*
Two *Pains de Veau.*
Two *Terrines*
Two Side-dishes of Ducks, with Oisters.
Two great Side-dishes of Roast-beef, garnish'd with Mutton-cutlets
And two other of Veal *de Riviere,* garnish'd with Cutlets of fried Veal and a Hash upon the Leg

The Out-works

Two Dishes of *Croquets*
Two of *Saucisses Franches.*
Two of *Saucisson Royal*
Two of Veal after the Italian Mode
Two of Pigeons with Fennel
Two of farced Chickens broil'd on the Coals

C 3

TWO

Two of Pigeons with sweet Basil
Two of Chickens *à la Tartre*
Two of young Pullets *à la Sainte Menehout.*
Two of *Bouillans*
Two of *Marinades* of Chickens.
Two Courses of Pigeons, with white Sauce.
And two of *Pain de Perdrix.*

The Second Course.

Twenty two Dishes of Roast-meat, consisting of all sorts of large Pieces of Beef, Mutton and Veal, and of all sorts of Poultry, wild Fowl, young Boars, sucking Piggs, Pheasants, &c. with Sallets.

The Intermesses.

Twenty four in number, viz.
Two Dishes of Gammon-pies.
Two of Pheasants.
Two of Salt-meats, Tongues and Sausages
Two Pies of Capons-breasts, garnish'd with little Tarts.
Two Pies made of crackling Crust filled with Marmelade of Apricocks
Two *Blanc-mangers* garnish'd with several Gellies.
Two Dishes of Veal-sweet-breads *à la Dauphine,* garnish'd with fried Sweet-breads of the same
Two of *Blanc-manger-fritters,* garnish'd with Water-fritters.
Two of Pigs-pettitoes, *à la Sainte-Menehout.*
Two of *Menus-droits.*
Two of *Hatlets*
And two of *Galantine.*

The Out-works.

Two Dishes of *Pain au Jambon.*
Two of Mushrooms in Cream.
Two of Cocks-combs and *Morilles.*
Two of Artichoke-bottoms.
Two *Omelets,* and a Gammon-hash thereupon.
Two *Omelets* with Sugar.
Two of Apple-fritters.
Two of burnt Cream.
Two of *Rissoles.*

Two

Two of Capons-livers.
And two of *Truffles* in a *Court-bouillon.*

An Entertainment of the like Nature was made by the Marquefs *de Louvois*, Aug 25, 1690, in his Caftle at *Meudon*, for the Dauphin, the Duke and Dutchefs of *Orleans*, the Duke of *Chartres* and his Sifter, and the whole Retinue of the Court. There were three Tables furnifhed with the fame Provifions; fo that almoft three Difhes of every Mefs were reiterated.

Another Entertainment that may be made during the fame Seafon, and in the following Months.

THree great Services of Pieces of Beef garnifh'd with *Marinade,* either in a *Cuvet* or in a large Difh.
   Twelve other Difhes, viz.
Three of fat Pullets and young Turkies.
Three of Carbonado'd Mutton.
Three of Pies after the Spanifh Mode.
Two of farced Lettice
And one of Pigeons with Fennel.

The Out-works.
   Four in number, viz.
Two of Veal-fweet-breads with white Sauce
And two *Filets* with Cucumbers.

On another Day.
   For the twelve Difhes,
Three of fat Chickens and young fat Pullets.
Three of Saufages and Partridges.
Three of Chicken-fricaffies
And three of Pies of Pheafants, Partridges and young Rabbets.

The Out-works
Three Difhes of white Puddings, Saufages and *Andou.lles*, and three others of Carbinadoes.

           For

For Tables of leß Strength

A great Dish of a Piece of Beef

Two leſſer of Pieces of Beef likewiſe, but diverſified, after ſome of the manners elſewhere deſcribed

A Pigeon-pye

And a Fricaſſy of Chickens.

For the Out-works

A *Filet*, with Cucumbers

A Diſh of Carbonadoe s.

A *Filet* with white Sauce

A Diſh of young Turkies, in a *Salmigund* or Hotch-potch.

At another time

For the Grand Diſh, a Piece of Beef.

  Two leſſer Diſhes, viz

One of *Filets* with Cucumbers, garniſh'd with Carbonadoe's; and the other of fat Pullets entire, with *Truffles.*

For the Out-works.

Four Diſhes of Sauſages, Puddings and *Andouillets.*

A Fillet of Mutton, with *Truffles.*

And a Fricaſſy of Chickens with Pies.

For Suppers

Three great Diſhes of Veal, garniſh'd with *Marinade* and Hatlets

  Twelve other Diſhes, viz

Three of Pullets and young Turkies.

Two of Pigeons, with Fennel

One of a Leg of Mutton, with Garlick

Two of young Turkies, with Gammon.

One of Pigeons, with ſweet Baſil.

And three Haſhes of Partridges.

The Out-works.

  Four in number, viz.

Two of *Filets* with Cucumbers, and two *Marinades* of Chickens

For

For another Table of less Strength.

A Quarter of Veal garnish'd with *Marinade* for the great Dish

Two other lesser *Dishes,* viz

One of a young fat Hen with Gammon, and the other of a Leg of Mutton

The Out-works.

A Dish of young Turkies, in a *Salmigund,* or Hotch potch.

One of Sweet-breads *en rond*

One of a Hash of Partridges,

And a *Filet* with white Sauce

Another Table

Three Quarters of Veal garnish'd with *Marinade,* for the great Side-dishes

Twelve other *Dishes,* viz

Three of fat Pullets, and young Turkies

Three of *Filets* of a short Rib of Beef in the Gravy

Three of young Turkies, with Gammon-sauce

And three of *Salpicons*

The Out-works

Two Dishes of fried Sweet-breads of Veal, and two of large fat Pullets, with white Sauce

Another Table

Two Side-dishes, viz

One of Calves-tongues, and the other of young Hens, with Gammon.

The Out-works.

A Dish of *Filets,* with Cucumbers

One of a Fricassy of Chickens

Another of a *Filet* in the Gravy

And of one *Marinade* of Chickens

The Order of all these first Courses is usually observ'd, during the same Season, in the Court of *France,* for the King's Table, and those of the Princes and the Comptroller of his Majesty's Houshold.

A

A List of what may be served up besides the abovementioned Messes during the Months of July, August *and* September.

Potages.

POtage of farced Quails
———— of Capons with Mushrooms.
———— of Capon with *Prunes de Brignoles.*
———— of Turkey-powts, with Cucumbers.
———— of a Shoulder of Mutton with Turneps.
———— of young Pheasants with *Truffles.*
———— of Wood-hens with white Succory.
———— of a Leg of Veal farced and larded
———— of Collops of Veal larded and broil'd.
———— of Thrushes, with brown Broth
———— of a Knuckle of Veal *à l' Epigramme.*
———— of Melons with little Chickens.
———— of green Geese with Turneps.
———— of the Gibblets of young Geese
———— of Partridges, in a *Capitolade.*
———— of young Partridges, with strained Broth.
———— of farced Chickens, with green Pease-soop
———— of large Pullets, with Cabbage.
———— of a boned Turkey.
———— of Ring-doves, with Mushrooms.
———— of Veal-sweet-breads.
And *Potage de Sante,* with a Knuckle of Veal and Capon.

Side-dishes

Beef *à la mode*
A sucking Pig after the German Way.
A *Civet* of a Hare.
A Leg of Mutton after the Swiss Mode
A Shoulder of Mutton, with Mushrooms.
Thrushes in a Ragoo.
A Breast of Mutton parboil'd, and afterwards fried.
Fresh Neats-tongues larded.
Calves-tongues, with sweet Sauce.
Young Rabbets in a *Casserole.*
A Loin of Veal hashed
Green Geese quartered,

A

A Fricaffy of young Pigeons.
Young Pigeons with Pepper and Vinegar.
A Breaft of Veal ragoo'd.
A Turkey in a *Pot-pourri*, or fort of Hotch-potch.
A boned Turkey.
A Fillet of Veal in a Ragoo.
A Loin of Mutton fried.
A Calve's Head fried.
A Calve's Udder, with fweet Sauce.

Roaft-meats.

Beccafigo's, young Quails, young Capons or fat Pullets, fucking Pigs, Pheafants and Pheafant-powts, Thruthes, Leverets, young wild Bores, *Mauviettes,* young Houfe-pigeons and Pullets of one Year.

Thefe forts of Meats are alfo proper for the enfuing Months; as likewife many of thofe that have been fet down for the Firft and Second Seafon, may be ufed at another time; if they are to be procured: Therefore we ought only to have regard to Convenience in this matter, and if that will allow it, to adhere in every thing to the Particulars of which the above-fpecified Entertainments are compos'd, rather than to thofe contained in the Lifts; which are more common Ragoo's, and lefs conformable to the new Mode

An Entertainment that may be made in the Months of Oƈober, November *and* December.

The Firft Courfe.

Potages and Side-diſhes.

A Great Diſh, four middling ones and four Out-works, *viz.*
A *Bisk* of Pigeons
A Potage of Ducks, with a Cullife of *Nantilles.*
  Three Side-diſhes, viz
One of a young fat Hen, *à la Saingaraz,* garniſh'd with Marinade.
One of a Rabbet-pye.

And

And a short Rib of Beef, with the *Filet*, garnish'd with *Fricandoe's.*

The four small Dishes, or Out-works are,

One of Partridges, with Sauce, after the Spanish Way.
One of *Filets* larded and Roasted
A Fricassy garnish'd with a Carbonadoe.
And a Dish of farced *Mauviettes* with Mustard.

The Second Course.

The Roast-meats and Intermesses.

Two middling Dishes of several sorts of Poultry and Wild Fowl, according to the Season
A great Pye of crackling Crust garnish'd with little Tarts and Fritters
A Dish of *Blanc-manger.*
And a Gammon-pye.

The four Out-works are,

A Dish of Cardoons, with Parmesan.
One of *Truffles* in a *Court-bouillon*
One of Veal-sweet-breads and farced Cocks-combs.
One of *Hatlets* and four Sallets

A Supper was served up in this manner at the Duke of *Chartres's* Palace, *December* the 1st, 1690.

Another great Entertainment for the Month of December.

The First Course.

Potages.

TWo *Bisks* of Pigeons.
Two *Casseroles*, with Parmesan.
Two Potages of farced Chickens, with green Pease-soop
Two of Ducks, with Turneps.

Two

Two of large fat Pullets, with Succory.
Two of farced Quails, with *Truffles.*
Two of *Cercelots,* or young Teals with sweet Basil.
And two of Partridges, with Cullises *à la Reyne.*

The Side-dishes

Three great Dishes, viz
A large Loin of Veal, garnish'd with *Marinade* and larded
with *Hatlets.*
A Piece of Beef, with the *Filet* garnish'd with Cutlets.
A Piece of Roast-beef and another of Mutton, garnish'd with
arced Cutlets.
Ten middling Dishes, viz.
Two of Slices of Beef roll d and farc'd.
Two of farced Water-fowl, with Oisters.
Two of Pheasants minc'd in a Pye.
Two of fat Pullets, with *Truffles*
And two of young Hens, with Cray-fish Cullises

The Out-works

Two Dishes of *Grenadins,* with large fat Pullets.
Two of Veal, *à la Bourgeoise.*
Two of Partridges, after the Spanish Mode
Two of Pheasants, with Carp-sauce
Two of Marinated Chickens
Two of roasted Wood-cocks, with Wine
Two of Quails broil'd on the Coals.
Two *Biberots* of Partridges
Two *Mirotons* of Veal, with Asparagus
Two Dishes of *Filets* of young fat Hens, with white Sauce.
Two of *Filets* of Beef, with Cucumbers.
Two of Pigeons with sweet Basil.
Two of Partridges, with Olives.
Two of *Saucisson Royal*

The Second Course.

For the Roast-meat.

Sixteen Dishes of all sorts of Wild Fowl and other Poultry,
articularly *Ortolans,* Pheasants, &c. with young wild Boars,
d twelve small Sallets.

The

The Intermeſſes.

The three great Diſhes are to conſiſt of three Gammon-pies.
  The middling Diſhes are ten in number, viz.
Two of *Blanc-manger.*
Two Pies made of Capons-breaſts
Two of Cakes farc'd with Marmalade
Two Pies of crackling Cruſt, garniſh d with Marmalade.
And two *Omelets,* with Gammon

The Out-works.

Two Diſhes of Apple-fritters.
Two of *Blanc-manger-*fritters
Two of *Riſſoles.*
Two of Muſhrooms in Cream.
Two of *Pain au Jambon.*
Two of burnt Cream.
Two of *Truffles* in a *Court-bouillon.*
Two of Artichoke-bottoms.
Two of fried Artichokes.
Two of iced Artichokes
Two of Aſparagus in a Sallet.
Two of *Menus-droits*
And two of *Galantine.*

A Feaſt of the like Nature was prepared at the Duke of *Aumont*'s Palace, *December* 27, 1690 The Table was fix'd with Horſe-ſhooes; and foraſmuch as there were forty two *Covers* or Services, it was requiſite to reiterate three Diſhes of ſeveral Particulars; as well for the Side-diſhes, as for thoſe of the Roaſt-meats and Intermeſſes

If theſe Models are not ſufficient for a due Variety of Entertainments on different Days; or if they do not ſuit with the Convenience of Perſons and Places; a more proper Choice may be made out of the following Liſt.

*A List of what may be served up, besides the abovemention-
ed Dishes, during the Months of* October, November
and December.

POtages of Larks, with Hypocras.
———— of *Andouilles,* with Pease
———— of Lambs-heads
———— of Ducks, with Cole-worts or Sprouts.
———— of Quails with Mushrooms.
———— of farced Mushrooms.
———— of Capons, with Colly-flowers.
———— of Capons, with Cardoons in white Broth.
———— of boned Capon, with Oisters.
———— of a farced Leg of Mutton, with Turneps.
———— of a farced Leg of Veal with white Sauce.
———— of a Leg of a Stag, or of a wild Boar.
———— of a fat Goose, with strained Pease.
———— of Partridges, with *Milan*-cabbage.
———— of farced Partridges.
———— of large Pullets farced and boned
———— of young Barn-door Chickens in a Bisk with *Truffles.*
———— of *Poupetons.*
———— of Teals, with Mushrooms.
———— of Teals, with Hypocras
———— of *Vermecelli,* after the Italian Mode.
And *Potage de Santé.*

Side-dishes.

Puddings of Calves-livers.
A *Capitolade* of Partridges and Capon.
A Duck in a Ragoo
A farced Duck, with sweet Sauce.
A fat Capon in a *Daube.*
A *Daube* of Veal, minc'd and larded.
Calves livers in a *Marinade.*
Calves-livers larded and roasted.
Hoggs-livers in a Ragoo.
A *Gallimafry* of a Shoulder of Mutton.
A *Haricot* of a Breast of Mutton.
A Neat's Tongue larded.

Sheeps-

Sheeps-tongues broil'd.
A *Marinade* of Partridges
A Partridge in a *Daube*
A Piece of Beef well larded
Sheeps-trotters, with white Sauce.
A Loin of Mutton *à la Croutade*
A Fillet of Veal, with Oisters.
A Calve's Head in *Mine-droit.*

For the Roast-meats, *fee* Page 15. becauſe the ſame Proviſions may alſo ſerve in this Seaſon, as it has been already
hinted   The Appurtenances of the Intermeſſes are much more
general, as being in uſe throughout the greateſt part of the
whole Year · Therefore it may not be improper here to make a
Collection of the different Meſſes, prepared for that purpoſe
in the above-ſpecified Entertainments for every Seaſon, adding
ſome others that may be ſubſtituted in their room, when Occaſion ſerves, and accordingly as particular Exigencies may
require

A general Table of the Intermeſſes.

ALmond-milk
  Apple-fritters
Artichokes, with white Sauce.
Artichokes fried.
Artichokes iced.
Artichokes, *à la Sangaraz*
Artichokes, with natural Butter.
Artichokes, *a l'Eſtoufade.*
Artichoke-bottoms put in Paſte and fried
Artichoke-bottoms, with Gammon-ſauce.
Aſparagus in Mutton-gravy.
Aſparagus with natural Butter.
Aſparagus in Cream
Aſparagus in a Sallet
Beans in Cream with Bacon.
Beatils in a Ragoo
Bignets, ſee Fritters
Blanc-mangers of ſeveral ſorts.

Calves·

Calves-kidneys, and others roasted.
Calves-ears farced.
Cardoons, with Parmesan.
Cheese-cakes.
Cocks-combs farced, and Capons-livers in a Ragoo.
Cocks-kidneys in a Ragoo
Colly-flowers, with natural Butter and Mutton-gravy
Creams of several forts
Cucumbers.
Echaudes or Simnels Iced
Eggs and *Omelets* after several manners.
Fritters of *Blanc-manger.*
Fritters of Apples
Fritters made with Water
Galantines
Gammon of Bacon in Slices and in a Hash.
Gruels.
Gammon-pies.
Heads of wild Boars
Hatlets.
Hogs-ears *à la Barbe-Robert.*
Hogs ears fried in Paste.
Hogs-tongues
Jellies of several forts
Kidneys of Cocks in a Ragoo.
Kidneys of Calves roasted.
Livers of Capons *a la Crepine;*
Livers of Capons roasted.
Livers of Capons with Mushrooms
Livers of Capons after other manners.
Livers of Rabbets in an *Omelet.*
Menus-droits
Moufferons or white Mushrooms and *Morilles,* farc'd and
ned.
Mushrooms in Cream.
Mushrooms fried.
Mushrooms in a Ragoo.
Mushrooms in a *Cafferole.*
6 Neats-tongues dryed.
Omelets
Pain au Jambon.

D Peafe,

Peafe, with Bacon and Cream.

Pigs-pettitoes, *à la Sainte Menehout*, and broil'd upon the Grid-iron.

Pyes of Pheafants, young fat Hens and feveral other forts, ferved up cold.

Poupelins

Rabbets-livers in an *Omelet*.

Riffoles of Capons breafts.

Salt-meats

Simnels iced

Tarts of feveral forts

Trouts and other Fifhes, on Fifh-days.

Truffles in a *Court-bouillon*.

Truffles broil d on the Coals.

Truffles in Mutton-gravy

Veal-fweet-breads farc'd, *à la Dauphine*.

Veal-fweet-breads and Cocks-combs farc'd.

Venifon-pafties.

Water-*Bignets* or Fritters.

Not to tire the Reader with too many Tables or Lifts of the like Nature, relating to Pafties, Pies and Tarts as well hot as cold, as alfo to the different forts proper for fome Things expreffed in the the preceding Table ; he is referr'd to the general Index or Table of the Meffes at the end of this Volume, where they are fet down at large , or elfe to every Letter in the Alphabetical Inftructions that treat of every Thing in particular, after having fpecify'd what relates to the Fifh-days.

Entertainments on Fifh-days throughout the whole Year.

IT were needlefs perhaps here to give a particular Account of the Services, becaufe it is an eafie thing to take meafures thereupon, from the Entertainments on Flefh-days that have been already defcrib'd However, that nothing may feem to be wanting, we fhall reprefent fome Models ; after having obferv'd what may be ufed, as well for the Potages and Side-difhes as for the Intermeffes ; the fried Fifh that are in Seafon fupplying the place of Roaft-meats. Let us then begin with the Potages.

T

The First Courſe.

Potages on Fiſh-days, for the Months of Januaiy, February *and* March.

POtages of Pike, with Turneps.
———— of farced Pike.
———— of Cardoons.
———— of *Milan*-cabbage
———— of Cray-fiſh
———— of Sturgeon
———— of Smelts, with brown Broth.
———— of Oiſters
———— of *Julians.*
———— of the ſoft Roes of Fiſh.
———— of Lobſters with Peaſe.
———— of Sea-ducks
———— of Onions with ſweet Baſil and otherwiſe.
———— of Parmeſan.
———— of *Profitrolle.*
———— of freſh Salmon.
———— of farced Soles.
———— of Soles in *Filets* with white Sauce, with ſweet Baſil, with Lentils, and with Cucumbers
———— of Soles, with Onions, in white Sauce.
———— of Turbot
———— of farced Tench.
———— of Tortoiſe

To theſe may be added Potages with Roots and Pulſe, hereafter mentioned , moie eſpecially the *Oil* for Fiſh-days, and alſo certain Fiſh-potages that are ſet down foi the enſuing Months.

Potages on Fish-days for the Months of April, May *and* June.

POtages of Afparagus.
——— of Muſhrooms.
——— of white Cabbage, with Milk.
——— of farced Cucumbers.
——— of Rasberries.
——— of Froggs.
——— of Gudgeons.
——— of Lampreys.
——— of farced Lettice.
——— of fried Mackerel
——— of *Morilles*
——— of young green Peaſe.

And *Potage de Santé* with Herbs, which is common for the following Months.

Potages on Fiſh-days for the Months of July, Auguſt *and* September.

POtages of Eels.
——— of Eel-powts, with brown Broth.
——— of farced Pike.
——— of farced Carps
——— of white Cabbage
——— of Citrulls, with Milk
——— of Frogs, with brown Broth.
——— of Milk, with Piſtacho's.
——— of Melons
——— of Muſcles.
——— of Muſcadine-grapes.
——— of Perches with white Broth
——— of Fiſh in a *Bisk.*
——— of Green Peaſe.
——— of Salmon with Muſhrooms.

Potages on Fiſh-days, for the Months of October, November *and* December.

POtages of Fiſh-*Andouillets.*
———— of Sandlings.
———— of Pike, with Cabbage
———— of Cardoons
———— of farced Muſhrooms.
———— of Smelts with white Broth
———— of a pickled Joll of Salmon
———— of Marbled-Milk.
———— of poach'd Eggs, with Parmeſan.
———— of Perches with brown Broth.
———— of young Pigeons.

There are alſo for all theſe Seaſons, Potages of Rice, of *Vermicelli,* of Almond-milk and others.

Side-diſhes of Fiſh for the whole Year.

A*Umar* in a Ragoo.
   Baſes.
Bouillans of Fiſh
Breams in a Ragoo and roaſted.
Burts
Carps in a Ragoo and *à la Daube.*
Carps in *Filets* ſtewed, with *Sauſſe-Robert.*
Carps farced in a Ragoo.
Carps in a *Demi-court-bouillon.*
Caſſeroles of Fiſh
Cervelats of Fiſh,
Cod-fiſh freſh and otherwiſe.
Congers cut into Pieces and fried, with Anchovies.
Congers *Marinated.*
Cray-fiſh in a Ragoo, with white Sauce.
Dabs.
Daubes of Eels.
Eels roaſted.

D 3   Eels

Eels broiled on the Grid-iron, with *Sauffe-Robert.*
Eels, with white Sauce
Eels fried
Eels, with brown Sauce
Filets of Carps, Soles, Perches, &c.
Fins in a *Casserole* and fried.
Flounders and Crabs.
Fricassies of Pikes, Quavivers and Soles.
Frogs fried.
Gold-fish in a Fricassy, in Pies, &c.
Gudgeons rolled in Paste and stewed.
Hashes of Carps, Cray-fish, Perches and Pikes.
Haricots of Fish.
Herrings, fresh and otherwise.
Kreelings.
Lampreys
Lobsters in a Ragoo, Hash, &c.
Mackerel.
Melwells
Mirotons of Fish.
Mullets fried, with Anchove-sauce and broil'd upon the Grid-
iron.
Oisters broiled, ragoo'd, fried or farced.
Pains of Fish
Perches, with Anchove-sauce.
Perches farced
Perches, with white or green Sauce, or with Cucumbers,
St. *Peter*'s Fish, with *Truffles*, with white Sauce, with Artichokes,
with Cucumbers, or with green Sauce.
Petits Patez or little Pies with white Sauce.
Plaice in a Ragoo
Pies of Fish, served up hot.
Pike with Pigeons-breasts
Pike farced
Pike in a *Casserole.*
Pike in a Fricassy
Pike farced, with Anchove-sauce.
Pike fried in Paste.
Pike cut in Pieces and put into a Ragoo.
Poupetons of Fish.
Pilchards.
Quavivers, or Sea-dragons in *Filets*, with Cucumbers, Ca-
pers, or *Mousserons.*   Qua

Quavivers, with Anchove-cullises.

Quavivers boned and stewed

Quavivers in a Fricassy of Chickens with white Sauce

Quavivers fried in a Ragoo

Raies or Thorn-backs fried, with *Sauffe-Robert*

Roches in a *Casserole.*

Roches broiled upon the Grid-iron and breaded.

Roches farced or in a Pie

Sandlings or Dabs and Eel-powrs in a Ragoo, in *Casseroles,* or in *Filets.*

Sandlings with Cream, or Anchovies

Salmon in a Ragoo, with Mushrooms

Sardins.

Sausages of Fish

Sea-ducks in a *Pot-pourri.*

Shads

Shrimps fried

Smelts with Anchovies and in a *Casserole.*

Soles broiled upon the Grid-iron, with Anchovies

Soles marinated, farced, in a Ragoo, with white Sauce, or with fine Herbs.

Soles in *Filets,* with Lentils, with sweet Basil, Cucumbers, *Sauffe-Robert,* or *Truffles,* after the Spanish Mode, with Cray-fish and with Capers, or Anchovie-cullises

Soles *à la Sainte Menehout*

Soles in a Fricassy of Chickens, or with burnt Butter

Soles in *Pigeons*

Soles with Laurel or Bay-leaves

Stock-fish of several sorts.

Tenches farced, in a Ragoo, in a Fricassy, or in a *Casserole.*

Tortoises in a Ragoo, or in a *Marinade*

Trouts in a Ragoo

Tunnies marinated, broiled, put into a Pie or baked in a Pot.

Tunnies cut into Slices, with poor Man's Sauce.

Turbot with Oil, or with Anchovie-sauce

Turbot in a Ragoo

Whitings in a *Casserole.*

To these sorts of Fish may be added Dishes of Spinage, farced Cabbage, Pease, and other Herbs or Pulse, according to the Season

The

The Second Course.

The abovementioned Fishes may be served up in a *Court-bouillon*, and fried, or broiled upon the Grid-iron, or Roasted: Among others, these that follow, *viz*

Shads roasted, and in a *Court-bouillon*.

Sandlings, in a *Court-bouillon*

Pike after the same manner ; or else larded with Eels and roasted

Carps in a *Court-bouillon*, broiled on the Grid-iron, or fried.

Sturgeon dress'd after the same manner.

Smelts fried

Mackerel broiled.

Plaice fried

Salmon, in a *Court-bouillon*.

Soles in a *Court-bouillon*.

Soles fried and broiled.

Tenches after the same manner.

Turbot in a *Court-bouillon*.

Quavivers broiled upon the Grid-iron, with Anchovie-sauce

There are also several Pies and Pastry-works of Fish, which are to be set down elsewhere ; and to these may be added divers Particulars belonging to the Intermesses on Flesh-days, such as Mushrooms, Artichokes, Asparagus, *Morilles*, Cucumbers, &c Moreover out of *Lent*, the use of Eggs is considerable, with which a very great number of Dishes may be varied , and even during that Season, a good Choice may be made out of those that belong to the Entertainments with Roots, which shall be hereafter described.

We shall only here subjoyn the Fish-sallets that likewise constitute a part of this Service

A List of the Fish-sallets.

SAllets of Sole-*filets.*
—— of fresh Turbot.
—— of fresh Sandlings.
—— of fresh Oisters.
—— of *Filets* of Smelts
—— of Salmon-trout
—— of Ray or Thorn-back
—— of Whiting-*filets.*
—— of Quaviver-*filets.*
—— of fresh Tunnies
—— of Anchovies and Pilchards
—— of fresh Salmon.
—— of Cray-fish.
—— of Lobsters and others.

A particular Account of the Root-sallets is to be hereafter inserted, and as for those of Herbs during the Summer, nothing is more easie than the manner of making them, for then there is so great an Abundance of all sorts of Garden-fruits, that they may be readily changed every Day, and several different sorts may be used at the same time

For several *Filets* of Fish 'tis requisite to prepare a certain Sauce call'd *Ramolade,* which is made of chopped Parsley, Chibbols, Anchovies and Capers, the whole mixture being put into a Dish, with a little Pepper, Salt, Nutmeg, Oil and Vinegar well temper'd together After having dress'd the *Filets* in a proper Dish, they are to be sprinkled with this *Ramolade,* and Lemmon-juice is usually added to some of the Dishes, which are to be served up cold

If any Persons are desirous to have Models of Entertainments on Fish-days, they may here take a View of a very remarkable Ordinary as it is prepar'd in the Duke of *Chartres's* Palace Whenever it shall be requisite to furnish greater Tables, due measures may be taken for the management of them, from the Entertainments that have been specify'd for Flesh days, and if more slender Provisions are only required, 'twill be less difficult to retrench the number of the Dishes, than to find means to match them and set them in good Order.

Mo-

Models of Entertainments on Fish-days.

For a considerable Ordinary or Dinner.

Potages

TWo middling Potages and four lesser.
The two middling ones consist of Cray-fish and farced Soles.
The four lesser are these, viz
The first *Potage de Sante*, the second with Cabbage, the third with Pease, and the fourth with Onions

The great Dish in the middle.

An Eel-pie.
Two Side-dishes, viz.
One of whole Perches, with white Sauce.
And the other of four Pikes.

The Out-works.

A Dish of Fricassied Oisters.
One of Spinage.
One of Soles in *Filets* with Cucumbers.
One of *Filets* of Perches, with white Sauce
One of Quaviver-*Filets*, with Capers
One a small Fricassy of Pike
And the last of Eels broiled upon the Grid-iron, with *Sausse-Robert*.

The Roast.

Two middling Dishes, each consisting of two Pikes and eight Soles.
The great Dish of a Carp and six Pickerils round about it
The rest of this Service consists of Particular Intermesses and *Filets* in a Sallet.

For the Supper.

Potages

Two middling Potages ; viz one of *Tortoises* and the other of farced Pike.
Two lesser, one of Sole-*Filets* with sweet Basil and the other of Soles, with Lentils.

The

The Side-dishes of the Table.

For the great Dish in the middle, farced Mullets.
  Four Side-dishes, viz.
A Pike-pye
A Dish of Gold-fish.
One of stewed Carps
One of Bases

Eight Out-works, viz.

A Hash of Carps.
One of Perches.
Tortoises.
Soles farced.
Sole-*Filets,* with *Sauffe-Robert.*
Others with *Truffles,* and others with Cray-fish.

For the Roast.

Two middling Dishes of Sturgeon and Roches round about
'em
  Two lesser, each of five Soles
  Several Intermesses for the rest of the Service.

The Second Table.

A great Dish in the middle, of Soles, with Anchovies.
  Four Side-dishes, viz
A Pie.
A Fricassy of Pike
Two Dishes of Gold-fish.
And two of Roast

An Ordinary for another Day.

Potages

TWo middling Potages and four lesser
  The two middling, are one of Perches with white Sauce,
and the other of Lobsters
  The four lesser are a *Potage de Santé,* one of Onions with
sweet Basil, one of *Profitrolles* and one of soft Roes

The

The Side-dishes.

A great Dish of Roches.

Two middling ones, *viz* the first of farced Perches and the other of whole Carps

Eight Out-works, viz.

A *Poupeton* of Tunnies
Filets of Perches, with green Sauce.
Farced Oisters.
A *Haricot.*
Filets of Soles, with *Truffles.*
Bouillans
Soles broiled on the Grid-iron, with Anchovies.
And a Pie with white Sauce.

For the Roast.

Two middling Dishes; each of six Pikes and four Soles.

Two others lesser, of two Sandlings and four Soles round a-bout

The rest of the Service consists of divers Intermesses and *Filets* in a Sallet.

For the Supper.

Two middling Potages, *viz* one of an *Oil* and the other of Muscles

Two lesser; one of Sea-ducks with Lentils, and the other of Soles with Cucumbers.

Side-dishes.

A great Dish of Thorn-back

Four others, *viz* one of Roches, one of Quavivers in a Fricassy of Chickens, one a Pie, and one of *Grenots.*

The Out-works.

Soles *à la Sainte Menehout*
Filets of Perches, with white Sauce.
Filets of Dabs, with Anchovies.
A Hash
Tenches.
A farced Cabbage.
Quavivers, with *Mousserons*
A *Casserole.*

For

For the Roaſt.

Two middling Diſhes; each of ſeven Soles
Two leſſer, one of a Carp and the other of a Pike.

An Ordinary for another Day.

Potages.

TWo middling Potages, one of farced *Grenots* and the other of Pike, with Oiſters

Four leſſer ones, *viz.* the firſt of Spinage, the ſecond of Lentils, the third of farced Soles upon the Edges, and the fourth of Onions, with a Loaf in the middle

The Side-diſhes

A Pike-pye, for the great Diſh.
Two others; the firſt of broiled Tunnies and the ſecond of Sandlings

The Out-works.

A *Miroton.*
Sole-*Pains*
Filets of Carps, with Cucumbers
Filets of Soles, with Culliſes of Capers.
Quavivers broil'd upon the Grid-iron
Roches farced.

For the Roaſt.

Two middling Diſhes; each of twelve Soles and two leſſer; each of two Sandlings.

The Supper.

Potages.

Two middling Potages, *viz.* one a *Julian,* and the other of Sole-*filets*

Two leſſer; one with Parmeſan, and the other of farced Crab-fiſh.

The

The Side-difhes

The great Difh of Whitings in a *Cafferole.*
  Four middling Side-difhes, viz.
One of Mackerel.
One of frefh Cod-fifh
One of a *Poupeton* of Tortoifes
And one of Roches breaded and broil'd upon the Grid-iron.

Eight Out-works, viz.

A farced Loaf.
A G-toe of Soles
Quavirers, with Cucumbers and *Moufferons.*
Soles after the Spanifh Way
Lobfters in a Hafh.
St *Peter's* Fifh, with white Sauce.

The Roaft

A large Difh of a Turbot and a Dab, garnifh'd with Roches.

Two middling Difhes, viz one of Shads and the other of frefh Salmon.

Thefe Models are more than fufficient for the regulating of a confiderable Ordinary As for others that are lefs fumptuous it were requifite only to provide as many Out-works, a there are Potages; to the end that the former may be ferved up, when the others are taken away. In like manner the reft of the Meffes may be proportioned for the fecond Courfe, every one accordingly as the Expences will admit of. Let us now take an Account of the Provifions of Roots.

Enter

Entertainments with Roots.

The First Course.

Potages.

SIx in number, four middle ones and two lesser, *viz*
A Potage of young Onions, with a Loaf in the middle.
One of Lentils with Oil, garnish'd with fried Bread.
One of Asparagus, with green Pease-soop.
And a Potage without Butter
The two lesser Potages are, one of Almond-milk, garnish'd
with crisp Almonds and the other of *Morilles*
An *Oil* or Potage of Roots may also be served up and Sallets
with Oil.

The Side-dishes.

A Dish of Lentils in a Ragoo, with fine Herbs.
One of Pease-soop, with fine Herbs.
One of French Beans.
One of Roots in a Ragoo.
One of Potatoes.
One of other different sorts of Herbs.
And four Dishes of Oisters.

The Second Course.

For the Roast

Take several sorts of Roots, as Parsnips, Carrets, Turneps,
Potatoes, Goats-bread, Parsley-roots, &c Let them be well
scrap'd and scalded: As soon as they are ready, take a Stew-
pan, with a sufficient quantity of good Butter and Onions shred
small. When the Butter turns somewhat reddish, throw in a
handful of fine Flower, as also the Roots, which are to be
fried and well seasoned. Afterwards the whole Mess is to be
chopped upon a Table to make a *Farce*, mixt with a little Parsley and *Chibbol*, all sorts of fine Herbs, some Pieces of *Truffles*
and Mushrooms, a Slice of Butter, a few Crums of Bread and
Milk-cream Thus this Farce is to be made delicious, not
too fat and seasoned according to Art.

With

With the fame Farce, all forts of Fifh may be reprefented upon Plates, at Pleafure, *viz* Soles upon one, a Turbot upon another, Flounders upon a third ; upon others, Roches, Qua-vivers, Mackerel, &c. A little Butter muft be put into every Plate under the Farce that is thus formed in the Shape of Fifh. Afterwards they are to be neatly breaded on the top and baked in an Oven As for the Soles in particular, they may be made upon a Leaf of Patience or Monks-rhubarb, which very much refembles their Shape, and fried with a great deal of eafe

Carrets may likewife be taken, and more efpecially red Beets which being well fcrap'd and boil'd according to Difcretion, each Root a-part, are to be cut into large Slices, fome in the Shape of Soles, others like Quavivers, and fo of the reft: Then they are to be left in a Pickle, for a little while, till, with fine Flower, Salt and white Wine a proper Batter be made, like that of Apple-fritters, to cover the Roots, before they are fried with frefh Butter and Oil; every thing a-part Thus they are to be fried as other *Marinades;* as well as Goats-bread and other Roots, of which one or two Difhes may be prepared for the Roaft

To diverfifie them, 'tis requifite to have feparate Ragoo's of feveral forts ; *viz.* fome of minced Mufhrooms, others of *Truffles,* others of Afparagus-tops and others of *Morilles* As alfo a good *Sauffe-Robert* a-part and white Sauce, without any Anchovies therein ; which may ferve chiefly for the Difhes that reprefent the fhape of Fifh and are made of a Farce They are to be garnifh d with a little fried Bread, fried Parfley, pickled Roots fried in Pafte, Artichoke-bottoms fried in Pafte, and fome Pieces of Cucumbers

For the Intermeffes.

A Difh of Afparagus in Cream
A Tart of Almond-milk and Cream.
A Difh of burnt Cream.
One of *Morilles* in Cream
One of Afparagus in a Sallet.
One of Jelly of Harts-horn.
A *Blanc-manger*
Mufhrooms breaded and baked.
Cabbage in a Sallet.
Spinage in Cream.

French

French Beans in the Cod preferv'd dry , fome ferved up in a Sallet and others in Cream

Pickled Artichokes, with white Sauce.

Dried *Truffles*, with Oil.

Apple-fritters.

This laft Entertainment was prepared as a Dinner for the Duke of *Orleans*, on Good-friday, *Anno Dom.* 1690.

To that purpofe, a fufficient quantity of Roots was provided the Day before, and three or four Tables were fill'd with them They were pick'd, fcrap'd and fcalded according to the ufual manner, as well for the Ragoo's and Side-difhes, as for the Roaft, fo that in the Morning, every thing was ready for the Farces.

A confiderable quantity of Peas was likewife boil'd in the Evening, which ferv'd to make a great deal of Onion-broth and to foak the Herbs and Roots for the *Oil*

Altho' there needs no great variety of Meffes on fuch Days, yet it will not be improper here to fhew, how the preceding Particulars may be diverfified or augmented , becaufe they may ferve upon other occafions during the whole Seafon of Lent.

For the Potages.

They may be made with,

Young Sprouts.

Ciboulets with Milk.

Moufferons and common Mufhrooms

Green Peas.

Truffles.

Turneps

And Artichoke-bottoms.

For the Side-difhes and Intermeffes.

Befides the ordinary Creams, Fritters, *Blanc-mangers* and Roots dipt in Butter and fried, which have been already defcrib'd, feveral Pies and Tarts may be made of fome , particularly of Spinage, *Truffles, Morilles, Moufferons,*common Mufhrooms, Plums, red Beets, &c. To thefe may be added Eggs and *Omelets,* difguifed after divers manners; and for thofe that are eaten with Butter, feveral forts of Roots may be drefs'd with white or red Sauce: Thus a very great Entertainment may be eafily prepar'd

E

par'd upon any emergent occasion, and such Materials as are at hand, may be managed so as to give satisfaction, as far as the Abstinence of the Season will admit

It remains only, that the particular Sallets be specified; because a greater quantity of them than ordinary, is requisite on that Day.

A List of the Sallets.

Artichokes,	Lettice,
Asparagus,	Mushrooms stewed,
Red Beets,	Olives,
Cardoons,	Oranges,
Celery,	Parsley of *Macedonia*,
Colly-flowers,	Pomegranates,
Cucumbers fried ,	Potatoes,
Escressionaire,	Purslain,
French Beans,	Young Sprouts,
Goats-bread,	Wild Succory,
Hops,	*Truffles*
Lemmons,	

Let us now proceed to the main Point of the Business, and to the practical Part of this Work   Indeed the general *Ideas* that have been already given may be sufficient for Stewards, Purveyors and Caterers, who are thereby plainly instructed as to the particular Provisions to be bought, and in the Method of Ordering the Entertainments committed to their Charge But some farther Directions are necessary for those that are Students in the Art of Cookery · Tis requisite to explain to them the Manner of Preparing every Mess, to the end that they may go on successfully in their Business without any difficulty; and this is what we undertake to do in the ensuing Treatise; without concealing any thing that is most *à-la-mode*, or most in use at the Court of *France*, and in the Houses of Persons of the greatest Quality: Such are the Entertainments that we have already produced for Models.

I N-

INSTRUCTIONS

IN

Form of a DICTIONARY,

DIRECTING

How to Drefs every particular Mefs, and how to Serve them up to Table, for the Side-difhes, Intermeffes and Roaft-meats, or otherwife, after the beft manner.

A.

ALMONDS.

Almonds ferve for feveral Ufes, particularly, to make Pafte, Potages, Almond-milk and Pies; and green Almonds are fometimes boil'd All thefe Things are prepared according to the following Method.

Almond-pafte.

Take Almonds that are well fcalded and wafh'd in fair Water · Pound and moiften them with a little White of an Egg and Orange-flowers, whipt together, and, as you are working them, continue to moiften them by degrees, that they may not turn to Oil, they cannot be pounded too much: The Pafte thus prepar'd, is to be fpread upon a large Difh, and dried with fine Sugar, as if it were ordinary Pafte, till it becomes very pliable. This Pafte may ferve to make the Bottom or Under-cruft for Pies, and all forts of fmall Paftry-works to garnifh them, but 'tis requifite to let it lye by a

E 2

little

little while, before you proceed to make ufe of it according to your Defign

The fame may alfo be done after another manner, thus: When the Almonds are fufficiently pounded and moiften'd as before, take a Copper-Pan, fuch as Confectioners ufe, and put into it a greater quantity of Sugar than of Pafte ; which Sugar is to be clarified with the White of an Egg, and boil'd till it becomes feathered Then put in your Pafte, and with a *Spatula* work all well together Set your Pan over the Furnace, and keep continually ftirring it as much as is poffible, until the Pafte be loofen'd from the Pan. Afterwards it muft be fpread upon a Difh, with fine Sugar underneath, and rolled up in large Rolls, that it may lye by for fome time, before it be us'd It may be workt feveral ways, that is to fay, fqueez'd thro' a Syringe, and form'd into divers Figures As for the Shreds or Remnants that are left, when dried, you need only put them into the Mortar, and pound them with a little White of an Egg, in order to foften them, and this will ferve to make fmall *Petits Choux* or other fine Ornaments for the garnifhing of the Difhes.

Almond-milk.

Almond-milk is us'd for the Intermeffes, and made thus: Take Almonds, and having fcalded them in order to Blanching, pound them in a Mortar, as before· Then take a little Milk, and be careful to ftrain all thro' a Sieve; which being done, take four Yolks of Eggs with the Whites, beaten together, and pour fome Milk upon them, by degrees, adding alfo a little Salt and Nutmeg. In order to boil it, fet a Kettle or Pot with Water upon the Furnace, and when it boils, put a Difh upon the Kettle, with a flice of very good Butter. Afterwards pour your Almond-milk into this Difh, and let it be continually ftirr'd, till it becomes a Cream, which muft be ferved up to Table hot without any Sugar.

Potage of Almond-milk.

Take a Pound or two of Almonds, according to the fize of your Difh; and let them be fcalded, and pounded all at once, moiftening them with a little Water· When they are well pounded, fet a Stew-pan on the Fire, with fome luke-warm Water,
and

and a very little Salt: Pour this Water into the Mortar, and strain all through a Sieve two or three several times Then put this Milk into a clean Pot, with a lump of Sugar and a little piece of Cinnamon, and boil all together by degrees To dress the Potage, cut the crummy part of a Loaf into Slices, and and put them in good order upon a Dish: When these Slices are toasted at the Fire, lay your Potage of the same Milk a soaking, and when 'tis ready to be serv'd up, moisten your Sippets with it, as much as is requisite

Some boil about two Quarts of Water in a Pot, and put into it the Crum of two small Loaves, which they mingle together with the Almonds in a Mortar, and afterwards let it soak in a Pot, for the space of three or four Hours, with Sugar and Cinnamon, as before · Then they strain and dress it in the same manner.

This Potage may be garnish'd with March-pane or crisp Almonds; the latter of which may be made after this manner, if you'll take the pains to do it Take Almonds that are well scalded and drain'd: Then Sugar them, and put them all at once into a Frying-pan that you have ready at hand, with good hot Oil: They must be continually stirred and turned, till they become of a Gold-colour. Then take them out speedily, and make four or five Heaps of them, because they are apt to stick together.

An *Almond*-Tourte *or Pon-pie.*

Take about two good Handfuls of sweet Almonds, and, as you are pounding them, sprinkle them with Orange-flower Water: Add thereto some candy'd Lemmon-peel, some Peel of green Lemmon and Sugar, and pound them all well together, with a very little fine Flower · Let the Whites of two Eggs be beaten up and pour'd therein, with three Yolks, and when the whole Farce is well mixt, let it be put into a little Dish In the mean while, a sort of Paste is to be made with Flower, Butter, the Yolk of an Egg and a little Salt, but great care must be taken that this Paste be duly prepared Then a piece for the Under-crust is to be rolled out and put into the Pie-pan, with a little Border round about it, made with the point of a Knife When 'tis time to have the Pie bak'd, the prepared Farce is to be put into it, so as to fill up the whole Bottom-crust Afterwards it must be iced with a little fine Sugar, and set into a Campain-

Oven; taking care of the Fire on the top, and continually fupplying that underneath

How to drefs green Almonds.

When you have green Almonds, fet a large Copper-Pan or Skillet upon the Fire, filled with Water and Afhes Scum off the Coals that rife on the top, and when this Liquor has boil'd a great while, and you perceive by the Tafte, that 'tis become fweet and flippery, as it were a perfect Lye, throw in your Almonds and let them have three or four Walms · Then take them out and put them into other frefh Water . Thus they are to be wafh'd in four or five Waters, and afterwards a Pan is to be fet on the Fire, with Water almoft ready to boil. Put the Almonds into that Water, and to prevent their fwimming on the top, thruft down into the Pan a Difh of almoft the fame breadth, yet fo as to be conveniently let into it ; by which means the Almonds will be hinder'd from becoming black A good Fire muft be continually kept underneath, and in cafe the Water inclines to boil, fome other cold Water is to be pour'd in by degrees to give it a check Thus your Almonds are to be drefs'd with a moderate Heat, and to know whether they are fufficiently fcalded, take a Pin and prick an Almond quite thro': If it ftick to the Pin, 'tis a fign they are not yet well fcalded, but if it be loofe, it denotes that they are. Then, having taken them out, put them again into fair Water, and afterwards into good Syrup of clarified Sugar. In order to ferve them up liquid, 'tis requifite that one half of your Sugar be in a Jelly ; and to keep them dry, as foon as your Almonds are fcalded in the aforefaid manner, take them out and let them be well drain d : Boil your Sugar till it be greatly feathered, and fee that it be not thick, but of a fine glofs, to the end that the Almonds which are put therein, may appear very green. The fame thing may be done with green Apricocks to preferve them liquid and dry.

A N C H O V I E S.

Anchovie-cullifes are frequently made, and put into feveral Ragoo's, as well for Flefh as Fifh-days, fo that it were need-lefs here to give a particular account of them, fince that is fufficiently done in the refpective places where they are to be us'd. We fhall only obferve at prefent, that the Bones of the Ancho-

vies,

vies, which have been already made ufe of, may be fried, after having put them into a Pafte made of Flower and white
Wine, with a little Pepper and Salt · So that you may either
garnifh another Difh with that Pafte, or ferve it up to Table
for an *Out-work*, with Orange and fried Parfley.

ANDOUILLES.

Andouilles or Chitterlings, are ufed for Side-difhes more than
for Intermeffes ; thofe of Hogs-guts are made after the following manner.

Andouilles de Cochon, *or Hogs-chitterlings.*

Take the great Gut of a Hog, and cut off the thick end of it,
to be fteep'd in Water for a Day or two When that is done,
let it be well wafh'd and parboil'd in other Water, with a little
Salt and fome Slices of Onions and Lemmons. Slit this Gut,
and put a little white Wine upon it, to take away the ill Savour When it is parboil'd, put it into frefh Water, and having brought it to the Dreffer, cut it according to the length
you would have your *Andouilles* or Chitterlings to be of. Take
fome part of the Hog's Belly, pare off the Fat and cut that
Meat into thick Slices of the fame bignefs with your Chitterlings · Thus you may make them, with half of one and half
of the other ; feafoning them as much as is needful Afterwards take the Skirts from the infide of which the fmall Gut
ought to be cut off, let them be well cleanfed and fcrap d likewife for fome time, to take away the ill tafte Then cut them
of the fame length with your Chitterlings, and having tied up
the ends of every one, put them neatly into the Skirts fo as they
may be cover'd and bound up therein When your Chitterlings are made, put them into a Kettle of Water with Slices of
Onion, an Onion ftuck with Cloves, two Bay-leaves and a
little Leaf-fat out of the Hog's Belly · Let them be gently
boil'd and well fcumm'd, pouring in, after the Scum is taken off,
a Glafs or two of white Wine Let them cool in the fame Liquor, and afterwards take them out, but be careful to avoid
breaking them They are ufually broil d upon a Grid-iron with
Paper under them and ferved up to Table all at once

A Potage of *Andouilles* may likewife be ferv d up with ftrained Peafe and good Broth, and to that end, each is to be made

apart ;

apart; that of the Chitterlings with a Faggot of Herbs and a Piece of green Lemmon: But you are to put into the Peaſe-ſoop, ſome fine Herbs chopt ſmall and toſs'd up in a Pan with Lard. The Chitterlings are cut into round Slices, to be laid upon your ſoaked Cruſts, with white Pepper, Mutton-gravy and Lemmon-juice, when ready to be ſerv'd up to Table, and are garniſh'd with fried Bread and Slices of Lemmon.

Andouilles de Veau, *or Calves-chitterlings.*

After having well waſh'd and prepar'd the larger Calves-guts, cut them according to the length you would have your Chitterlings to be of, and tye up one of the ends: Then take a ſufficient quantity of Bacon, Calves-udder, and Calves chal-dron, all parboil'd, and cut them into ſmall pieces in form of a Die: Put them into a Stew-pan and ſeaſon them with Spice beaten ſmall, and a Bay-leaf. There muſt be alſo ſome Pep-per and Salt, with a few minc'd Shalots, and you may add about a Gallon of good Milk-cream Set the whole Mixture over the Furnace, and afterwards draw back the Pan; into which you are to put four or five Yolks of Eggs, and a few Crums of Bread: Thus all being well thicken'd, proceed to make your Chitterlings hot, with a Funnel, and tye up their ends. Afterwards let them be parboil'd in Water and dreſs'd in the ſame manner as the Hogs-chitterlings · They are like-wiſe to be boil'd and left to cool in their Liquor; then let them be broil'd upon a Grid-iron, with Paper, and ſerved up to Table. Theſe ſorts of Chitterlings may be made in Summer, when Pork is out of Seaſon; as alſo in thoſe Countries, where no Hogs are kill'd throughout the whole Year, as it happens at *Paris.*

ANDOUILLETS.

Veal-*Andouillets* are made of minc'd Veal, Bacon, fine Herbs and the Yolks of Eggs, with Pepper, Salt, Nutmeg and beaten Cinnamon, ſo as to give them a fine colour, and in ſerving them up, ſome beaten Yolks of Eggs are to be added, with Verjuice and Lemmon-juice. Theſe *Andouillets* are to be roaſt-ed on a Spit between Slices of Bacon, and baſted with their Dripping, with the Yolks of Eggs and Crums of Bread, ſome-times one and ſometimes another, to produce a fine Cruſt upon
them:

them : When they are ready to be ferv'd up, add fome Mutton-gravy, or of another fort, with the Juice of a Lemmon and fried Parfley to garnifh them

Andouillets are likewife made of Fifh, with the Flefh of Eels and Carps minc'd or pounded in a Mortar, and feafon'd according to the ufual manner : With part of this Flefh, a *Cervelas* is to be made in a Linnen-cloth, and boil'd with white Wine, Butter and a Faggot of fine Herbs ; and *Andouillets* are made with the reft, which are likewife to be boil'd in Butter, with Broth and a handful of fine Herbs   Then tofs up fome Mufhrooms in a Pan, with Carp-roes and a little fine Flower, and after having caus'd them to boil a little while, with fome Fifh-broth and green Lemmon ; put them to your *Andouillets*   Thus they may be ferv'd up for Side-difhes, or elfe in Potage ; dreffing them on your foaked Crufts, garnifh'd with *Cervelas* in Slices and with fome Slices and Juice of Lemmon.

A R T I C H O K E S.

There are feveral Ways of dreffing Artichokes to be ferv'd up for Intermeffes, and amongft others thefe are the chief, *viz.*

Artichokes with white Sauce.

Let fome fmall Artichokes be boil'd in Water, with a little Salt. When they are fufficiently boil'd, put the Bottoms into a Pan, with Parfley feafon'd with Salt and white Pepper, and prepare a Sauce for them, with the Yolks of Eggs, and a little Vinegar and fome Broth.

Artichokes dreß'd with natural Butter.

When your Artichokes are boil'd, as before, take off the Chokes, and make Sauce for them, with natural Butter, Vinegar, Salt and Nutmeg

Fried Artichokes.

Take away the Chokes, cut them into Slices and let them boil three or four Walms   Let them be fteep'd in Vinegar, with Pepper, Salt and Chibbols   Then, having flower'd them, fry them in Lard or refined Butter, and ferve them up to Table with fried Parfley.

Arti-

Artichoke-bottoms fried in Paste.

The Artichokes being boil'd and freed from their Chokes, make a Paste, with Flower, Water, Pepper and Salt, and put them into it in order to be well fried Let them also be ferv'd up, with fried Parfley and a little Rofe-Vinegar.

Other Ways of Dreffing them.

Artichokes in Cream are likewife prepar'd after the fame manner as Afparagus, others *à la Saingaraz* and with Gammon-fauce, on Flefh-days, for which fee Gammon-effence under the Letter G. and young Rabbets *à la Saingaraz* under R. And laftly, others *à l'Eftoufade* or ftew'd and iced. Artichokes are of very great Ufe throughout the whole Year, for almoft all forts of Ragoo's Potages and Side-difhes; fo that 'tis requifite to provide good ftore of them, obferving the following Directions.

The manner of preferving Artichokes.

Take fo much Water, according to the quantity of your Artichokes, as will be fufficient to cover them, and let them boil, with Salt proportionably, then take them off from the Fire, and let them lye by, to the end that the Drofs of the Salt may fink to the Bottom. Afterwards pour the Liquor, into the Pot, wherein you would have your Artichokes put, which ought to be well turn'd and only fcalded, to take off the Chokes and Scum. They are to be wafh'd in two or three Waters, and afterwards put into a prepared Brine or Pickle, pouring Oil or good Butter thereon, to hinder the Air from penetrating them; you may, alfo if you pleafe, add a little Vinegar They muft be carefully cover'd with Paper and a Board over it, that the leaft Air may not be let in Thus they may be kept for a whole Year, but before they are us'd, the Salt muft be taken away, by foaking them in frefh Water.

Artichokes may alfo be preferv'd dry; and to that purpofe, when they are Scalded, and the Chokes taken off as before, you are to fpread them upon Grates or Hurdles of wattled Oziers, in order to drain them; then they are to be dry'd in the Sun, or in an Oven moderately heated; till they become

as

as dry as Wood. Before they are us'd, they are to be fteept in Luke-warm Water during two Days, by which means they'll return to the fame Condition as when they were frefh, and will relifh much better than when prepared after the other manner. They are to be fcalded in Water, with a little Verjuice Salt and new Butter, on Fifh-days, and with good Beef-fat on Flefh-days.

Asparagus.

Afparagus is eaten feveral Ways, and Potages are made of it, with different forts of Fowl, or with green Peafe-foop; of which divers Examples have been already produced. 'Tis alfo ufually ferv'd up in Inter-neffes, Out-works and other Difhes; fometimes in a Sallet, fometimes in white or thick Gra-and fometimes in Cream.

Afparagus in Cream

Let your Afparagus be cut into fmall Pieces, and fcalded a little in boiling Water. Then let them be tofs'd up in a Stew-pan with frefh Butter, or with Lard, if you have no very good Butter, taking care that the whole Mefs be not too fat. Then put into it fome Milk and Cream, and feafon it well, adding alfo a Faggot of fine Herbs. Before this Difh is ferv'd up to Table, it would be requifite to beat up one or two Yolks of Eggs, with Milk-cream, in order to thicken your Afparagus

The fame thing may be done in dreffing Artichoke-bottoms and green Peafe, but for the latter fome Sugar is to be ufed, with a little chopt Parfley, and then they may be order'd in the fame manner

Afparagus may alfo be ferv'd up among green Peafe, with a green Cullis of Peafe-cods or fomewhat elfe. Then put a Cruft of Bread in the middle, and garnifh your Difh round a-bout, with *Pain de Jambon.*

Afparagus in Gravy.

Drefs your Afparagus cut into Pieces, with Lard, Parfley, Chervil chopt fmall and a *Ciboulet* Seafon them with Salt and Nutmeg, and let them foak in a Pot over a gentle Fire. Then take away the Fat, put therein fome Mutton-gravy and Lem-mon-juice, and ferve it up, with fhort Sauce.   *A-*

Asparagus with natural Butter.

Boil your Asparagus in Water, with a little Salt, prepare a Sauce with Butter, Salt, Vinegar and Nutmeg or white Pepper, continually stirring it, and pour it upon the Asparagus, when they are dress'd. There is nothing in this Article, that is not sufficiently known, as well as what relates to Asparagus in a Sallet For the Potages, you may observe by means of the General Table, those that are hereafter mentioned and under the Article of *Tourtes* or Pan-pies, the manner of making one of Asparagus.

To preserve Asparagus.

Cut off the hard Stalks, and give them one seething with Salt and Butter: Throw them again into fresh Water, and let them be drain'd. When they are cold, put them into a Vessel, in which they may lie at their full length, with some Salt, whole Cloves, green Lemmon, and as much Water as Vinegar · Cover them with melted Butter, as 'tis usually done to Artichokes, putting a Linnen-cloth between, and keep them in a temperate Place In order to make use of them, let them be steept and boil'd as the others.

B.

French BEANS or Kidney-beans.

The best Manner of Preserving and Dressing them.

FRench Beans may be preserved two several Ways, *viz* either pickled with Vinegar, Water and Salt, as Cucumbers, or else dried, after they have been well pickt and scalded. They are usually dry'd in the Sun, and set in a Place that is not moist To recover them, they are only to be steep'd in luke-warm Water for the space of two Days, and they'll resume almost the same Verdure that they had when first gather'd: Then let them be scalded and dress'd after the usual manner As for those that are Marinated or Pickled, when they are sufficiently season'd in a Pot, with some Cloves and a little Pepper, they must be well cover'd, lest they should be
spoil

ſpoil'd, and ſome melted Butter may be put upon them: As often as you have Occaſion to uſe them, let them be ſoak'd in Water, as the others; to the end that all their Saltneſs may be taken away, and then they may ſerve either for Sallets or for Intermeſſes, after they have been ſcalded and put into Cream.

B E E F.

Foraſmuch as Beef is a Thing no leſs common than neceſſary in Entertainments, 'tis requiſite to deviſe ſeveral Ways of dreſſing it to the beſt Advantage, in order to make it delicious and graceful even on the moſt ſumptuous Tables.

A ſhort Rib of Beef, à la Godard.

Let the firſt ſhort Rib of Beef, be Spitted and one half of it larded, with thick Slips of Bacon: When it is half roaſted, take it off from the Spit, and put it into a Pot, after it has been well ſeaſon'd, with good Gravy, a few *Truffles, Morilles,* common Muſhrooms and Artichokes, only to give it a Reliſh · In the mean-while prepare another Ragoo of *Truffles,* Muſhrooms, *Morilles,* Artichoke-bottoms, Veal-ſweet-breads, and Cocks-combs, all well thicken'd, which you are to put upon the ſhort Rib; garniſhing it with a *Marinade* of Chickens or marinated Cutlets.

A ſhort Rib of Beef dreſs'd after the Engliſh Way.

Take a large ſhort Rib of Beef, and let it lie two Days in Salt · Afterwards Spit it, and when 'tis well roaſted, bread it and put a good Ragoo both on the top and underneath. Let this Diſh be garniſh'd with *Hatlets, Marinades* or roaſted *Poupiets.*

A ſhort Rib of Beef with Cucumbers.

Another middling Side-diſh may conſiſt of a ſhort Rib of Beef, with a good Ragoo of Cucumbers, a few Shalots and fine Herbs chopt ſmall, ſo as to give all a good Reliſh. It muſt be ſet out with marinated Veal-culets, fried Bread, or ſome other convenient Garniture.

A

A short Rib of Beef farced.

It may be farced with a *Salpicon*, of which fee the manner under the letter S Or elfe, when the fhort Rib is almoft roafted, take fome of the Flefh out of the middle, to be minced fmall with Bacon, Beef-fewet, fine Herbs, Spice and good Garnitures Then farce your fhort Rib between the Skin and the Bone, and fow it up again neatly, left the Meat fhould fall into the Dripping-pan, whilft you are making an end of roafting it. This Difh is to be garnifh'd with *Fricandoe's* or Scotch Collops in form of larded Cutlets, with fried Bread, and when ferv'd up to Table, the Skins are to be taken off, to have the Liberty of earing the Meat with a Spoon

A great Side-difh of a Buttock of Beef.

Take a Buttock of Beef, as large or fmall as you fhall think fit; lard it with Gammon and other Bacon, that is well feafon'd with Pepper, Salt, Coriander-feed, Cinnamon, Cloves and grated Nutmeg ; as alfo Parfley, Onions and fmall Shalots, all well mixt together. Stuff as much of thefe as you can into the Bacon, and lard your Meat both on the top and underneath Seafon it again with all your Ingredients, and put it into a Stew-pan to be marinated a little while, with Onions, Parfley, Shalots, Garlick, fweet Bafil, Thyme, Verjuice, Slices of Lemmon and a little Broth. It muft be left therein two Hours, and boil'd in the Evening for the next Day · It muft be put in a Napkin, with thin Slices of Bacon, and the Napkin is to be wrapt up clofe, fo that no Fat may enter In the mean while, you are to choofe a Pot that is fit for it, and a Silver-Plate is to be laid on the Bottom, to keep the Napkin or Meat from being burnt For the feafoning of it, you may put therein about two Pounds of Leaf-fat taken out of a Hog's Belly, or of frefh Beef-fewet, according to the bignefs of the Piece of Beef, adding fome Verjuice, white Wine, Ginger, Cinnamon, long Pepper, Slices of Lemmon, Nutmeg, Onion, Parfley Bay-leaves, as much Salt as is requifite, fweet Bafil and Coriander whole, Fennel and Anis. Having put all into the Pot, cover it, and let your Piece of Beef be ftew'd very gently When 'tis fufficiently boil'd, let it cool in its own Fat; then make a great *Godivee*, which is to be put into the Difh, in which the Piece

of

of Beef is to be dress'd, cover it with the same *Godivoe*, and set it into the Oven for an Hour In order to bring it to Table, a well seasoned Beef-cullis is to be prepar'd; then make a round Hole on the top of the *Godivoe*, to pour in your Cullis, so as to penetrate into every part, and the Juice of a Lemmon thereupon. This sort of Beef may be serv'd up cold in thin Slices instead of Beef *à la Royale*.

A Side-dish of a Piece of Beef.

Take the hinder part of a Buttock, larded with thick Slips of Bacon, and having put it into a Pot or Kettle with two Pounds of Lard, some good Slices of Bacon and the necessary seasoning Ingredients, let it boil very gently, about two Hours. Take care that it be corned, and that no Air comes to it, when 'tis boiling At least, you may put a little Brandy thereto, and garnish it with *Marinade*.

Another Side-dish of a Piece of Beef.

Let a Buttock of Beef, moderately corned, be put into a Pot, with all sorts of fine Spices and Onions. Having fill'd the Pot with Water, let it boil and be well scumm'd: Then some good Meat-gravy is to be put therein to enrich it. When 'tis boil'd and ready to be dress'd in its Dish, you must take away a little of the Fat from the top, and put upon it a Gammon-hash, garnish'd with a *Marinade* of larded Veal fried, and farc'd Cucumbers, according to the Method hereafter describ'd; or else with Artichoke-bottoms cut into two pieces, and Veal Sweet-breads, all fried and steept in the same manner as the Cucumbers.

A Side-dish of Beef-stakes rolled.

Having cut some good Slices or Stakes of Beef, beat them flat on the Dresser, with a Cleaving-knife · For example, Take three or four large Slices, according to the size of your Dish, and make a farced Meat of Capons-flesh, a piece of a Leg of Veal, Bacon, tried Sewet, boil'd Gammon, Parsley and Chibbols, with some Veal-Sweet-breads, *Truffles* and Mushrooms, all minc'd and well season'd with Spice and fine Herbs. To these are also to be added three or four Yolks of Eggs with a little Milk-cream,

cream, and when your Farce is well minc'd, lay it upon the Beef-ftakes, which are to be neatly roll'd up, till they become ve-firm and compact, and of a convenient thickness Thus they are to be ftew'd over the Fire for a confiderable time, then take them out of the Pot, drain off the Fat, cut them into two pieces, and drefs them in a Difh, on the fame fide that they were cut, which is uppermoft When they are fet in order fome Ragoo or Cullis may be put upon them, and nothing elfe.

This Farce may ferve for feveral forts of Fowl, when in great Entertainments there are many to be faiced. It may alfo be ufed for fcollop d Veal, farced *Fricandoes* and other Things Side-difhes and Out-works of the like nature, are ufually made with Veal-ftakes drefs'd after the fame manner.

A Side-difh of a Piece of Beef, with Cucumbers.

Take a Piece of good tender Beef and roaft it, barded or cover'd with thin Slices of Bacon, and wrapt up in Paper, but let it not be over-done : Then cut it into *Filets* or fmall thin Slices, and put them into a Difh In the mean while, fome Cucumber are likewife to be cut into Slices, according to the quantity of the *Filets*, but they muft be marinated Squeeze them, and put them into a Stew-pan with fome Lard to be well ftew'd over the Furnace Afterwards drain off all the Lard, throw in a little Flower and tofs them up again a little while : Laftly, Soak them with good Gravy, proportionably to the quantity of your *Filets* When they are ready, fome good thickening Liquor muft be put in, to make the Ingredients incorporate well toge-ther; a Spoonful of Gammon effence, would be excellent for that purpofe : Add to thefe, a little Verjuice or Vinegar, and let not your *Filets* boil any longer left they fhould grow hard. They are to be ferv'd up hot to Table, and garnifh'd with fried Bread, Marinades, or *Riffoles*

All other forts of *Filets*, with Cucumbers, may be made in the fame manner.

Another Side-difh of Beef-Filets.

Another Side-difh may be prepar'd with Beef-*Filets* larded, and marinated with Vinegar, Salt, Pepper, Cloves, Thyme and Onions, which are to be roafted by a gentle Fire When
they

they are ready, put them into good Gravy with *Truffles*, and garnish them with marinated Chickens or Pigeons, or with *Fri-candoes.*

Other Courses of Beef.

Some small pieces of Beef may be serv'd up for Out-works, which are to be a little corn'd and garnish'd with Parsly; but if it be a middling Side-dish, it may be garnish'd with what you shall think fit   They are also put into Gravy, when minc'd very small, with a Shalot, or a Clove of Garlick, and chopt Parsly

A piece of Brisket-beef may be put into a Pot, and when par-boil'd, larded with thick Slips of Bacon season'd with Salt, Pepper, beaten Cloves and Nutmeg, and the boiling of them may be finish'd in an Earthen Pan, with thin Slices of Bacon at the Bottom, Pepper, Salt, a Bunch of Herbs, a little White-wine, green Lemmon, Bay-leaves and Broth   When 'tis boil'd, put thereto a Ragoo of Mushrooms, Oisters, Capers and stoned Olives, all well thicken'd; as also Lemmon-juice, when ready to be serv'd up to Table, and let it be garnish'd with Slices of the same.

For the Sauce with Vinegar and Pepper; take a Beef-stake, let it be well beaten, larded with thick Slips of Bacon, and boil'd in Water, with a Glass of White-wine, seasoning it high with Pep-per, Salt, Cloves, Bay-leaves and a Faggot of Herbs   Let the Broth be well soaked, and when cold, the Stake being in the same Pot, it may be serv'd up with Lemmon-slices and a little Vinegar.

Beef-stakes may also be put into a Pie; to which purpose see that of a Fillet of Veal, under the Letter P, and observe the same Method; except that the Beef-stake Pie requires longer time in baking   But you must by no means forget to make a Hole therein, when put into the Oven, and to stop it up, when taken out

Beef à la Mode, ought to be well beaten, larded with thick Slips of Bacon, and, if you please, stew'd in a Pan, before it be boil'd, with Pepper, Salt, Bay-leaves, green Lemmon, half a douzen of Mush-rooms, a Glass of White-wine and two Glasses of Water: It may likewise be stew'd in its own Gravy, close cover'd over a gentle Fire.   When 'tis boil'd, fry some Flower in a Pan, with Lard, which may be put thereto with Lemmon-juice.

F   The

The Palate of an Ox is frequently used in *Mine-droit*, or *Menus-droits*, for which see the Letter M.

BISKETS.

The Manner of Making Savoy-biskets.

There are several sorts of Biskets very common, but for those that are call'd *Savoy*-biskets, take three or four new-laid Eggs, more or less according to the quantity of Biskets you intend to make: Then having provided a pair of Scales, put the Eggs into one, and some baked Flower into the other. Lift them up to render the Weight equal on both sides, for example, if four Eggs were put in, you are to take out one, and leave the three others. Weigh out as much fine Sugar pounded to Powder, as the weight of the Eggs amounts to, and take away the four Whites, to make as strong a Snow of them as possibly can be. Having minc'd some green Lemmon-peel, reduce it as it were to Powder, and mix it with the Flower that was weigh'd a little before. Beat them up a little, put some Sugar thereto, after having beaten them again, add some Yolks of Eggs, and whip all together for some time. Afterwards let the Biskets be made upon Paper, either in a round or long Form, at pleasure, and they may be neatly iced with Sugar beaten to Powder. They are to be bak'd in an Oven, taking care that it be not too hot, and as soon as they are done, cut them off from the Paper, with a thin Knife. They are us'd for Fruit or to garnish certain Pies.

Another sort of Biskets.

Take three or four Eggs, according to the quantity of Biskets you are desirous to make, and beat them up a little while; to which add as much rasped Sugar as you can take up between your Fingers at four or five times, with some Lemmon-peel, and mix all together, with four or five Spoonfuls of baked Flower. This Compound is to be laid upon Paper that has been strew'd thick with Sugar, and some Sugar being likewise strew'd on the top, set into the Oven, to be dried. When it is drawn out, cut the Biskets, all at once, with the Paper underneath, according to the bigness and shape, you would have them to be of, and with a Pen-knife cut off the Paper gently,

for

for fear of breaking any of them, which may be eaſily done, becauſe they ought to be very dry. Theſe Biſkets ſerve, as the former, either for Fruit, or to garniſh Pies

There are ſeveral other ſorts of Biſkets, but beſides that they ſcarce differ in any thing, except the Name, it is the peculiar Province of the Confectioner Therefore the inquiſitive Readers are referr'd to the Inſtructions that have been already publiſh'd for the uſe of thoſe Perſons.

B I S K S.

Theſe ſorts of Potages are made with Quails, Capons and large fat Pullets, and moſt commonly Pigeons; ſo that we ſhall firſt ſhew the manner of preparing the laſt

To make a Biſk of Pigeons

Take Pigeons newly kill'd; ſcald, pick and parboil them, and let them be ſtew'd, in clear Broth, with ſeveral *Bards* or thin Slices of Bacon, an Onion ſtuck with Cloves, and two Slices of Lemmon, all well ſcumm'd. Set them on the Fire, only one Hour before they are us'd, according to their bigneſs, and when they are dreſs'd, lay them aſide for a while. In order to make a proper Ragoo for them, 'tis requiſite to take ſome Veal-Sweetbreads cut into two parts, Muſhrooms cut into ſmall pieces, *Truffles* in Slices, Artichoke-bottoms cut into four quarters, and one whole, to be put into the middle of the Potage You muſt carefully fry this Ragoo, with a little Lard, fine Flower, and an Onion ſtuck with Cloves, and need not ſtay till it grows brown. When 'tis thus dreſs'd, put a little good Broth therein and ſtew it, with a Slice of Lemmon In the mean while, cauſe to be boiled a-part in a little Pot, ſome Cocks-combs well ſcalded and pickt, with thin Slices of Bacon, Veal-ſewet, ſome clear Broth, a Slice of Lemmon and an Onion ſtuck with three Cloves, but care muſt be more eſpecially taken, that the whole Mixture be well parboil'd: To which purpoſe, ſtrain a little Bread-crum, with only two Spoonfuls of good Broth thro' a Sieve. Your Pigeons, Cocks combs and Ragoo being ready, make Sippets, with Cruſts of Bread toaſted at the Fire, and lay the Potage a ſoaking with good Broth: Then dreſs the Pigeons therein, and the Artichoke-bottom in the middle, the Ragoo being put between the Pigeons, and the Cocks-combs

upon

upon their *Stomacks* · When the Fat is throughly taken away, pour in the reft of the Ragoo. At the fame time you are to provide a piece of Beef or Veal half roafted, which is to be cut in a Stew-pan or on a Difh, and to be fqueez'd hard, to get all the Gravy : It ought to be fet at a diftance from the Fire, to the end that it may become white, and when the Potage is drefs'd, fprinkle it with this Gravy, that it may be well marbled. It muft be garnifh'd with Lemmon, one half of which may be fqueez'd thereupon, and ferv'd up hot to Table

Bisks of Quails and others

Trufs your Quails neatly in the fame manner as Chickens, and drefs them with burnt Butter till they acquire a fine Colour : Then put them into a little Pot, with fome good Broth, Slices of Bacon, a Bunch of Herbs, Cloves, and other Things proper to feafon them ; as alfo a piece of a beaten Beef-ftake, another of lean Bacon and fome green Lemmon, and let all boil over a gentle Fire. This Bisk muft be garnifh'd as the other, with Sweet-breads of Veal, Artichoke-bottoms, Mufhrooms, *Truffles*, *Friciandoes* and Cocks-combs, with the fineft of which you may make a Ring or Border round about the Difh ; marbling the Potage with a Veal-cullis and Lemmon-juice, as it is a ferving up to Table.

The Bisks of Capons and fat Pullets are made after the fame manner as the preceeding, as well as thofe of young Barn-door Chickens.

As for Bisks of Fifh, chop fome Mufhrooms very fmall, and lay them upon the Crufts of Bread that are to be foaked with good Fifh-broth   The Ragoo may be made with Carp-roes, Pike-livers, the Tails and Claws of Cray-fifh, and Juice of Lemmon, garnifh'd with the fame

B L A N C - M A N G E R S.

Blanc-mangers are us'd in Intermeffes, or for middling Difhes or Out-works, and may be made thus : Take Calves-feet, and a Hen that is not very fat, let them be well boil'd without Salt and ftrain'd, taking care that it be not too ftrong nor too thin. If you have too great a quantity of Jelly, take out fome of it, putting fome Sugar, Cinnamon and Lemmon-peel to the reft, and let all boil a little while over the Fire, in a Stew-pan ; after

ter having taken off the Fat In the mean while, some sweet Almonds are to be provided, and if you please, seven or eight bitter ones among them, according to the quantity of your *Blanc-manger* These are to be well pounded, and well moisten'd with Milk, that they may not turn to Oil. Then strain the *Blanc-manger*, that is not too hot, twice or thrice with the Almonds; wash the Sieves well, and strain them again once more, to the end that the Liquor may become very white. After having pour'd it into a Dish, ice it neatly, and pass over it two Sheets of white Paper, to take off the Fat Let a little Orange-flower-water be put thereto, and when 'tis well congeal'd, serve it up cold to Table, garnishing it with Lemmon.

To make *Blanc-mangers* of divers Colours, see what is hereafter declar'd under the Article of *Jellies.*

A Blanc-manger *of Harts-horn.*

Take about a Pound of rasped Harts-horn, proportionably to the quantity you design to make, and let it boil for a considerable time; so that, dipping your Finger therein, you perceive that the Liquor is become as it were clammy, which is a sign that 'tis sufficiently boil'd. Strain this Jelly thro' a very fine Sieve, and pound the Almonds, moistening them with Milk and a little Cream Then you must strain the same Jelly with these Almonds, three or four times, to render it very white, and put thereto a little Orange-flower-water

If the Entertainment be made on Fish-days in Lent, for the Evening-course, the *Blanc-manger* must only be strain'd with pounded Almonds; squeezing a little Lemmon-juice therein, and no Milk is to be put into it. When 'tis ready it may be serv'd up in Ice.

B O A R's H E A D, *see* H E A D S.

B O U C O N S.

To make *Boucons,* take a Fillet of Veal cut into small Stakes or Slices, that are somewhat long and thin, and beat them on a Table or Dresser Then having prepar'd some small Slices of fat Bacon, with as many of raw Gammon, dispose them in Ranks a-cross your Veal-slices, that is to say, first one Slice of

F 3 Bacon,

Bacon, and then another of Gammon   Strew them with a little Parsley and Chibbols, and season them with Spice and fine Herbs   The Veal-stakes being thus cover'd with these Slices, are to be neatly roll'd up, as if they were *Filets Mignons* and broil'd upon the Coals   When they are dress'd, let the Fat be drain'd off, and serve them up hot, with a good Cullis, and a Ragoo of Mushrooms.

BOUILLANS

Are made thus ⋅ Take the Breasts of roasted Pullets or Capons, with a little Marrow, about the thickness of an Egg, some Calves-udder parboil'd, as much Bacon and a few fine Herbs, and put the whole Mixture well minc'd and season'd upon a Plate : Make some fine Paste and roll out two pieces, as thin as Paper. Wet one of them lightly with a little Water, and lay your farced Meat upon it in small heaps, at a convenient distance one from another: Cover them with the other piece of rolled Paste, and with the tips of your Fingers, close up every Parcel between the two Pastes; then with an Instrument proper for that purpose, cut them off one by one, and set the uppermost underneath; dressing them neatly, as if they were so many little Pies. Thus they are to be bak'd, and may be used for Out-works, or to garnish Side-dishes; but they must be serv'd up hot to Table.

BOUTON.

A Side-dish of a small Bouton.

Prepare a good well-season'd *Godivoe*, as for the *Poupeton*, according to the Method hereafter, described under the Letter G. Let it serve as it were for a Lay upon broad thin Slices of Bacon, that are capable of wrapping up your whole *Bouton*, and add thereto a good Ragoo of Mushrooms, Veal-Sweet-breads, Artichoke-bottoms, Cocks-combs, *Mousserons, Truffles* and Asparagus-tops dress'd with white Sauce. Then cover it again with another Lay of *Godivoe* and Bacon-slices, and let it be bak'd between two Fires, or dress'd otherwise   When 'tis ready to be serv'd up to Table, after the Fat is taken off, put some Lemmon-juice therein, garnish it with little farced Rolls, *Fricandoes* and *Marinades* intermixt.

The

The same thing may be done on Fish-days, making the *Godi-vve* of the Flesh of Carps, Eels, Tenches and other sorts of Fish, well minc'd and season'd

BRAISES.

We shall not here enlarge upon every Thing that may be bak'd or stew'd *à la Braise*, that is to say, between two Fires, *viz.* one on the top and the other underneath, which is a manner of Dressing that extremely heightens the Relish of Meat, and is very much in vogue. Some Examples of it have been already produc'd in the Article of *Beef*, and many others will be found hereafter, which shall be likewise explain'd in the respective Places to which the Things themselves belong, and if this be not always done, you need only consult the Articles that come near them, and have recourse for that purpose, to the Table of the principal Matters at the end of this Volume.

BROILING *upon a Grid-iron, see* GRILLADE

BROTHS.

Altho' this Article might be referr'd to that of Potages, as properly belonging thereto, nevertheless we have judg'd it necessary to take notice of it in this place, to the end that the Reader may be freed from any Doubt that might arise concerning the different sorts of Broths which he has already observ'd or may meet with hereafter, or from the Pains he might otherwise take in searching for some Light in the matter elsewhere: Therefore we have here set down what is most remarkable, with respect to the Broths that are requisite, as well for the Potages, as for the Side-dishes

Fat Broth.

Boil some part of a Buttock and Leg of Beef, with other Meats, and take out the Gravy and Broth; straining it thro' a Linnen-cloth. Let the same pieces be put a second time into the Pot, and having caus'd them to be well boil'd, take out the Broth again, keeping both these sorts hot apart. The first will be of good use to be put to Capons, young Turkeys, Chickens, Quails, Veal and other farced Meats, that are to be serv'd up

in white Potage. Capon or Veal-broth ought to be taken to
foak young Pigeons for Bisks, and with the Broth of the Bisks,
a Cullis may be made, for the Potages *a la Reine* and *a la Roy-
a'e* Laftly, The Broth of farced Meats will ferve to make a
Cullis for the fame forts of Meat, *viz* young Turkeys and Pullets, Knuckles and Breafts of Veal, and other Joynts of Meat
that ought to be farc'd and parboil'd.

The fecond fort of Broth taken out of the great Pot, is to
be put into the brown Potages, particularly, thofe of Ducks,
Teals, Rabbets, Ring-doves, Larks, Pheafants, Thrufhes, Cabbage, Turneps and others, and the brown Ingredients which
ferve to thicken them, are to be mixt with the fame Broth,
without confounding that of one of thefe forts, with the others
This Broth is alfo proper for the Side-difhes, and fome of it
may be ufed in boiling the Pickings of Mufhrooms, of which
the Pulp is to be taken out, to ferve for that Cullis, for all the
Potages, Side-difhes and Intermeffes

N B *The other forts of Cullifes are hereafter defcrib'd under
the Letter* C, *and the Gravies under* G.

Morning-broth for Breakfaft.

'Tis ufually made with a piece of Buttock-beef, the fcraggy
end of a Neck of Mutton, a Neck of Veal and two Pullets.
Take the Breafts of the Pullets when they are boil'd, pound
them in a Mortar with a piece of Bread-crum, fteept in fome
Broth ; and all being well feafon'd, ftrain it thro' the Sieve, to
be laid upon the Crufts foak'd in the fame Broth that is then
made.

The particular Broths for Potages *de Santé* and others are to
be found in their proper Places, under the Letter P ; only in
favour of fick Perfons, it may not be improper to fubjoyn what
may tend to their Advantage.

Jelly-broth for Confumptive Perfons.

Put a Joynt of Mutton into an Earthen Pot, with a Capon,
a Fillet of Veal and three Quarts of Water; which is to be
boil'd over a gentle Fire, till one half be confum'd. Then fqueez
all together and ftrain the Liquor thro' a Linnen-cloth.

The Reftaurative Broth is ranked among the Potages, under
the Title of *Potage without Water.*

N. B.

N B *The following Liquors tho' not falling under the Order of the Alphabet ought to be inserted in this place,* viz

Veal-liquor.

Having cut a Fillet of Veal into very thin Slices, let them boil in an Earthen Pot full of Water over a gentle Fire, for the space of an Hour ; and then strain this Liquor thro' a Linnen cloth, without squeezing the Meat.

Chicken or Pullet-liquor

Put two or three Chickens or young Pullets into a Pot, with Water, and when they have boil'd two Hours over a gentle Fire, strain the Liquor thro' a Linnen-cloth ; to which may be added Buglofs, Borage, Succory and other cooling Herbs, according to the Circumstances of the Patients and the Prescriptions of the Physicians.

Capon-liquor.

Let a Capon be set over a gentle Fire, in an Earthen Pot, with three Quarts of Water. When the Capon is boil'd, and one Pint of the Water wasted, take it out without squeezing.

Fish-broth.

This Broth is the chief Ingredient of all sorts of Fish-potages that can be prepar'd with the several Distinctions that are made for every one. To that purpose, cleanse Tenches, Eels, Pikes and Carps from their Slime, and cut off their Gills : Then put all into a great Kettle or Pot, with Water, Butter, Salt, a Faggot of fine Herbs and an Onion stuck with Cloves When they have boil'd an Hour and half, strain the Broth thro' a Linnen-cloth, and pour some of it separately into three Pots In one of them put the Pickings of Mushrooms, which afterwards are to be pass'd thro' the Sieve, with a Cullis, fried Flower and a piece of green Lemmon · This thickening Liquor may serve for the brown Potages, as also for the Side-dishes and Intermesses In the second, may be put pounded Almonds, with the Yolks of hard Eggs, if the time will permit, and this is proper for white Potages, particularly those of *Profitrolles,* Smelts,

Smelts, Perches, Soles and other Fish drefs'd in white Broth and for fome Ragoo's of the like Nature   Laftly, in the third Pot, the Fish of all the Potages as well White as Brown, both for the Side-difhes and Intermeffes may be boil'd together, and fome Jelly may alfo be made of them

Another fort of Fifh-broth may likewife be prepared thus, Take a great Kettle or Pot, of a fize proportionable to the quantity of Potage that is to be made   Hang it over the Fire, and put Water therein, with Parfly-roots, Parfneps, whole Onions, a handful of Parfly and Sorrel, all forts of fine Herbs and good Butter, all well feafon'd   Add to thefe, the Bones and Carcaffes of Fifhes, whofe Flefh has been taken to make Farces, and even the Entrails of thofe that have been farc'd, after having been well cleanfed, and, if you pleafe, fome Cray-fifh-tails pounded, with four or five Spoonfuls of Onion-juice   The whole Mefs being well feafon'd and fufficiently boil'd, ftrain it thro' a Sieve, put it again into the Pot, and keep it hot, to lay the Soops a foaking, to prepare the Fifh for the Potage, and for other Ufes.

Broth on Fifh-days, for the Potage with Herbs.

Let all forts of good Herbs be put into a Pot, with two or three Crufts of Bread, feafon'd with Salt, Butter and a Bunch of fine Herbs: When they have boil'd an Hour and half, ftrain the Broth thro' a Linnen-cloth, or a Sieve. This will ferve for the Potage *de Santé* without Herbs, and for many others, particularly for thofe of Lettuce, Afparagus, Succory, Artichokes, Cardoons, &c.

A fort of Broth may likewife be made on Days of Abftinence, with Roots without Fifh, and with clear Peas-foop; ftraining the whole Mefs, as before.

B R U S O L E S.

Take fome Stakes, or Meat cut into Slices, beaten a little while with the back of a Knife, and put them into a Stew-pan, with feveral thin Slices of Bacon laid in order underneath Strew them with Parfly, chopt Chibbols and Spices ; continuing to make a Lay of the like fort of Seafoning, and another of Stakes, till at laft you cover them well with broad Slices of Bacon, and fet them between two Fires, on the top and underneath,

neath, after having caus'd the Pan to be clofe cover'd. When they are ready, a Cullis may be prepar'd with the Carcaffes of Partridges: Then, having taken off all the Fat, put thefe Stakes into a Difh and pour the Cullis upon them · They are commonly call'd *Brufoles* or *Burfoles* in *French*, and are ufed for Side-difhes.

They may alfo be farc'd with a good *Godivoe*, minc'd and well pounded in a Mortai, with fine Herbs, Yolks of Eggs, Cream and the ufual feafoning Ingredients, putting this farc'd Meat upon very large *Fricandoes* or *Scotch* Collops, that are to be wrapt up in broad Slices of Bacon and bak'd in a Pie-pan. As foon as they are ready, pour a Ragoo upon them, made of *Truffles*, *Moufferons* and a Veal-cullis to thicken them

See under the Letter F the Manner of Dreffing farc'd *Fricandoes*, which have fome relation to thefe *Brufoles*.

B U R T S or *Bret-fifh.*

In dreffing Burts, you may endeavour to imitate the Method hereafter explain'd for Soles, for as to the Way of ordering them with natural Butter, or of making a Ragoo, by frying them in burnt Butter, after having cut off their Heads, 'tis fo very common, that none can be ignorant of it

Neither fhall we infift on the Manner of ftewing Bafes, or other Appurtenances belonging to them; becaufe 'tis only requifite to take Meafures in thofe Cafes, from other Things of the like Nature.

C.

C A B B A G E S *and* C O L E W O R T S.

AMong the Potages you may obferve the Manner of thofe that are drefs'd with Cabbages or Coleworts, for different forts of Fowl, *viz.* Pigeons, Partridges, Wood-hens, Stock-doves, Pullets, Capons, Chicken, Ducks, *&c* They may alfo be prepar'd with farc'd Cabbage, according to the following Directions; or elfe they may be ferv'd up for Side-difhes, garnifhing them with farc'd *Fricandoes*

The

The Manner of Dreſſing a farc'd Cabbage for a Side-diſh.

Take a good Cole-cabbage; cut off the Stalk, with a little of the Body, and let it be well ſcalded. Then take it out of the Water, ſpread it on the Dreſſer, ſo as the Leaves may lye together, and lay ſome farced Meat upon them, made of the Fleſh of Fowls, a piece of a Leg of Veal, ſome parboil'd Bacon, Fat of boil'd Gammon, *Truffles* and Muſhrooms chopt, Parſly, Chibbol and a Clove of Garlick; the whole Mixture being ſeaſon'd with fine Herbs and Spice, with ſome Bread-crum, two whole Eggs, and two or three Yolks, all well minc'd. Your Cabbage being ſtuff'd with this Farce, let it be clos'd, neatly tied up and put into a Pot or Stew-pan. At the ſame time, take part of a Leg of Veal or of Beef cut into Stakes and well beaten; put them in order in a Pan, as it were to make Gravy: When they are colour'd, throw in as much Flower as you can take up between your Fingers, and let them be brought to a colour all together: Afterwards ſoak them with good Broth and ſeaſon them with fine Herbs and Slices of Onion: When they are half boil'd, let the Cabbage, Stakes and Gravy be intermixt and all ſeathed up together, but be careful not to put too much Salt therein All being thus made ready, dreſs them in a Diſh without Broth, put a Ragoo upon them, as it may ſtand with your convenience, either *à la Saingaraz* or ſome other ſort, and ſerve them up hot to Table

A Cabbage may likewiſe be farced on Days of Abſtinence, with ſome Fleſh of Fiſh and other Things to garniſh it; as if it were a Carp, Pike, or other Fiſh prepared to be farc'd.

How to make certain Ornaments call'd Petits-choux, *i. e. Small Coleworts.*

Take ſome Cheeſe that is very fat, ſuch as the beſt ſort of Cream-cheeſe, as much as you ſhall think fit. Let it be put into a Stew-pan, with two handfuls of Flower, propoitionably to the quantity of Cheeſe, adding thereto ſome green Lemmon-peel minc'd, and ſome candy'd Lemmon-peel likewiſe cut very ſmall: Then, taking a *Spatula* in your Hand, ſtir all together with a little Salt: When 'tis well mixt, put four or five Eggs therein, and make a ſort of Paſte or Batter like that of Fritters. Afterwards take ſome ſmall Pie-pans, butter them on the inſide, and

put

put a little of this Farce into every one of them · But before they are set into the Oven, they muſt be waſh'd over with the Yolk of an Egg beaten up. As ſoon as they are bak'd, they may be ic'd over with fine Sugar, or a proper white Ice may be made for them, which is elſewhere deſcribed

CAPONS.

It were needleſs here to make a Collection of the different ſorts of Capon-potages ; becauſe they are particularly expreſs'd in the General Table of the Meſſes   The Reader is alſo re-ferr'd for the other Meſſes, that are made with Capons-breaſts, ſuch as *Tourtes* or Pan-pies, *Riſſoles* and *Bouillans* to the reſpective Letters of the Alphabet to which thoſe Articles properly belong. And for roaſted Capons, it may be obſerv'd with what Sauce they ought to be dreſs'd, under the Letter R ; where every Thing is ſet down that relates to *The Roaſt* Recourſe may alſo be had, for thoſe that are dreſs'd in a *Daube* to the Letter D ; where Examples are to be found for other ſorts of Fowl, which may be follow'd, without any difficulty, and ſo of the reſt.

CAPONS-LIVERS, *ſee* LIVERS.

CARDOONS.

Pick your Cardoons very well, and leave nothing on them but what is good · Then, having cut them into pieces, let them be waſh'd and ſcalded in Water, with a little Salt, Slices of Lem-mon, Beef-ſewet and *Bards*, or thin broad Slices of Bacon   On Fiſh-days, ſome Butter is uſually put to them thicken'd with a little Flower. When they are ſcalded, let ſome good Gravy of a fine colour be prepared in a Stew-pan, drain the Cardoons and put them into that Gravy, with a Bunch of fine Herbs, ſome minced Beef-marrow and a little raſped Parmeſan, and let them be ſtew'd in this manner, after they have been well ſeaſon'd. Before they are ſet on the Table, a little Vinegar or Verjuice muſt be pour'd upon them, and care muſt be taken, that they do not turn black. They ought alſo to be well clear'd from the Fat, and ſo ſerv'd up hot for Intermeſſes, after having given them a colour with the red-hot Fire-ſhovel
Cardoons are alſo broil'd in Broth and Gravy, with a thicken-ing Liquor of a reddiſh colour . They are to be ſet in order in

a

a Dish or Plate, with a Cruft of Bread underneath to make the *Dome* or Coronet Strew them with rafped Cheefe and a little grated Cinnamong and bring them to a good colour.

CARPS.

A Side-difh of a Carp.

Leave the Carp with its Scales on, and make a Ragoo of *Moufferons,* or elfe of common Mufhrooms, Fifh-roes and Artichoke-bottoms: Then fry fome Crufts of Bread, to be put into the Sauce as it is ftewing, with Onions and Capers. When 'tis ready to be fet on the Table and your Carp is taken up, without being broke, put the Ragoo upon it, and garnifh it with fried Bread and Lemmon-juice

Carp in a Daube.

Take a couple of Soles with a Pike; unbone them, and with their Flefh make farced Meat, chopping it fmall with a little Chibbol, beaten Spice, Pepper, Salt and Nutmeg. Then thicken this Farce with Yolks of Eggs, if the time will allow it, and you may try to do it with an *Andouillet* ready drefs'd Take one of the fineft Carps you can get, ftuff it with this Farce, feafon it with fine Herbs, and boil it with white Wine in an oval Stew-pan, over a gentle Fire In the mean while, prepare a great Ragoo of *Moufferons, Morilles,* common Mufhrooms, *Truffles,* Artichoke-bottoms and Cray-fifh-tails ftrained. Keep your Ragoo a-part for a confiderable time, and then pour it upon the Carp, which is to be drefs d upon an oval Difh, when ready to be fet on the Table. It muft be garnifh'd with Crayfifh and Slices of Lemmon, and may ferve for a great Sidedifh

Another Side-difh of Carps.

They are to be ftuff'd with a well-feafon'd Farce foak'd in Cream, and then bak'd in an Oven: Garnifh your Difh with Bread and Parfly fried, or with *Marinades.*

A Carp larded with Eel in a Ragoo.

When the Carp is scal'd, lard it with thick Pieces of Eel and fry it in a Pan with burnt Butter. Then put it into a Dish, with the same Butter, a little fried Flower and Mushrooms; seasoning it with Pepper, Salt, Nutmeg, Cloves, a Bay-leaf, a piece of green Lemmon, and a Glass of white Wine. As soon as it is dress'd, put thereto some fresh Oisters and Capers, and let them soak together for a little while. This Dish may be garnish'd with Slices of Lemmon.

Farced Carps.

Let the Carps be scal'd, and the Skin separated from the Flesh; leaving the Head and Tail Make a Farce with the same Flesh and that of an Eel, season'd with fine Herbs, Pepper, Cloves, Nutmeg, Thyme, Mushrooms and Butter. Farce your Skins likewise and sow or tie them together: Then bake them in an Oven or otherwise, with burnt Butter, white Wine and Broth, pouring upon it some Butter well mixt with fried Flower and Parsly cut very small. Let them be garnish'd with Carproes, Mushrooms, Capers and Slices of Lemmon.

Carp-Filets.

They may be mixt with Cucumbers and *Mousserons*, and 'tis only requisite to follow the Directions set down for the Pike, under the Letter P, or those for the Soles under S. The same thing ought to be observ'd with respect to the other sorts of Fish, which we shall refer to their proper Places, to avoid needless Repetitions.

A Carp in a Demi-court-bouillon.

Cut a Carp into four quarters, leaving the Scales on, boil it with white Wine, or some other sort of Wine, a little Verjuice and Vinegar, Pepper, Salt, Nutmeg, Cloves, Chibbols, Bay-leaves, burnt Butter and Orange-peel. Let the Broth be boil'd to a very small quantity, add some Capers as it is a dressing, and Lemmon-slices to garnish it

Carps

Carps in a Court-bouillon.

Cut off the Gills and Entrails of your Carps and put them into a *Court-bouillon au bleu*, which is hereafter defcrib'd for the Pike under the Letter P : Then boil them in white Wine, with Ver-juice, Vinegar, Onions, Bay-leaves, Cloves and Pepper, and ferve it up to Table on a Napkin, with green Parfly and Slices of Lemmon, among the Intermeffes.

Carps broil'd upon the Grid-iron.

Let your Carps be fcal'd, and broil'd upon the Grid-iron, with Butter and Salt, whilft a Sauce is making for them, with burnt Butter, Capers, Anchovies, green Lemmon or Orange, and Vinegar, feafon'd with Pepper, Salt and Muftard. They may alfo be drefs'd with white Sauce

Potages of farced Carps and otherwife.

'Tis fufficient to have recourfe to the preceding Article of *a farced Carp*, or to what is elfewhere fpecified concerning the Potage of a farced Pike. The latter may be garnifh'd with Artichoke-bottoms, fried Oifters, Capers, Mufhrooms in a Ragoo and in Slices, and Lemmon-juice

Potage of *Profitrolles* is made with Carp-flefh minc'd , after the manner that fhall be declar'd among the Potages for Fifh-days.

For Carp-hafhes, fee the firft Article of the Letter H, and look for Carp-pies, among thofe of Fifh under P

CASSEROLES.

Cafferoles, take their Name from the Stew-pan in which they are drefs'd, call'd *Cafferole* by the *French,* and are generally u fed for Side-difhes and Potages : For the former, take a large Loaf wafh'd over with Eggs, which muft not be chipt on the upper fide ; bore a Hole therein underneath, and take away the Crum or Pith Afterwards prepare a good Hafh of roafted Chickens, fat Pullets, or fome other fort of Roaft-meat, and put this Meat well minc'd into a Stew-pan, with good Gravy, as if it were to make a Hafh. When it is drefs'd, put fome

of

of it with a Spoon into the Loaf, that was toasted at the Fire ;
on the crummy side : After having thus pour'd in a little of
this Hash, add some small Crusts of Bread, and proceed to fill
up the Loaf alternately, with the Hash and small Pieces of Crust.
Then take a Stew-pan that is no bigger than your Loaf, put
a Sheet of Paper into it, or rather, some *Bards* or thin Slices of
Bacon, and afterwards the Loaf on that side where it was farc'd ;
covering the bottom of it, with the same Loaf. Let it lye a
soaking in this manner, with good Gravy, but it must not be
too much press'd, nor too long steept, so that it may be kept
altogether entire, and well cover'd. A little before 'tis serv'd
up to Table, turn it out dextrously into a Dish, take away the
Bacon-*Bards*, drain off the Fat, and cover your Loaf with a
good Ragoo of Veal-sweet-breads, Artichoke-bottoms and *Truffles*; small tops of Asparagus being also spread round about the
Dish, according to the Season.

A Casserole *with Cheese.*

The only difference is, that a little rasped Parmesan must be
put into the farced Loaf, and when the same Loaf is dress'd
in its Dish, it must also be strew'd with Parmesan. 'Tis usually
brought to somewhat of a colour in the Oven, and the Ragoo
put round about it This is call'd a *Casserole* with Parmesan.

A Casserole *with Rice.*

Boil your Rice in a Pot, and make a Ragoo with *Morilles*,
common Mushrooms, *Truffles*, Veal-sweet-breads, Cocks-combs
and Artichoke-bottoms If you please, the Combs and *Morilles*
may be farc'd and dress'd a-part, and afterwards put into the
Ragoo. Then make an Essence, with two or three Cloves of
Garlick, sweet Basil, Cloves and Wine ; let all boil together,
strain the Liquor thro' a Sieve and pour it into the Ragoo. If
you have a large fat Pullet, or any other tame or wild Fowl,
to be serv'd up with your Soop, lay it in a convenient Dish,
put the Ragoo to it, and cover it neatly with Rice; leaving a
little Fat on the top, to render it smooth and cause it to come
to a colour in the Oven; it must be serv'd up hot to Table.
If there be no Fowl at hand, but only a good Loin of Mutton
boil'd, put it in like manner into a Dish, when it is well dress'd,
and cover it very thick with Rice: Then bread it, or rather
G   spread

fpread on the top of it, fome Fat, with Bacon and a few Chippings of Bread, to give it a colour.

See under the Letter S a Tail-piece of Salmon in a *Cafferole*,
and obferve the fame Method in ordering other forts of Fifh,
that are to be dreffed after the like manner.

CHEESE-CAKES.

To make Cheefe-cakes, take fome white Cheefe that is very
fat, and pound it well in a Mortar with a Lump of Butter as
big as an Egg, and a little Pepper When 'tis well pounded, put
in a handful of Flower, a little Milk and two Eggs, and take
care that this Mixture be not too thin. In the mean while, a fine
Pafte is to be made, and fmall pieces of it to be roll'd out, according to the bignefs you would have the Cheefe-cakes to be
of. Put fome of this Farce upon the pieces of Pafte rolled out
for the Under-cruft , raife the fides with three Corners, as it
were in form of a Prieft's Cap, and pinch thofe Corners well
with your Fingers, to the end that they may not fall or give way
as they are baking : Then wafh them over with an Egg well
beaten, and fet them into the Oven. They may be ufed in garnifhing feveral Difhes.

CHICKENS.

We are now come to an Article that affords fufficient Materials for the making of a great number of different Side-difhes,
let us then begin with the chief of them.

Chickens with Gammon.

Take Chickens, draw and trufs them, but let them not be
fcalded : Cut fome Slices of Bacon for every Chicken, beat them
a little, and feafon them with chopt Parfly and Chibbols· Loofen
the Skin over the Breaft of your Chickens, to let in that Slice
of Gammon, between the Skin and the Flefh, but more efpecially take care, that the latter be kept entire. Sindge them at
the Fire, cover them with a good *Bard*, or thin Slice of Bacon,
and let them be well roafted When they are done enough
take off the *Bard*, pour fome good Gammon-Sauce upon them,
and ferve them up hot to Table.

Chickens farced with Oisters

Take young Chickens, dress them as it were for roasting, and make a small Farce to stuff them with, between the Skin and the Flesh To that purpose get some Oisters, a little Veal-sweet-bread, Mushrooms, *Truffles*, Parsly and Chibbols chopp'd, all well season'd and dextrously toss'd up in a Stew-pan, with a little Flower and strain'd Broth The Chickens must be farc'd in the Body, well tied up at both ends, and roasted with a *Bard* on their Breasts When they are ready, dress them in a Dish, pour a small Cullis of Mushrooms upon them, and serve them up hot to Table.

Chickens à la Mazarine.

Cut your Chickens, as if it were to make a white Fricassy, and set them a broiling upon the Coals ; as the broil'd or fried Pigeons mentioned under the Letter P, with all sorts of fine Herbs: All being well dress'd, let them be neatly breaded and afterwards broil'd upon a Grid-iron They may serve either for separate Dishes, or to garnish others, and are set hot upon the Table for a Side-dish , but they are not commonly fry'd, as Pigeons may be order'd Many call these Chickens, Pigeons and other Fowls that are dress'd in this manner, *Pieces à la Sainte Menehout* 'Tis requisite that the Bread, with which Chickens are breaded, be fine and white, to the end that it may take a good colour when they are broil'd.

A Side-dish of Chickens, with a Cullis of Cray-fish.

Take good fat Chickens, let them be well truss'd and roasted : If you are desirous to have them broil'd upon the Coals, they must be larded with thick Slips of Bacon and Gammon, accordingly as it shall be judg'd convenient When they are dress'd either way, 'tis requisite to have a good Ragoo, made of all sorts of Garniture, and well season'd, *viz.* Veal-sweet breads, *Truffles*, Asparagus-tops and Artichoke-bottoms, according to the Season. As soon as your Ragoo is made ready, the Chickens are to be put into it, which ought to have their Breasts somewhat beaten, to the end that they may imbibe the quintessence of the Sauce Then take some Cray-fish, and let all their Legs

be

be well pounded, but neither their Thighs nor their Tails; because otherwife the Cullis would not be very red. Having pounded thefe in a Mortar, with a fmall Cruft of Bread, foak them with fome Gravy, or only the Legs, to the end that the Liquor may become more reddifh To thicken the Ragoo, prepare a Bread-cullis, and when all is drefs'd, pour that of the Cray-fifh into it : You may alfo add fome Cray-fifh-tails, and, if you pleafe, an Anchovie. Take away the Fat from the whole Mefs, and ferve it up to Table.

Chickens à la Brochette.

Take Chickens, and cut them in the fame manner as for a white Fricaffy : Let fome Lard be put into a Stew-pan, with a little Flower and afterwards the Chickens When they are well feafon'd, foak them with good Gravy, and make an end of ftewing them ⋅ Then prepare fome Mufhrooms and *Truffles*, as alfo a Glafs of good *Champagne*-wine, a few Capers and minc'd Anchovies If the Sauce be not fufficiently thicken'd, put a little good Cullis into it The Chickens being thus well order'd and clear'd from the Fat, drefs them neatly in a Difh, and pour the Sauce upon them Let them be garnifh'd with Cutlets, or any thing elfe, at pleafure, and ferv'd up hot to Table.

Farced Chickens, with a Cullis of Mufhrooms.

Take Chickens and trufs them well, but do not parboil them. To make the Farce, take fome raw Bacon, Marrow, Veal-fweet-breads, *Truffles*, Parfly, Chibbols, all forts of fine Herbs, Capons-livers and Mufhrooms, all chopt fmall, pounded together and well feafon'd The fame Farce may ferve for Partridge-pies and all forts of ftuff'd Fowls, that are to be broil'd or roafted : Let the Sauce be thicken'd with two Yolks of Eggs Roaft your farc'd Chickens, well tied up and cover'd with Paper, and at laft prepare your Mufhroom cullis, to which ought to be added a little Gammon, with fome Capers, *Truffles* and Anchovies. Let the Chickens be drefs'd in a Difh, with the Cullis pour'd upon them, and garnifh'd with white Bread.

Chickens are likewife farced on their Breafts, after having taken out the Flefh, which is to be ufed for that purpofe; but before they are ferv'd up, they muft be breaded, bak'd and brought to a fine Colour.

Chicken

Chickens à la Civette.

Take fat Chickens and truſs them well, in order to be roaſted ; parboil them, and cut off their Legs   Then let them be ſteept in good Lard, about three or four Hours, with ſome Slices of Chibbol, and ſeaſon'd with all ſorts of beaten Spice and a little Salt · Afterwards they muſt be roaſted and baſted with the ſame Lard   When they are dreſſed, put to them a good Ragoo, or a Muſhrooms-cullis, or a Pepper and Vinegar-ſauce, and let all be ſerv'd up hot   The ſame thing may be done for ſeveral ſorts of Fowl and even for fat Pullets *à la Sainte Menehout.*

Chickens dreſs'd with Garlick.

Lard your Chickens with Bacon in Rows, and roaſt them, after having firſt ſtuff'd them with ſmall pieces of Garlick. Then make a good Pepper and Vinegar-ſauce, or a Muſhroom-cullis, or a Ragoo of *Truffles*, putting a Clove of Garlick into it, and before the Diſh is ſerv'd up, ſqueez the Juice of two Oranges into the ſame Sauce.

Chickens in a Fricaſſy.

Fricaſſies of Chickens are made with white and red Sauce. For the latter, let the Limbs of the Chickens be flea'd, and fry'd with Lard   Then ſtew them in a little Butter, Broth or Water, and a Glaſs of white Wine, ſeaſon'd with Pepper, Salt, Nutmeg, Chervil chopt very ſmall and whole *Ciboulets.* Make a thick'ning Liquor, with ſome of the ſame in which the Chickens were dreſs'd, with a little Flower ; putting into it ſome Veal-ſweet-breads, Muſhrooms, Artichoke-bottoms and other Ingredients.   Let them be garniſh'd with *Fricandoes* and roaſted *Poupiets*, or Slices of Lemmon, and ſerved up with Mutton-gravy and Lemmon-juice

The Fricaſſy of Pullets or Chickens with white Sauce is dreſs'd with a good Thickening of three or four Yolks of Eggs, and Verjuice or Lemmon-juice   It may be garniſh'd with marinated Chickens and fried Bread and Parſly in the Intervals.

As for the Fricaſſy of Chickens with Cream ; when they are dreſs'd as before, a little of the Fat is to be taken away, and Cream put to them, as they are ſerving up to Table.

A Side-dish of Chickens à la Gibelote.

Take Chickens and cut them as if they were to be fricaffied: Then put them into a Stew-pan, and feafon them, in the fame manner as ftew'd Carps Let Mufhrooms and other Garnitures be put to them, with a piece of Lemmon and fome Gravy in ferving them up to Table

Another Side-dish.

Another Side-dish may be made of Chickens larded and roafted: When they are ready, put them into a Difh, cut their Joints and Legs, and pour upon them, a Ragoo of *Moufferons,* common Mufhrooms, Artichoke-bottoms, Veal-fweet-breads, Capons-livers and Capers.

Chickens drefs'd à la Braife *or between two Fires.*

Cut your Chickens thro' the Back to the Rump, and feafon them with Pepper, Salt, Chibbols, Parfly chopt very fmall and Coriander. Then let them be laid between thin Slices of Bacon, with their Breafts downwards, and heated, before they are fet between two Fires; one above and the other underneath. You may alfo add a little Gammon, a piece of Lemmon and a Faggot of fine Herbs · Chop the raw Gammon very fmall, ftrew it over your Chickens, and when they are ready, put their own Gravy upon them, as alfo fome Lemmon-juice at the very inftant of ferving them up. Thefe Chickens may alfo be farced, before they are drefs'd.

A Side-dish of boned Chickens.

Let the Chickens be farc'd with a good *Godivoe,* and drefs'd with red Sauce; whilft you are a preparing for them a Ragoo of Veal-fweet-breads, *Truffles,* Mufhrooms and Artichokes cut into fmall pieces: Let all be well feafon'd and fet out with *Marinades* or fome other proper Garniture, and Gravy put to them, as they are ferving up to Table.

Chicken-

Chicken-Filets, *for Out-works.*

They may be dreſs'd with white or red Sauce, and a Liquor to thicken them is to be made of Bread-crum fried in Lard with fine Herbs, Broth and Lemmon-juice   Let all be ſtrain'd thro' the Hair-ſieve, with a little Gravy.

Chickens with Wood-cock Sauce.

They are to be dreſs'd with reddiſh-brown Sauce and a little Liquor to thicken them, or a Cullis of Wood-cocks: Then add an Anchovie chopt very ſmall, with a *Rocambole*, or Clove of ſmall Garlick, ſome Lemmon-juice and a little Wine. They are alſo us'd for Out-works and Side-diſhes, as well as the following Meſſes.

Chickens in Gravy.

They are to be ſerv'd up without being either breaded or larded, only with a little fine Salt ſtrew'd upon them , and may be garniſh'd with ſmall Cruſts of Bread.

Chickens with Pike-ſauce.

Let them be dreſs'd with brown Sauce, as in a Fricaſſy, and a chopt Anchovie put to them, with a Shalot, a few Capers, a little Vinegar, black Pepper, and Lemmon-juice, as they are ſerving up to Table.

Chickens, call'd Poulets-mignons.

After having farc'd your Chickens, lard them neatly, and cover them with a *Bard* or thin Slice of Bacon, and a Sheet of Paper.   Then roaſt them on a Spit, and ſerve them up, with good Sauce.

Chickens dreſs'd after other manners.

Fat Chickens are likewiſe dreſs'd with *Truffles*; others *à la Tartre*, and others *à la Polacre*, with a *Ramolade*-ſauce. Beſides theſe, there are *Marinades* of Chickens; for which ſee the Let-

G 4

ter

ter M, and Chickens in *Civet* under C, as also Pies and Potages of Chickens, which are explain'd elsewhere under P, and Chicken-pies, with which we shall conclude this Article.

A Chicken-Tourte *or Pan-pie.*

Take Chickens and cut them as it were for a white Fricaffy · Drefs them with all forts of good Garnitures, and make your Pie in the fame manner as that of Pigeons, under the Letter P. Let a good Cullis be pour'd in, before it be ferv'd up, and let it be well clear'd from the Fat

When young Chickens are in feafon, let them is pickt and trufs'd, as it were for boiling, but they muft not be fo much as parboil'd   Take away the Breaft on the fide of the Throat, as alfo all the Bones, if you pleafe; but be careful neverthelefs to keep the Skin entire: Take the Flefh with fome pieces of Veal and chop them together, with a little Bacon, Marrow, *Truffles,* Mufhrooms, Chibbols and Parfly; the whole Mixture being well feafon'd and bound with two Yolks of Eggs: Let this Farce be put into the Skin of the Chickens, that they may appear as it were quite whole, and let them be fcalded a little in Water: Afterwards let them be laid in Pafte, with all forts of proper Garnitures.   This Pafte may be made very fine, with fweet Butter, Flower, Salt and two or three Yolks of Eggs Some call this fort of Pie a *Tourte à la Parifienne* · As for the Cullis, it may be prepar'd according to your convenience. When the Pie is ready, take away the Fat carefully, and let it be ferv'd up hot, garnifh'd with its own Cruft.

C H I T T E R L I N G s, *fee* Andouilles.

C I V E T S.

Side-difhes of Chickens in Civet.

Let your Chickens be broil'd a little upon the Coals, and cut into Quarters   Then drefs them with red Sauce, and put them into a little Pot with fome Broth, or if that be wanting, with boiling Water   Pour in as they are boiling, a red thickning Liquor a little Wine and a Clove of Garlick, or a Rocambole; alfo fome Lemmon-juice, when they are ferv'd up, and let them be garnifh'd with *Marinade* and fried Parfly.

A *Hare*-Civet.

Take away the Legs and Shoulders entire, and cut the reft into pieces. Lard them with thick Slips of Bacon, fry them with Lard, and afterwards boil them with Broth and white Wine, a Bunch of fine Herbs, Pepper, Salt, Nutmeg, Bay-leaves and green Lemmon. Then fry the Liver, and, having pounded it, ftrain it thro' a Sieve, with fried Flower and a little of the fame Broth ; putting into it fome Lemmon-juice and Slices of the fame.

A Civet *of a Hind,* Stag *or Roe-buck.*

Let the Hind or Stag be cut into pieces of the bignefs of a Hare's Shoulder, lard them with thick Slips of Bacon, fry them as it is exprefs'd in the preceding Article, and let them alfo boil after the fame manner. The Sauce is to be thicken'd with fried Flower and a little Vinegar.

COCKS-COMBS.

Befides the great ufe of Cocks-combs in the moft exquifite Ragoo's and Bisks, particular Courfes are made of them for the Intermeffes ; more efpecially farced Cocks-combs, either alone, or with Veal-fweet breads, Capons livers, *Morilles* and common Mufhrooms.

Farced Cocks-combs.

Take fome of the beft and largeft Cocks-combs, let them be parboil'd and afterwards open'd at the thick end, with the Point of a Knife : Then, having made a Farce with the Breaft of a Pullet or Capon, Beef-marrow, pounded Lard, Pepper, Salt, Nutmeg and the Yolk of an Egg, fry your Cocks-combs, and ftew them in a Difh, with a little thick Broth and four or five Mufhrooms cut into Slices   To thefe add the Yolk of an Egg raw, and when the Difh is ready to be ferv'd up, fome good Gravy and Lemmon-juice.

To preserve farced Cocks-combs.

Let them be well cleansed, put into a Pot with Lard, and kept upon the Fire a little while, without boiling: About half an Hour after, throw in a little fine Salt, an Onion stuck with Cloves, a Lemmon cut into Slices, some Pepper and a Glass of Vinegar: When the Lard begins to coagulate, take them out, pour in some melted Butter, and cover them with a Linnen-cloth, as it is usually done to other Things that are to be pre-served

C O D - F I S H.

It were needless to take any notice of the ordinary ways of dressing Cod-fish, either fresh or salted, as being sufficiently known, so that we shall here insist only on what may contribute to enrich them, and to heighten their Relish; such are the follow-ing Directions.

Fresh Cod in a Ragoo.

Scale your Cod, and boil it in Water, with Vinegar, green Lemmon, a Bay-leaf or two, Pepper and Salt: Prepare a Sauce for it, with burnt Butter, fried Flower, Oisters and Capers; adding thereto when serv'd up, some Lemmon-juice and black Pepper.

A Cods-tail in a Casserole.

Take a good Cod's Tail, and having scal'd it, loosen the Skin, so as it may fall off from the Flesh Take away the *Filets*, and fill up the void space with a good Fish-farce, or with fine Herbs, Butter and Chippings of Bread. Afterwards put the Skin upon the Tail again, and having neatly breaded it, set it into the Oven, to give it a fine colour Lastly, make a Ragoo for it with proper Garnitures, and serve it up to Table

If you would have it fry'd, it must be scalded in hot Water, without boiling, to the end that it may remain altogether en-tire, and when 'tis drain'd, it must be flower'd and fry'd in refined Butter. Let it be serv'd up with Orange-juice and white Pepper. It may be garnish'd with some Pieces taken off from the Cod's Back put into Paste and fry'd; unless your
Ordi-

Ordinary be fo mean, as not to afford a feparate Difh of them

COLLY-FLOWERS.

Colly-flowers are ufually eaten with Butter, or Mutton gravy. For the firft Way, when they are well pickt, let them boil in Water, over a quick Fire, with Salt, Butter and Cloves · Then let them be well drain'd and put into a Difh, with Butter to keep them hot When they are drefs'd, make a thick Sauce for them, with Butter, Vinegar, Salt, Nutmeg, white Pepper and Slices of Lemmon.

For the other Way, when your Colly-flowers are boil'd as before ; tofs them up in a Pan, with Lard, Parfly, Chervil, Thyme a whole Chibbol and Salt, and let them foak together. When you would ferve them up, put fome Mutton-gravy into them, with a little Vinegar and white Pepper. Both thefe forts of Difhes properly belong only to the Intermeffes.

Colly-flowers are alfo eaten in a Sallet, and all that has been faid on this Subject is fo common, that it ought not be infifted upon ; were it not that our Defign leads us as well to inftruct the meaner fort of People in what may be ufeful, as to fhew what is ufually practis'd in Noble-mens Kitchens.

COURT-BOUILLON

Forafmuch as the *Court-bouillon* is common to many forts of Fifh, the Reader is referr'd to the Articles of *Pike* and *Carp*, directing what ought to be obferv'd in that way of Dreffing , to the end that unprofitable Repetitions of the fame thing in feveral places may be avoided, as much as is poffible.

CRAY-FISH.

Cray-fifh may be drefs'd after feveral manners, that is to fay, they may be put into Ragoos, Hafhes, Pies and Sallets , and Potages may be made of them, as well for Flefh-days as for thofe of Abftinence.

For a Ragoo, boil your Cray-fifh in Wine, Vinegar and Salt Then take the Tails, Claws and infide of the Body and tofs them up in a Pan, with burnt Butter, fine Herbs chopt fmall, a piece of green Lemmon, Pepper, Salt, Nutmeg and a
                                                                littlc

little fry'd Flower; adding fome Mufhroom-juice and Lemmon, when they are ready to be ferv'd up to Table

A Hafh of Cray-fifh is to be garnifh'd with their Leggs marinated and fried, after having taken away the Flefh, and a Ring or Border may be made with them round about the Difh.

For a Cray-fifh-*Tourte* or Pan-pie, fee the Letter T, and Page 41, for a Sallet of the fame Fifh; for which, you may make the *Ramolade*-fauce there fpecified, after having boil'd them in Wine, with Vinegar, Pepper, Salt, Cloves, Bay-leaves and Chibbols: They are to be ferv'd up entire with green Parfly.

Cray-fifh may alfo be ferv'd up in a Pan, with white Sauce, in the fame manner as many other Things.

Cray-fifh-Potage.

The Broth for this Potage, is that of Fifh, which has been already defcrib'd Having boil'd your Cray-fifh according to the ufual Method, take them out, and put all the Tails a-part into a Stew-pan, with *Truffles*, Mufhrooms, Artichoke-bottoms and Afparagus-tops, fuch as are then in feafon: Drefs this Ragoo with frefh Butter and a little fine Flower, and lay it a foaking, with good Fifh-broth, or fome other: Afterwards put your Roes into it, with a Faggot of fine Herbs, all well feafon'd, and let it boil over a gentle Fire.

To make the Cullis; all the Thighs and Legs of the Cray-fifh muft be pounded, and ftrain'd thro' a Sieve, with a little Broth and a fmall Cruft of Bread: If you would have the Cullis redder, take only the Legs of your Cray-fifh, and when all things are duely prepar'd, fet them a-part Some other Cray-fifh are likewife to be provided; leaving their Tails and only taking the Shells and fmall Legs to thicken your Potage. Then take the Flefh of a good Carp, and make a well feafon'd Hafh of it, which may ferve for the fame Potage Let it foak with good Broth, and if you have a Loaf farc'd with the fame Carp Hafh, and fome fmall Garnitures, they may be opportunely put into the Potage; garnifhing it with the Cray-fifh, difpofing of your Ragoo round about the Loaf, and foaking it all at once with the Cullis.

To garnifh a Potage of the like nature; the Shells of the Cray-fifh, may be ftuff'd with a good Fifh-farce, that is fomewhat thick, and flower'd a little. When the Difh is ready to be fet on the Table, they may be fry'd in frefh Butter, and ferve

to

to garnish your Potage, as well as the above-mention'd Messes; more especially the Cray-fish-hash.

Thus all sorts of Cray-fish-potages for Flesh-days, that are found in this Book, may be easily prepar'd, by following what is even now express'd in this Article, for what relates to the Cullis, without making use of Gravy or Broth.

CREAMS.

There are several sorts of Creams; particularly of Almonds and Pistachoes, burnt Cream, crackling Cream, fried Cream, Cream after the Italian Mode and some others; of which in their Order.

Pistachoe-cream.

Take Pistachoes well scalded, and pound them in a Mortar, with some candy'd Lemmon-peel, and a little green Lemmon-peel: When they are well pounded, take as much Flower as you can get up between your Fingers at once or twice, with three or four Yolks of Eggs: Mix them together in a Stew-pan of the size of your Dish, and put some Sugar therein proportionably, afterwards pouring in some Milk by degrees, to the quantity of somewhat more than a Pint: Then take your pounded Pistachoes, and having temper'd them with the rest, strain all thro' a Sieve twice or thrice: Let it boil in the same manner as other sorts of Cream, and when it is ready, pour it into a Dish, to be kept cold for Intermesses. If you would have it serv'd up hot, you may, when 'tis cool'd, make a white Ice upon it, and set it into the Oven to be dried

Almond-cream.

Almon'd-cream is made after the same manner as the former, but when it is to be prepar'd for Fish-days, on the Evening before the Collation, after having pounded the Almonds, strain them with Water thro' the Sieve, to make Almond-milk, to which purpose, a considerable quantity of Almonds is requisite. As soon as the Almond-milk is duely prepar'd, make your Creams, either of Pistachoes, Chocolate or others, with nothing but a little Flower, some Sugar and Orange-flower-water, without Eggs or Milk; only a little Salt and a great deal of Sugar.
When

When the whole Mixture is well boil'd, let it be serv'd up to
Table, and if you design to make Pies of it, they are to be
made with crackling Crust, hereafter describ'd, and garnish'd
with *Savoy*-bisket, *Meringues*, or other Things of the like Nature.

Cream after the Italian Mode.

Take about a Pint of Milk, according to the bigness of your
Dish, and boil it with some Sugar, a small Stick of Cinnamon,
to give it a good Relish, and a little Salt: Then taking a large
Silver-dish, with a Sieve, put four or five Yolks of new-laid
Eggs into it, and strain the Milk and Eggs all at once, three or
four times Afterwards the Dish is to be set into a Campain
or portable Oven, that is very straight, with Fire on the top
and underneath, till the Cream be well coagulated and ready
to be serv'd up hot. If some Milk-cream be put into all these
sorts of Creams, it will render them much more delicious

Pastry-cream.

If you would have a sufficient quantity for several Courses,
it would be requisite to beat up the Whites and Yolks of a
douzen Eggs, and having put to them, half a Pound of Flower,
rather more than less, let all be well mixt together, to these
another douzen of Eggs must be added and temper'd with the
rest At the same time, take about five Pints of Milk and put
it into a Pan of a proportionable bigness, to be boil'd: When it
begins to boil, turn the whole Mixture into it, and let it be
continually stirr'd: Then having added a little Salt, about half
a Pound of Butter, and a little white Pepper, let it be well
boil'd, but take care that it do not stick to the bottom. Your
Cream being thus thicken'd and duely prepar'd, pour it into a-
nother Pan and let it cool therein When you have a mind to
make Pies or Tarts of it, take as much as is requisite, according to the bigness you would have them to be of, and put it into another Pan Let it be well mixt with the *Spatula*, and add
thereto some Sugar, with Lemmon-peel cut small, both green
and candy'd, a little Orange-flower-water, some Yolks of Eggs,
and on Flesh-days, some Beef-marrow or fried Beef-sewer
The whole Mixture being well strain'd and clear'd, make your
Pies of Puff-paste, with a little Border round about, and pour

in your Cream. When thofe Pies or Tarts are almoft bak'd, they muft be iced, and ferv'd up for Intermeffes. On Fifh-days, melted Butter is generally us'd inftead of Beef-marrow.

Burnt Cream.

Take four or five Yolks of Eggs, according to the bignefs of your Difh or Plate, and beat them well in a Stew-pan, with as much Flower as you can take up between your Fingers; pouring in Milk by degrees to the quantity of about a Quart: Then put into it a fmall Stick of Cinnamon, with fome green Lemmon-peel cut fmall and likewife fome candy'd Orange-peel may alfo be minc'd as that of Lemmon, and then 'tis call'd *Burnt Cream with Orange* To render it more delicious, pounded Piftachoes or Almonds may be added, with a little Orange-flowei-water. Then fet your Cream upon the Furnace, and ftir it continually, taking care that it do not ftick to the bottom When it is well boil'd, fet a Difh or Plate upon a Furnace, and having pour'd the Cream into it, let it boil again, till you perceive it to ftick to the fide of the Difh. Then it being fet afide, and well fugar'd on the top, befides the Sugar that is put into it; take the Fire-fhovel heated red-hot, and at the fame time, burn the Cream with it, to give it a fine Gold-colour. To garnifh it make ufe of *Feuillantins* fmall *Fleurons* or *Meringues*, or other cut Paftry-works of crackling Cruft. Ice your Cream if you pleafe, or elfe let it be ferv'd up otherwife, but always among the Intermeffes.

Crackling Cream.

Take a Difh with four or five Yolks of Eggs, according to the quantity of Cream you would have prepared: Beat up thefe Yolks with a Spoon, and as you are working them, pour in fome Milk by degrees, till the Difh be almoft full: Then fome rafped Sugar muft be put into it with Lemmon-peel, and the Difh being fet upon a Furnace, the Liquor is to be continually ftirr'd about with a Spoon, till the Cream begins to be made. Afterwards having caus'd the Heat of the Furnace fomewhat to abate, ftill keep ftirring the Cream without intermiffion, and turn it upon the fides of the Difh, fo as very little or none may remain in the bottom, and that a Border may be form'd round about· Care muft be taken that it be not burnt

to,

ro, but only continue ſticking to the Diſh   When it is ready, you may give it a fine colour, with the red-hot Fire-ſhovel, and with the Point of a Knife, looſen the whole Border, that it may remain entire: Let it be put again into the ſame Diſh, and ſomewhat more dried in an Oven, ſo as very little be left in the Diſh, and that it crackle in the Mouth.   This ſort of Cream is often ſerv'd up to the Duke of *Chartres*'s Table.

Virgin-cream.

Having taken five Whites of Eggs, let them be well whipt and put into a Pan, with Sugar, Milk and Orange-flower-water.   Then ſet a Plate upon the Furnace, with a little Cinnamon, and pour in your Cream that is well beaten, and which, when made, may be brought to a colour by paſſing the red-hot Fire-ſhovel over it.

Fried Cream

Take about a Quart of Milk, and let it boil upon the Fire, putting into it four beaten Yolks of Eggs with a little Flower Stir all together over the Furnace, till the Cream be made, adding a little Salt, a ſmall Lump of Butter and ſome minc'd Lemmon-peel: When your Cream is ſufficiently boil'd, pour it into a flower'd Diſh, ſo as it may ſpread it ſelf, and that, when cool'd, it may become as it were a fried *Omelet* or Pan-cake Cut it into pieces, of what thickneſs you ſhall think fit, and fry them with good Lard; taking care that they do not ſquirt in the Frying-pan   When they are colour'd, take them out, ſtrew them with fine Sugar, and ſprinkle them with Orange-flower-water: Dreſs them in a Diſh, and having ic'd them (if you pleaſe) with the red-hot Fire-ſhovel, let them be ſerv'd up hot.   Otherwiſe, when this ſort of Cream is ſpread in a Diſh upon the Dreſſer, you may put ſome Butter into a Frying-pan, and fry it in the ſame manner as an *Omelet*   As ſoon as it is colour'd on one ſide, turn it upon the Diſh, and let it ſlip thence gently into the Frying-pan to give it the like colour on both ſides.   Then it may be ſugar'd, ic'd and ſerv'd up hot among the Intermeſſes

To render all ſorts of Creams more delicious, inſtead of ordinary Flower, that of Rice may be us'd, which is much better for that purpoſe, and good Creams may be made even altho' no Eggs

Eggs were put therein, *viz.* with Milk, if they are to be eaten with Butter, and with Almond-milk, if eaten only with Oil. A Quart of Milk must always be reduc'd to a Pint, in the boiling, to the end that the Flower may not be tasted.

Chocolate-cream.

Take a Quart of Milk with a quarter of a Pound of Sugar, and boil them together for a quarter of an Hour Then put one beaten Yolk of an Egg into the Cream, and let it have three or four Walms · Take it off from the Fire, and mix it with some Chocolate, till the Cream has assum'd its colour Afterwards you may give it three or four Walms more upon the Fire, and, having strain'd it thro a Seve, dress it at pleasure.

Sweet Cream.

Take three Quarts of Milk newly milk'd from the Cow, and let it boil; but when it rises, take it off from the Fire, and let it lye by a little while Then take off all the Cream that appears on the top, to be put into a Plate; set the Pan or Skillet again upon the Fire; and continue to do the same thing, till your Plate be full of such Cream Afterwards put some scented Waters into it, and forget not to sugar it well, before it is serv'd up to Table.

White and light Cream.

Take three Gallons of Milk, with half a quarter of a Pound of Sugar, and let it boil half a quarter of an Hour: Then take it off from the Fire, and put in two Whites of Eggs well whipt, stirring all together without intermission Set your Milk or Cream upon the Fire again, and let it have four or five Walms, continually whipping it Afterwards you may dress it as you please, sprinkling it, as soon as it is cold, with Orange-flower-water, and strewing it with fine Sugar It may also be brought to a colour, with the red-hot Fire-shovel.

Cinnamon-cream is made after the same manner, as that of Chocolate.

As for the Sauces with Cream, see the Articles of Artichokes, Asparagus, Mushrooms, &c as also the *Omelets*, with Cream of several sorts, and other Messes mentioned in the General Table.

H CRE-

CREPINES.

Take some part of a Fillet of Veal, with a piece of Bacon, and let them be parboil'd together in a Pot · When they are cold, mince them with Leaf-fat out of a Hog's Belly, Chibbols, two or three Rocamboles and other seasoning Ingredients. Then beat them all in a Mortar, with a little Cream or Milk, and some Yolks of Eggs, and put this Farce into Veal-cauls after the manner of white Puddings They are usually bak'd in a *Tourtiere* or Pie-pan, in an Oven moderately heated, and brought to a fine Colour ; to be serv'd up for the Out-works of Side-dishes.

CROQUETS.

Croquets are a certain Compound made of a delicious Farce, some of the bigness of an Egg and others of a Walnut.   The first sort may be us'd for Side-dishes, or at least for Out-works, and the others only for garnishing.   To that purpose, take the Breasts of large fat Pullets, Chickens and Partridges, and mince this Meat with some Bacon, Calves-udder, Veal-sweet-breads, all parboil'd , *Truffles*, Mushrooms, Marrow, the crummy part of a Loaf, steept in Milk, and all sorts of fine Herbs, as also a little Cream-cheese , and as much Milk-cream , as shall be judg'd requisite : When the whole Mixture is well minc'd and season'd, let four or five Yolks of Eggs be put into it, and one or two Whites With this Farce, the *Croquets* are to be form'd of a round Figure, then roll'd in a beaten Egg, breaded at the same time , and set by in a Dish , in order to be fried afterwards with sweet Lard, and serv'd up hot to Table.   The same Farce may also serve to stuff *Fricandoes* or *Scotch*-Collops, and for the *Filets-Mignons* hereafter-mention'd

As for the lesser *Croquets*, they may be made with the same Farce, or with any other that is somewhat delicious and thick, and are usually dipt into a certain Paste or Batter, like that of Apple-fritters, before they are fried · They may also be Flower'd or breaded, to garnish all sorts of Dishes, in which there are any Services of wild Fowl, and ought always to be serv'd up hot to Table.

C u-

CUCUMBERS.

Cucumbers are ufually farced to ftuff great Joints of Beef, as it has been already obferv'd, and are alfo drefs'd after feveral other manners, particularly *a la Matelotte*, and in a Sallet. Potages are often garnifh'd with them, *Filets* of Cucumbers are fometimes prepar'd, and they are one of the principal Ingredients of the *Salpicon*. We have elfewhere explain'd what relates to the Cucumber-*Filets*, and the *Salpicon* fhall be defcrib'd in its proper Place. Therefore it will be fufficient here to give fome account of the farced Cucumbers and of thofe *à la Matelotte*, in regard that all the reft may be very eafily prepar'd, fuch as Potages, Sallets and Legs of Mutton with Cucumbers.

Farced Cucumbers.

Take Cucumbers, fuch as are not too thick, let them be clear par'd from their Seeds and kept whole. In the mean while, a Farce is to be prepar'd of all forts of Fowl, and if you pleafe, a piece of Veal, all well minc'd, with fome parboil'd Bacon, a little tried Fat, fome boil'd Gammon chopt, Mufhrooms, *Truffles* and all forts of fine Herbs, the whole Mixture being well minc'd and feafon'd. Then your Cucumbers, being fcalded a little while, are to be ftuff'd with this Farce, and boil'd in good Gravy or fat Broth, but not too much. Having taken them out, let them be cut into two pieces and fet by to cool, whilft a fort of Pafte or Batter is preparing, as it were for Apple-fritters. This Pafte is to be made of Flower mixt with white Wine or Beer, a little melted Lard and fome Salt. Afterwards certain fmall Skewers are to be neatly cut out, of the bignefs of a writing Pen, and the pieces of Cucumbers are to be pierc'd thro' with them, fo as all the ends may be on one fide, that they may be conveniently thruft into a piece of Beef. The Cucumbers are to be dipt in the faid Pafte, and brought to a fine Colour with melted Lard, and the piece of Beef being drefs'd with a Gammon-hafh, and the *Marinades* put upon it, is to be ftuff'd with thefe farced Cucumbers. If there be any Farce left, you may roll it up, with your Fingers dipt in Flower, and make round pieces of the thicknefs of an Egg, which are to be boil'd at the fame time with the Cucumbers, but very gently, that the

H 2 Farce

Farce may hold together : They muft alfo be fried in the fame manner.

Cucumbers dress'd à la Matelotte, *or after the Sea-fashion.*

They are to be farced as the former, and boil'd in good Gravy : Take care that the Fat be well taken away, and that too much Sauce be not put to them · Then thicken them with fome good Cullis and pour in a little Vinegar, before they are ferv'd up hot to Table : They ought to be all of a fine red Colour.

Farced Cucumbers are alfo put into a Ragoo and white Sauce

To preferve Cucumbers.

Take the beft fort of Cucumbers, that are not too ripe, and fet them in good Order in a Pail, earthen Pan, or fome other Veffel, in which is put an equal quantity of Water and Vinegar, with fome Salt; fo as they may be thoroughly fteept : They muft be well cover d, and not touch'd for the fpace of a whole Month. Thus when Cucumbers are out of Seafon, thefe may be us'd, after they have been well par'd and foak'd. If you would garnifh Potages with them, they muft be fealded, alfo when they are us d for *Filets*, as well on Days of Abftinence as on Flefh-days, they muft be cut after the ufual manner, and drefs'd, as if they were frefh. Indeed they will be of great ufe throughout the whole Winter, and during the time of Lent. To thofe that are to be eaten in a Saller, fome Pepper is ufually added, with fome Handfuls of Salt, and they may be ftuck with Cloves, at leaft one for every Cucumber They are commonly call'd Girkins or pickled Cucumbers ; and to this purpofe, the leffer fort is to be chofen, fuch as grow in the latter Seafon. They are generally pickled with the Stalks or Leaves of Purflane, and more efpecially with Samphire, which ferves inftead of fweet Herbs for that fort of Saller.

CULLISES.

A Cullis for different Potages on Flesh-days.

This fort of Cullis may ferve for feveral fmall Potages on Flefh-days, particulaily, of *Profitrolles*, Partridges, Quails, Larks, Wood-cocks and Teals, all which may be garnifh'd with *Fricandoes* and Veal-fweet-breads To make this Cullis, take a piece of Buttock-beef, and having caus'd it to be roafted very brown, let all the browneft part of it be pounded hot in a Mortar, with Crufts of Bread, the Carcaffes of Partridges and of other Fowls that are at hand The whole Mafs being well pounded and foak'd with good Gravy, put it into a Stew-pan with Gravy and ftrong Broth, and feafon it with Peppei, Salt, Cloves, Thyme, fweet Bafil and a piece of green Lemmon. Let it have four or five Walms, ftrain it thro' the Hair-fieve, and make ufe of it to be pour'd upon youi Potages with Juice of Lemmon

A Gammon-cullis.

Take one half Veal and the othei Gammon, put it into a Stew-pan and order it, without Lard, as if it were for Veal-gravy When it is fufficiently boil'd, add thereto fome dry Crufts, Chibbol, Parfly, fweet Bafil and Cloves, with the beft fort of Broth Let it be well feafon'd, ftrain'd thro' a Sieve and kept fomewhat thick

A Capon-cullis.

Take a roafted Capon, and pound it in a Mortar, as much as is poffible : Then fry fome Crufts of Bread in Lard, and when they are become very brown, put to them fome Chibbol, Parfly, fweet Bafil, and a few *Moufferons* well chopt : Mix thefe with the reft, and make an end of dreffing them over the Furnace. Afterwards poui in as much of the beft Broth, as you fhall judge requifite, and ftiain it thro' the Hair-fieve,

A Partridge-cullis.

Take two roasted Partridges, and pound them well in a Mortar, with the Birds or thin Slices of Bacon with which they were dress'd · Then taking as many green *Truffles* as you can get up between your Fingers, with the like quantity of Mushrooms, fry them in Lard with fine Herbs, Chibbol, sweet Basil and Marjoram: Afterwards mix your pounded Meat together in the same Stew-pan, with two good Spoonfuls of Veal-gravy; let them soak over a gentle Fire, and strain them thro' the Sieve with Lemmon-juice.

A Cullis of Ducks

Take a roasted Duck, and let it be well pounded in a Mortar: Then cause some Gammon to be fried brown in a Silver-dish, and put it into a Pot, with a Handful of Lentils to be stew'd all together; adding two or three Cloves, a Clove of Garlick, some Savoury and Chibbol: When they are all boil'd, pound them with the Duck-meat, and dress them in a Pan with Lard, as also afterwards with clear Broth, to the end that your Cullis may come to a lively fair colour Lastly, let it be strain'd thro' the Hair-sieve with Lemmon-juice, and kept for use

A Cullis of large Pigeons.

Let two or three large Pigeons be roasted, and pounded in a Mortar: Then mince three Anchovies, with as many Capers as can be taken up between your Fingers, a few *Truffles* and *Morilles*, two or three Rocamboles, some Parsly and Chibbols all chopt very small; mix them with the Pigeon-meat, and fry them in a Pan, with Lard: Let some of the best Gravy that you have be put thereto, strain it thro' a Sieve with the Juice of a Lemmon, and keep it as thick as you shall think fit.

A Cullis made with the Breast of a fat Pullet.

Take the Breast of a large fat Pullet, with a piece of Veal boil'd very white and pound them in a Mortar · Then provide a quarter of a Pound of sweet Almonds, which are likewise to
be

be pounded together, with the crummy part of a white Loaf soak'd in good Broth made of the Pullet's Bones, that was pounded before. The same Broth may be us'd to lay the Meat and Almonds a soaking in a Stew-pan, giving them a Walm or two. In straining it thro' the Sieve, a little Milk or Cream may be put to it, to render it white, and care must be taken, that it do not turn as it is heating.

A white Cullis for Fish-days.

Take as many Almonds, as you shall judge requisite, and pound them in a Mortar: You are also to provide some Bread-crum soak'd in Cream or Milk, and some Fish-*Filets*, dress'd as white as is possible. Add thereto some fresh *Mousserons*, white *Truffles*, sweet Basil and Chibbols, and take some of the clearest Broth you can get, to boil all for the space of one quarter of an Hour. Afterwards this Cullis is to be strain'd thro' the Hair-sieve and may serve for all sorts of Messes that require white Broth.

Other Cullises for Fish-days.

Some Onions and Carrets are to be fried as it were for a sort of Broth, and when they are turn'd brown, let a Handful of Parsly be thrown in, with a little Thyme, sweet Basil, Cloves, Crusts of Bread, Fish-broth and a little Vinegar.

A Cullis of Roots

Take Carrets, Parsly-roots, Parsneps and Onions cut into Slices, toss them up all for a little while in a Stew-pan, and pound them in a Mortar, with a douzen and half of Almonds and a piece of Bread-crum soak'd in good Peas-soop · Let the whole Mixture be boil'd in a Pan, and well season'd as the others. Then strain it hot thro' the Sieve, and make use of it for all the Potages of white Onions, Leeks, Cardoons and Goats-bread that are fried, marinated, or put into Paste, as also for the Potage of Skirrets.

A Cullis of Lentils.

Take some Crusts of Bread, Carrets, Parsneps, Parsly-roots and Onions cut into Slices, fried in Oil or very hot Butter If it be for

Flesh-

Flesh-days, you may put thereto some burnt Lard, and throw in your Pulse and Crums of Bread Let all be fried brown, till that which sticks to the bottom of the Pan becomes very red : Then put some Lentils therein, with Broth, and let it be well season'd. When it has had four or five Walms, with a piece of Lemmon, let it be strain'd thro' a Sieve; so that it may serve for Lentil potages, Crusts farced with the same, Crusts farced with Pike and Lentils, and several others ; as Soles, Qua-vivers, Carps, &c. On Flesh-days 'twill also be of good use for Potages of Pigeons, Ducks, Partridges, &c

There are also many other sorts of Cullises, that are made for different Things ; as Cullises of Anchovies, Carps, *Truffles*, *Mousserons*, *Morilles*, common Mushrooms, Peas, Yolks of Eggs, and others that may be found by means of the General Table of the Messes, at the end of this Volume.

CUTLETS.

Farced Cutlets.

Take a Quarter of Mutton or Veal, and boil it in a Pot with good Broth : Then take it out and cut off all the Flesh, keeping the Bones of the *Cutlets* or small Ribs. This Flesh serves to make a Farce, with parboil'd Bacon, Calves-udder boil'd, a little Parsly and Chibbol, Mushrooms and *Truffles*, all chopt together, and pounded in a Mortar, with the necessary Spices and seasoning Ingredients , also the Crum of a Loaf soak d in Milk or Gravy, and a little Milk-cream. Let the whole Farce be thicken'd with the Yolks of Eggs, so as it may not be too liquid Then take *Bards* or broad Slices of Bacon according to the bigness of your Cutlets ; put some of this Farce upon those *Bards*, with the Bones of the Cutlets, and do the same thing to every Cutlet which is to be made round, with a Knife steept in whipt Eggs, as if it were a real Cutlet. After-wards they are to be wash'd over and breaded on the Top, and when put in good Order in a Baking-pan, they are to be set into the Oven, to give them a fine colour. These are call'd *Farced Cutlets, with Cream*, and may serve to garnish all sorts of Side dishes and for Out-works.

Veal-Cutlets farced with nothing but Fennel are likewise in use, and some Gravy is to be put in the bottom of the Dish, as they are serving up to Table for Out-works.

Ano-

Another Side-difh of Cutlets.

Take the Cutlets of Veal or Mutton, that are very tender and well cut ; lard them with thin Slips of young Bacon, as it were *Fricandoes* , and drefs them in the fame manner ; feafoning them, as much as is needful. If thefe Cutlets ferve for a feparate Difh, all forts of Garnitures ought to be put to them ; but if they are to be us'd only for the garnifhing of fome other Side difh, it would be only requifite to ftew them in their own Gravy , becaufe a particular Ragoo is to be pour'd upon the Mefs in the middle of the Difh.

Cutlets in Haricot *and otherwife.*

Mutton-cutlets may be in *Haricot*, with ftew'd Turneps, and a well-feafon'd Liquour to thicken them, as they are dreffing : Some Chefnuts may be added , before they are prepar'd for Out-works. As foon as they are drefs'd, they may alfo be fteept in Lard, breaded and broil'd upon the Grid-iron , putting to them fome good Gravy and Lemmon-juice, when ready to be ferved up. Otherwife they may be marinated, fried till they come to a fine colour and garnifh'd with fried Parfly ; or elfe a good Cullis and Gravy may be pour'd on them, with a piece of Lemmon and *Truffles* ; fo as they may be laid a foaking together for a while, and fome Lemmon-juice fqueez'd in, as they are ferving up to Table.

D.

D A B S *or* S A N D L I N G S

A Side-difh of a marinated Dab.

LEt your Dab be cut thro' the Back, to the end that the *Marinade* may penetrate it, and when it is fufficiently pickled let it be well breaded with Bread-crum and feafon'd Chippings : Then let it be bak'd and garnifh'd with *Petits-patez* or little Pies.

A

A Dab or Sandling in a Sallet.

Boil this Fish in a *Court-bouillon,* and when it is cold, cut it into *Filets;* with which, and some small Sallet-herbs, you are to dress a Plate; seasoning them, with Pepper, Salt, Vinegar and Oil: Or else you may make the *Ramolade*-sauce, mention'd Pag. 41. and serve them up for Intermesses

Other manners of dressing Dabs.

If you have no other Dish with white Sauce, leave your Dab entire, and let it be serv'd up hot with white Sauce and Cream, for a Side-dish.   Sometimes they are dress'd in *Filets,* with Anchovie-sauce, and in a *Court-bouillon,* to be serv'd up, when cold, upon a Napkin for Intermesses, and they may also be put into a Pie, as the Turbots, but they ought not to take up so long time in Baking.

DAUBES.

We have already explain'd the manner of preparing a Fish-*Daube,* under the Second Article of Carp, let us now shew how it ought to be order'd for Flesh.

A Daube of a Leg of Veal.

Having taken off the Skin from the Leg, let it be parboil'd, larded with small Slips of Bacon, and steept in white Wine, with Verjuice, a Faggot of fine Herbs, Pepper, Salt, a Bay-leaf or two and Cloves Then let it be roasted, and basted with the same Wine, Verjuice and a little Broth When it is ready, make Sauce for it, with the Dripping, a little fried Flower, Capers, Slices of Lemmon, Mushroom-juice and an Anchovie, and let your Leg of Veal soak therein for some time, before it is serv'd up to Table, which may be done for a Side-dish.

A Leg of Mutton may be dress'd in a *Daube* after the same manner.

Daubes of green Geese and others.

Let your Geese be larded with middle-fiz'd Slips of Bacon; feafon'd with Pepper, Salt, Cloves, Nutmeg, Bay-leaves, Chibbols and
green Lemmon; and wrapt up in a Napkin· Then let them
be boil'd in a Pot, with Broth and white Wine, and left till
they are half cold, in their own Broth; in order to be ferv'd
up to Table upon a Napkin, with fome Slices of Lemmon.

In like manner, you may drefs Turkeys, fat Capons, Partridges and other forts of Fowl.

D E E R

The Manner of Dreffing it.

If you would have it roafted, let it be larded with thick
Slips of Bacon, feafon'd with Pepper, Salt and beaten Cloves,
and fteept in Vinegar, with Bay-leaves and Salt: Then let it
be roafted by a gentle Fire and well bafted When it is ready,
put fome Anchovies, Capers, Shalots cut fmall, and green
Lemmon into the Sauce, which may be thicken'd with fried
Flower It may likewife be larded with fmall Slips of young
Bacon, and put into a *Marinade*, with five or fix Cloves of
Garlick· Let it be roafted, cover'd with Paper, and eaten with
Pepper and Vinegar

The Fawn of a Deer may be drefs'd after the fame manner,
except that the *Marinade* or Pickle for it, ought not to be fo
ftrong

You may alfo prepare for a great Difh, the Leg of a Fawn,
with the Rump, one half larded and the other breaded, garnifh'd, with *Petits-patez* or little Pies, and having Vinegar and
Pepper for Sauce; of which fee an Example, Pag 16 Or elfe
being larded with thin Slips of Bacon, it may be eaten, with
fweet-four Sauce made of the Dripping, Sugar, Cinnamon,
white Pepper, green Lemmon, a little Salt, fried Flower and a
minc'd Shalot· Let all be boil'd over a gentle Fire, with Claret or Vinegar, let the Fawn be turn'd therein, from time to
time, to take the whole relifh; and let fome Capers be added,
as it is ferving up to Table.

D U C K S

DUCKS.

Potages are fometimes made with Ducks, they are alfo roafted and ferv'd up with Sauce, and drefs'd after feveral other manners, of which thefe that follow, are moft remarkable

To drefs Ducks with Oifters.

Take wild Ducks, let them be well trufs'd; and make a Ragoo, with Veal-fweet-breads, *Truffles* and Oifters, feafon'd with fine Herbs, chopt Parfly and Chibbols · Care muft be taken that this Ragoo be fomewhat thick; but 'tis no matter whether it be red or not: When it is almoft ready, the Ducks muft be farced with it, well ty'd up, and roafted a little while. Afterwards a Mufhroom-cullis, or Sauce after the *Spanifh* Mode, fuch as is ufually made for Partridges, may be pour'd upon them, and they are to be ferv'd up hot, for a Side difh. Other forts of Water-fowl may be drefs'd in the fame manner

Other Side-difhes of Ducks.

A Ragoo may be prepar'd for them, with Veal-fweet-breads, Artichoke-bottoms, *Truffles*, Mufhrooms, a Clove of Garlick, a little Vinegar and a Bunch of fine Herbs, and they may be garnifh'd with *Fricandoes*, and Lemmon-juice, before they are ferv'd up to Table.

At another time, when your Ducks are roafted, cut them into *Filets*, and put them into a Ragoo of Cucumbers, with Rocamboles, Lemmon-juice and a little Vinegar; fo as they may be ferv'd up for Out-works.

Ducks may be alfo drefs'd in a Ragoo; and Turneps boil'd with them, may ferve for their Garniture.

Potages of Ducks

Ducks may be us'd in Potages with Peas, a Cullis of Lentils, Cabbage, Turneps and other Roots. But forafmuch as this is common to them, with feveral other Meffes, a particular Enumeration of which, would lead us too far and even to little purpofe out of the Way; the Reader is referr'd to the refpective Potages of thofe different forts of Pulfe under the Letter P. where

he

he may find general Inftructions, as to what ought to be obferv'd, with refpect to all forts of Wild-fowl and Poultry, for
the avoiding of tedious Repetitions. So that this one Inftance
may be his future Direction, whenever any Matters fhall occur
of the like Nature.

See likewife under the Article of Pies, what relates to thofe
of Ducks, as well hot as cold.

S E A - D U C K S.

They may be put into a *Daube*, after the very fame manner
as green Geefe or Ducks, and being well drefs d, may be ferv'd
up to Table, upon a white Napkin, garnifh d with Parfly and
Slices of Lemmon.

A Side-difh may alfo be made of them, with Cucumbers,
as well as many others, or elfe they may be drefs'd after the
following manners.

A Sea-duck in a Court-bouillon.

After having pickt and drawn your Sea-duck, let it be larded or ftuff'd, with thick Slips of Eel-flefh, and boil'd four or
five Hours over a gentle Fire, in Water, with Pepper, Salt, a
Bunch of Herbs, a Bay-leaf or two, Cloves, a little white Wine
and a Lump of Butter · Then prepare a Sauce for it, with natural Butter, fine Flower, white Pepper, Salt, green Lemmon
and Vinegar, and let the bottom of the Difh, in which it is
drefs'd, be rubb'd with a Shalot

A Sea-duck with Chocolate in a Ragoo.

Having pickt, cleans'd and drawn your Sea-duck, as before,
let it be wafh'd, broil'd a little while upon the Coals, and afterwards put into a Pot; feafoning it with Pepper, Salt, Bay-
leaves and a Faggot of Herbs. Then a little Chocolate is to be
made and added thereto, preparing at the fame time a Ragoo
with Capons-livers, *Morilles*, *Moufferons*, common Mufhrooms,
Truffles and a quarter of a hundred of Chefnuts When the
Sea-duck is ready drefs'd in its proper Difh, pour your Ragoo
upon it; garnifh it with what you pleafe, and let it be ferv'd
up to Table.

A

A Sea-duck in Haricot

Let it be drefs'd as before, and let a Ragoo of Turneps be made, which are to be fried fomewhat brown Then let all be foak'd with the Sauce of your Sea-duck, which, when ready, muft be cut into pieces and laid upon the Turneps Laftly, let it be prepar'd and ferv'd up to Table at a convenient time, garnifh'd, as you fhall think fit.

Sea-ducks in a Pot-pourri *or Hotch-potch*

Lard your Sea-ducks with thick Slips of Eels-flefh, and tofs them up in a Pan with burnt Butter Then put them into a Pot or Earthen Pan, with a little of the fame Butter, Flower and Water, feafon'd with Pepper, Salt, Nutmeg, Cloves, Mufhrooms a Faggot of Herbs and green Lemmon Let them boil over a gentle Fire, during four or five Hours, as it were in a *Court-bouillon*, and when you would have it ferv'd up, add fome Oifters, Capers and Lemmon-juice.

A roafted Sea-duck

Let the Sea duck be bafted as it is roafting, with Butter and Salt, and then let a Sauce be made for it with the Liver, which is to be minc'd very fmall and put into the Dripping, with Pepper, Salt, Nutmeg, Mufhrooms and Orange-juice

A Sea-duck Pie

Take Sea-ducks that are well pickt and trufs'd, let them be beaten a little on the Breafts broil'd on the Coals and tied up at the ends Take the Liver, with fome minc d *Truffles*, Mufhrooms, Parfly and Butter, a few Chibbols and Capers, with an Anchovie, all being well chopt, enrich'd and feafon'd . Then the Body of the Sea-duck is to be ftuft d with this Farce, and a little of the fame kept, to be put underneath In the mean while, roll out your Pafte for the Under and Upper-crufts, and let the Pie be bak'd when fill d with the Sea-ducks If you would have it ferv'd up hot, a good Ragoo muft be made with Carps roes, Cray-fifh-tails, Mufhrooms and *Truffles*, or one of Oifters, but if it be defign d for a cold ftanding Difh, you
have

have no more to do, but to let it cool after it is bak'd, and to set it on the Table, as you shall find an occasion.

Potage of Sea-ducks.

As for the Potages of Sea-ducks, 'tis requisite that they be boil'd with good Fish-broth, and afterwards laid a soaking with the same. Then a good Fish-hash is to be prepai d, to be pour'd upon the Sea-ducks, as soon as they are put into the Soop, which has been sufficiently soak'd Let them be garnish'd with Sole-*Filets*, Whitings, Cray-fish, or other sorts of Fish; with a well season'd Ragoo, and a good Cullis of Cray-fish or Mush-rooms Thefe are all to be ferv'd up hot, and Potages may be made of Sea-ducks with Lentils.

E.

EARS.

Calves-ears farced.

Calves-ears farced are commonly us'd for Intermesses; to which purpofe, fome entire Ears are to be well scalded or par-boil'd a little Then a good thick Farce being made, stuff the Insides of them, and sow them up neatly round about They are to be boil'd, as Pigs-pettitoes, *à la Sainte Menehout*, and insow'd, when ready, but so as the Farce may not fall out. Af-terwards, roll them up in Eggs lightly whipt, bread them at the same time, fry them in Lard, as it were *Croquets*, and garnish them with fried Parsly

Hogs-ears.

Hogs-ears may be dress'd with Herb-*Robert* Sauce, after they are cut into Slices, and fried in a Pan with a little Butter You must also fry in the same Butter fome Chibbols cut very small, feason'd with Pepper, Salt, Nutmeg, Vinegar, Capers and a little Broth, and when you would have them ferv'd up, add some Mustard ⋅ The fame Slices may be put into Paste, fried and set on the Table with white Pepper and Lemmon-juice

For a *Soufce* of Hogs-ears and Feet, fee the last Article of the etter S.

E E L S.

E E L S

How to farce them.

The Bones of Eels may be farc'd in form of a white Pudding: To that purpose, a good *Godivoe* is to be made with the Flesh of the Eels, which you must pound in a Mortar, mixing with it some Cream, Bread-crum, two or three Rocamboles and half a Clove of Garlick: When the *Godivoe* is well season'd, farce your Bones neatly with it, bread them well with Bread-crum, and bake them in a Pie-pan, till they come to a fine colour.

Eels with white Sauce.

When the Eels are skinn'd, cut them into pieces, and let them be scalded in boiling Water: As soon as they are dried with a Napkin, tofs them up in a Pan, with natural Butter, and stew them with Pepper, Salt, Cloves, Nutmeg, a Bay-leaf and a piece of Lemmon; some add a Glass of white Wine to these Ingredients. In like manner dress some Artichoke-bottoms, Mushrooms and Asparagus tops, with sweet Butter and fine Herbs, and make a white Sauce, with the Yolks of Eggs and Verjuice; accordingly, as the time will allow it, or when they are ready to be set on the Table: Let them be garnish'd with fried Bread and Slices of Lemmon, and serv'd up with the Juice of the same.

Eels with brown Sauce.

Let them be tofs'd up in a Stew-pan with burnt Butter, fine Herbs chopt very small, Chibbols, Pepper, Salt, Cloves, Nutmeg and Capers; adding also a little Verjuice and white Wine, if you think fit, with fried Flower. Afterwards let all be stew'd together in a Dish or earthen Pan, and garnish'd with Lemmon, as they are serving up to the Table.

Fried Eels.

They must not be skinn'd, but the Bones being only taken away, let them be cut into pieces, and marinated with Vinegar, Pepper, Salt, Bay-leaves, Chibbols and Lemmon: Then they are

are to be flower'd and fried in refined Butter Before they are serv'd up, let a Sauce be made for them with Parsly, Rose-vinegar and white Pepper.

Eels broil'd upon the Grid-iron.

After having skinn'd your Eels and cut them into pieces, let them be marinated as before, and let a Sauce be prepar'd for them, with burnt Butter, Flower, Capers, Pepper, Salt, Nut-meg, Cloves, Vinegar and a little Broth When the Eels are sufficiently broil'd upon the Grid-iron, let them be stew'd a little in that Sauce : They may also be dress'd with *Robert*-Sauce and sweet Sauce.

Eels in a Daube.

Let some of the Flesh of Eels and Tenches be minc'd, and season'd with, Pepper, Salt, Cloves and Nutmeg : Then let *Lardoons* be made of the other part of the Eels-flesh ; of which one Lay is to be put upon the Skins, and another Lay of the minced Flesh, continuing so to do alternately Then let all be wrapt up in a Linnen-cloth, and boil'd in the same manner as Fish-gammon, that is to say, in one half Water and the other red Wine ; seasoning them with Cloves, a Bay-leaf or two and Pepper When they are cool'd in their own Broth, let them be serv'd up in Slices for Intermesses, rather than Side-dishes.

-Eel-potage.

When your Eels are skinn'd and cut into pieces, fry them in a Pan with burnt Butter, fine Herbs, Flower, and the proper seasoning Ingredients. Afterwards put them into a Pot with Fish-broth, the manner of preparing which is explain'd under the Letter B. As soon as the Crusts are soak'd, let your Po-tage be dress'd and serv'd up, with Capers and Lemmon-juice.

An Eel-pie and a Tourte or Pan-pie of the same.

An Eel-pie is generally serv'd up hot for a Side-dish : When the Eels are cut into pieces and their Skins pull'd off, let them be season'd after the usual manner, with Pepper, Salt, Cloves,

I Nut-

Nutmeg, fine Herbs, Chibbols, Butter, Capers, Bay-leaves and Bread-chippings The Pie muſt be made with fine Paſte either of an oval or round Figure · When it is half-bak'd, a Glaſs of white Wine may be pour'd into it, and ſome Lemmon-juice, when ready to be ſerv'd up to Table

As for the *Tourte* or Pan-pie ; the Eels may either be minc'd, after they have been skinn'd and the Bones taken out, or they may be cut into ſmall Slices, ſeaſoning them as before, with pieces of Muſhrooms, the Yolks of Eggs and Lemmon-juice as they are ſerving up, in order to make a white Sauce.

E E L - P O W T S.

The Eel-powt is both a Lake and River-fiſh. They may be dreſs'd in Ragoo and *Caſſerole* , or they may be put into a Pie, and a Potage may be made of them, with brown Broth.

A Ragoo of Eel-powts.

Let the Eel-powts be cleans'd from their Slime, with hot Water, and afterwards flower'd, and fried · Then being put into a Diſh, with burnt Butter, Flower and diſſolv'd Anchovies, let all be ſtew'd together ; ſeaſoning them with Salt, Nutmeg, a Chibbol and Orange-juice or Verjuice   Let them be garniſh'd with fried Parſly, and Slices of Lemmon, and ſerv'd up for Side-diſhes, as all other Fiſh-ragoo's.

Eel-powts in Caſſerole.

Cleanſe your Eel-powts from their Slime, laying the Livers a-part, and fry them in a Pan, with burnt Butter : Then put them into an earthen Pan, with the ſame Butter, a little Flower and white Wine ; ſeaſoning them with Pepper, Salt, Nutmeg, a Faggot of fine Herbs, and a piece of green Lemmon   In the mean while, prepare a ſeparate Ragoo, with the ſame Sauce as that of the Eel-powts, as alſo with their Livers and ſome Muſhrooms, and garniſh your Diſh with it, adding the Juice of Lemmon ; when ready to be ſerv'd up to Table.

Eel-

Eel-powt Potage and Pie.

For the Potage, after having wash'd the Eel-powts, let them be fried whole in a Frying-pan, with burnt Butter and a little Flower. Then let them be stew'd in an earthen Pan, with Pepper, Salt, a Bunch of fine Herbs, some Fish-broth or Pease-soop, and a little white Wine. When they are ready, dress them upon your soaked Crusts, and garnish them with Mushrooms and Capers.

For the Pie, skin your Eel powts, and make a fine Paste, to put them in, with their Livers and Roes, Mushrooms, Cray-fish-tails, Oisters and Artichoke-bottoms: Let them be seafon'd with Pepper, Salt, Nutmeg, fine Herbs and Chibbols, adding some Lemmon-juice, when they are brought to Table.

EGGS.

There is not any one Particular throughout the whole Practice of Cookery that affords greater Variety of Dishes, than Eggs, which are us'd even on Flesh-days, and serve altogether for the Out-works of Intermesses the principal ways of dressing them, are as follows *viz.*

Eggs with Orange-juice.

Let some Eggs be whipt, according to the bigness of the Dish you would have prepar'd, at the same time squeezing in the Juice of an Orange and taking care that none of the Kernels or Seeds fall into it. When they are all well beaten and seafon'd with a little Salt, take a Stew-pan, and put a slice of Butter therein, if it be a Fish-day, or a little Gravy on a Flesh-day. Pour in your Eggs, and keep continually stirring them, as if it were Cream; lest they stick to the bottom. As soon as they are ready, turn them into a Plate or Dish, garnish them if you think fit, with fried Eggs, and let them be serv'd up hot to Table.

Farced Eggs.

Take two or three Cabbage-lettices, scald them, with Sorel, Parsly, Chervil and a Mushroom, and let all be chopt very small, with some Yolks of hard Eggs, seafon'd with Salt, and

I 2   Nut-

Nutmeg: Then ftew them with Butter, adding alfo fome natural Cream, when they are fufficiently ftew'd ; and covering the bottom of the Dish with them　Let the Sides be garnish'd with fine Herbs and the Whites of the Eggs ftuff'd with another Farce, giving them a Colour with a red-hot Fire-shovel.

Farced Eggs may alfo be fried, after having dipt them into a clear Pafte or Batter, and ferv'd up with fried Parfly.

Eggs with Tripe.

Let the Whites of Eggs only be cut into long or round Slices, and tofs'd up in Butter with Parfly and Chibbol chopt very fmall: Then thicken them a little, feafon them with Salt and Nutmeg, adding alfo fome Cream ; and let the Yolks be fried to garnish your Dish.

Petits Oeufs *or fmall Eggs.*

Take a Gallon of new Milk, and heat it till almoft ready to boil, with a little Salt and pounded Sugar, a piece of Cinnamon, a Slice of Lemmon, and fome Orange-flower-water · Break four or five new laid Eggs, take away the Whites of fome of them, and beat them up with your Milk or Cream fcalding hot: Then heat a Plate upon a Chafing-dish, and when it is very hot, pour in fome of your prepar'd Mefs, after having ftrain'd it thro' a Sieve　Let it run about, fo as the Plate may be cover'd all over, and let it be brought to a Colour with the red hot Fire-shovel.　Afterwards beat your Yolks without Whites and a little Flower to thicken them, with the reft of the Milk · Set the Plate again upon the Fire to be heated, fo as the Eggs may become, as it were a Cream, and put the Yolks into it : Laftly, let the whole Mefs be ftrew'd on the Top with Sugar, adding the Juice of a Lemmon and fome Orange-flower-water, as it is ferving up to Table.

Eggs after the German Mode.

Break fome Eggs into a dish, as it were *au Miroir,* and put a little Peas-foop therein : Mix two or three Yolks with a little Milk, and ftrain them thro' a Sieve : Then take away the Broth in which the Eggs were drefs'd, put the Yolks upon them with fome fcraped Cheefe and give them a good Colour.

Egg

Eggs after the Burgundian Way.

Take a piece of red Beet, that has not an earthy or unfa-
voury taste, and pound it well with a Slice of Lemmon, a few
Macaroons, Sugar and beaten Cinnamon: Then taking four or
five Eggs, without the Sperm, mix all together very well, and
strain them thro' the Hair-sieve, with a little Milk and Salt Afterwards they may be dress'd in the same manner as Eggs with
Milk, and brought to a fine colour.

Eggs fried in Hogs-ears.

The Yolks must not be us'd in this Fricassy, which is to be
garnish'd with Mustard, if you please, and Lemmon-juice, when
serv'd up to Table.

Eggs with Bread.

Let some Bread-crum be well soak'd in Milk during two or
three Hours, and afterwards strain'd thro' a Sieve, or fine Cullander ; putting thereto a little Salt, Sugar, candy'd Lemmon-
peel cut very small, grated Orange-peel and Orange-flower-
water Then rub the inside of a Silver-dish with Butter somewhat heated, pour in your Eggs, keeping a Fire on the top and
underneath, that they may take a fine colour, and let them be
orderly serv'd up to Table.

Eggs after the Swiß Way.

Having dress'd your Eggs as it were *au Miroir*, bread them
with Crum . Then let them be cover'd with a Pike-hash and
some scrap'd Cheese, and brought to a fine colour.

Eggs with Gravy or à la Huguenotte.

Let some Mutton-gravy or any other sort be put into a hollow Dish, and when 'tis hot, break your Eggs into it either
au Miroir or mingled together Season them with Salt, Nutmeg and Lemmon-juice, and pass the red-hot Fire-shovel over
them, to give them a good colour.

I 3

Eggs

Eggs after the Portuguese Way.

Let some Sugar be diffolv'd, with Orange-flower-water, the Juice of two Lemmons and a little Salt. Then set it upon the Fire with your Yolks and stir all with a Silver-spoon. When the Eggs flip from the sides of the Dish, they are sufficiently boil'd, and may be left to cool. Afterwards let them be dress'd in form of a Pyramid and garnish'd with Lemmon-peel and Merchpane.

They may also be serv'd up hot in a Dish, after they are ic'd over with Sugar, and colour'd with the red-hot Fire-shovel.

At another time, they may be mix'd in a Mortar with some Goofeberry-jelly or Beet-juice boil'd in Sugar, and then fqueez'd thro' a Syringe, or a Hair-fieve, to be serv'd up dry in a green or red Rock.

Eggs with Piftachoes.

Pound your Piftach er with a piece of candy'd Lemmon-peel; be a fufficient quantity of Sugar with Lemmon-juice, and when the Syrop is half made, put the Piftachoes into it, with the Yolks of Eggs. Let them be ftirr'd as before, till they leave ft cking to the Skillet, and ferv'd up with fweet Water.

Eggs with Orange-flower-water.

Let Sugar and Orange-flower-water be put into a Dish or Skillet, with fome natural Cream, candy'd Lemmon-peel grated, and a little Salt. Then pour in eight or ten Yolks and ftir them about after the manner of mingled Eggs.

Eggs in Filets.

Prepare a Syrop of refin'd Sugar and white Wine, and when it is above half done, beat your Eggs therein : Then taking them up with a Skimmer, to the end that the *Filets* may be well made, let them be dried at the Fire, and ferv'd up with Musk or fome other Perfume.

Eggs after the Italian Mode.

Let a Syrup be prepar'd with Sugar and a little Water : When it is above half made, take the Yolks of Eggs in a Silver-spoon, one after another, and hold them in this Syrop to be poach'd. Thus you may dress as many as you shall think fit, continually keeping your Sugar very hot, and they may be serv'd up to Table garnish'd and cover'd with Pistachoes, Slices of Lemmon-peel, and Orange-flowers boil'd in the rest of the Syrop, with Lemmon-juice sprinkled upon them.

Eggs with Rose-water.

Having temper'd your Yolks with Rose-water, Lemmon-peel, Macaroons, Salt and beaten Cinnamon , let them boil in a Pan over a gentle Fire, with refined Butter When they are ready, ice them over with Sugar and Rose-water or Orange-flower-water, and put to them some Lemmon-juice, with Pome-granate-kernels, as they are serving up to Table.

Eggs with Sorrel-juice.

As your Eggs are poaching in boiling Water, pound some Sorrel, and put the Juice of it into a Dish, with Butter, two or three raw Eggs, Salt and Nutmeg · Let this thick Sauce be pour'd upon the Eggs, when served up to Table.

Eggs with Verjuice.

Beat up your Eggs with good Verjuice and season them with Salt and Nutmeg · Then let them be poach'd with a little Butter, and garnish'd with fried Bread or fried Paste.

Eggs with Cream

When your Eggs are poach'd whole with Butter in a Stew-pan, take them out, and dress them upon a Plate : Then put to them some natural Cream, with a little Salt and Sugar, and serve them up hot with Pomegranate-kernels or other sorts of Garniture

I 4

An

An Egg-ſeller.

'Tis uſually made with Anchovies, Capers, Fennel, Lettice, red Beets, Purſlain and Chervil, either of all theſe Herbs, or of every one of them in particular, and ought to be well ſeaſon'd.

There are alſo many other ſorts of Eggs, which it will be ſufficient here only to mention, *viz*.

Eggs with young Chibbols and other fine Herbs
—— poach'd with *Robert*-Sauce
—— with Milk
—— dreſs'd *au Miror.*
—— dreſs'd whole with green Sauce
—— in a Haſh, poach'd with fine Herbs and garniſh'd with ſmall round Pellets of fried Eggs.
—— with raſped Cheeſe
—— Eggs put into a Paſte and fried.
—— fried in a Pan with burnt Butter
—— poach'd in Water, with thick Butter.
—— poach'd with Sugar.
—— with Anchovies
—— with Sorrel, &c.

Counterfeit or artificial Eggs

Artificial Eggs of ſeveral ſorts may be made uſe of during the time of Lent, and more eſpecially on Good-friday. To that purpoſe, take two Quarts of Milk, and let it boil in an earthen Pot or a Silver-pan, continually ſtirring it with a wooden Ladle, till it be reduc'd to a Pint: Then pour one third part of it into a Diſh, by it ſelf, and ſet it on the Fire again, with ſome Rice-cream and a little Saffron: When it is thicken'd and become ſomewhat firm, you may make with it, as it were Yolks of Eggs, which are always to be kept Luke-warm. With the reſt of the Milk fill up ſome Egg-ſhells that you have open'd, after having waſh'd and topt them, and in order to ſerve them up to Table, put your artificial Yolks into thoſe Shells, as alſo on the top, a little Almond-cream, or raw Milk-cream and Orange-flower-water. Theſe are uſually ſerv'd up, on a ruffled Napkin and call'd *Artificial ſoft Eggs.*

As

The Court and Country Cook. 121

As for the other sorts, you are to mix at first with your Milk some fine Flower or Starch, and make as it were a kind of Pastry-cream, without Eggs, season'd with Salt. When it is boil'd, take some part of it to make the Yolks, adding some Saffron, and put these Yolks into certain half Egg-shells wash'd and steept in Water or white Wine. Afterwards fill up other whole Shells with the rest of the Cream, which being cold, these Whites and Yolks may be taken out of their respective Shells, to make such sorts of artificial Eggs, as you shall think fit. As for example.

For *farced Eggs*, after having taken away the Shell, cut the Whites into two equal parts, and hollow each of them with a Silver-spoon, in order to be stuff'd with the above-mention'd Farce. Then let them be dress'd in the same manner and garnish'd with artificial Yolks, that have been flower'd and fried for that purpose.

For *Eggs with Tripe*; after having cut and made them hollow, as before, stuff them with Yolks and cut them again into Quarters; then let them be flower'd and well fried. Having dress'd them upon a Plate, let a Sauce be prepar'd for them, with burnt Butter, fine Herbs, Mushrooms boil'd and chopt, Pepper, Salt, Nutmeg and Rose-vinegar. They may be garnish'd with Bread, Parsly and Mushrooms fried.

For *Eggs with Milk*; take boil'd Milk, and Almond-cream, and temper them with Marmelade of Apricocks. Let all these be put with Butter into a Plate over a gentle Fire and afterwards the Compound of Eggs. Then cover them with a Tin or Copper-lid with Fire upon it, to give them a colour like that of a Custard, and let them be serv'd up with Orange-flowers and Sugar.

Artificial Eggs *au Miroir* are made after this manner. Fill the bottom of a Plate with your Cream, and let it boil with Butter, cover'd with a Lid having Fire upon it. As soon as you perceive it to grow firm, take away the Fire, make ten or twelve hollow places, with a Spoon, and fill them up with artificial Yolks. Afterwards prepare a Sauce, with thick Butter, fine Herbs chopt very small, Pepper, Salt, Nutmeg and a little Vinegar, or otherwise, and when you would have the Dish serv'd up to Table, pour it in hot upon the Eggs. The same thing may be done with several other sorts.

F.

F.

FARCES.

The number of Farces is very great; so that it would be difficult to give a particular account of them after a better manner, than in speaking of every Thing in which they are us'd. For example, Directions have been already given how to make those of *Croquets*, Veal and Mutton-cutlets, &c And so of the rest Therefore the Reader is referr'd to every one of these Articles, to observe the nature of every Farce, and we shall here only explain that of Fish

To make a good Fish-farce.

Take Carps, Pikes and other Fishes that are at Hand, and let all be well minc'd upon the Dresser. Let an *Omelet* be like-wise prepar'd, that is not fried too much, with Mushrooms, *Truffles*, Parsly and Chibbols cut small, and let all be put upon the Farce, when it is well order'd and season'd: To these may be added the Crum of a Loaf soak'd in Milk, with Butter and Yolks of Eggs, and in a Word, care must be taken that the -Farce be well thicken'd It may serve to farce Soles and Carps, as also Cabbage; to make small *Andouillets*, *Croquets*, and every Thing else that you shall judge expedient, as it were on Flesh-days.

FAWN, see *Deer*.

FEET.

A Side-dish of Lambs-feet.

The Lambs-feet must be well scalded, boil'd and farc'd, af-ter having taken away the Bone in the middle: Then they must be dipt in a beaten Egg, well breaded and fried in the same manner as *Croquets* This Dish is to be garnish'd with fried Parsly.

They may also be us'd for Out-works, or to garnish a Side-dish of a Lambs-head, with white Sauce; as if they were Pi-geons with white Sauce: Lastly, they may be of further use

to

to garnish the Potage of Lambs-heads, and ought to be serv'd up hot to Table

For Hogs-feet in a *Soufce*, fee the Letter S.

Pigs-feet, fee Pigs-pettitoes

FILETS.

We have already explain'd what relates to the Manner of Dreffing a *Filet* of Beef with Cucumbers, and we have obferv'd in that Place, that the fame thing may be done with all other forts of *Filets* Let us now give fome Account of the *Filets Mignons* that are ferv'd up both for Side-difhes and Out-works.

To make Filets Mignons.

Take good *Filets* of Beef, Veal or Mutton, cut them into large Slices, and beat them well upon a Table or Dreffer : Then a Farce is to be made of the fame Ingredients as thofe of the *Pain au Veau*, except that it muft be thicken'd with Yolks of Eggs; confifting particularly, of Bacon, part of a Fillet of Veal, a little Gammon-fat boil'd, and fome Flefh of Fowl, with Parfly, Chibbols, *Truffles* and Mufhrooms; as alfo fome Bread foak'd in Broth or Milk, and a little Milk-cream. Your Farce being thus prepar'd, fpread it upon the *Filets*, according to the quantity that you would have, and roll them up very firm Afterwards, having provided a Stew-pan that is not too large, let feveral thin Slices of Bacon be laid in order on the bottom of it, with fome Slices of Veal well beaten, as alfo your farced *Filets* well feafon'd with all forts of fine Herbs, and fome Slices of Chibbol and Lemmon : Cover them on the top as well as at bottom, and fet the Pan between two Fires, but fuch as are not too vehement, to the end that they may boil gently When they are ready, let them be taken out, clear'd well from the Fat, and ferv'd up hot, with a good Cullis, according to difcretion, and fome Lemmon-juice A fmall Ragoo of *Truffles* may alfo be added, if you think fit If any other Side-difh of farc'd Fowl be requir'd, you may make ufe of the fame Farce, and bake them likewife between two Fires with your *Filets*, but to diftinguifh them, when they are all ready, different Ragoo's or Cullifes ought to be made for them : Then they are to be well drain'd drain'd from the Fat, and every Thing a-part ferv'd up to Table.

Filets *of a fat Pullet, with Cream.*

Take the *Filets* of large fat Pullets roafted, and cut them into pieces: Then put into a Stew-pan a little Lard and Parfly, and, having tofs'd it up with a little Flower, add Artichoke-bottoms cut into quarters, Mufhrooms and Slices of *Truffles,* a Faggot of fine Herbs, and a little clear Broth, all well feafon'd When they are fufficiently ftew'd, put your *Filets* to them, and a little before they are ferv'd up, pour in a little Milk-cream, taking care to keep them hot. To thicken them, let one or two Eggs be beaten with Cream, and having brought it to a due confiftence, let all be fet on the Table at once, as well for Side-difhes as Intermeffes.

The *Filets* of a fat Pullet are likewife drefs'd with white Sauce, Oifters and Cucumbers; the *Filets* of Mutton with *Truffles*; others in Slices, with Gammon; and fo of feveral others that may be found by means of the General Table.

As for the *Filets* of Fifh that may be ferv'd up in a Sallet during the time of Lent, fee Page 41.

F R I C A N D O E S.

Fricandoes or Scotch Collops ferve not only to garnifh very fumptuous Side-difhes; but alfo to make particular Difhes· When they are us'd for garnifhing, 'tis requifite only to lard them; but when farced for a feparate Difh, they are to be prepar'd in this manner.

To make farc'd Fricandoes *or Scotch Collops.*

Cut a Leg of Veal into fomewhat thin Collops, and having larded them fet them in order upon a Table or Dreffer, with the Bacon underneath. Then put on the middle of every one, a little of fome good Farce, and ftroak the Sides of it with your Fingers dipt in a beaten Egg, to the end that the *Fricandoe* or Collop when put thereupon, may ftick to it and be as it were incorporated with it; but care muft be taken that the Bacon appear on all fides. Having put thefe *Fricandoes* in due order into a Stew-pan, let them be well cover'd and fet over a Fire that

15

is not too quick ; neither muft there be any on the top   They
are to be brought to a colour on both Sides, then taken out
and drain'd a little from the Fat, to the end that they may be
render'd fomewhat brown,with a little Flower : Afterwards you
muft foak them in good Gravy that is not black , and put
them again into the Stew-pan to be thoroughly drefs'd   If they
are defign'd only for Garniture, they may be left in this manner ; but if you would have a particular Difh made of them,
it would be requifite to add fome *Truffles*, Mufhrooms and Veal-
fweet-breads, with a good Bread-cullis, and to take care that
all be well clear'd from the Fat   When they are ready, fprinkle
them with a little Verjuice ; drefs them in a Difh, pouring your
Ragoo on the top, and let them be ferv'd up hot   Some call
this fort of *Fricandoes*, by the Denomination of *Scollop'd Veal*

The manner of preparing *Fricandoes* to make a *Grenade*, will
be explain'd hereafter under the Letter G.

F R I T T E R s.

Fritters are made feveral Ways, that is to fay, with Apples,
Blanc-mangers, Milk, or Water ; and all thefe forts are us'd for
Intermeffes.

Intermeffes of Water-fritters.

Let fome Water and a little Salt be put into a Stew-pan, with
green and candy'd Lemmon-peel minc'd very fmall   Let it
boil over a Furnace, and having put therein two good Handfuls of Flower, with a little Butter, ftir it about, as much as
is poffible, till it be loofen'd from the Pan · Then, drawing it
afide, put in the Yolks of two Eggs and mix them well together ; continuing to put in two Eggs at once fucceffively, to
the number of ten or twelve, till your Pafte or Batter become
very rich.   Afterwards, having flower'd the Dreffer-board, dip
your Fingers likewife into Flower, and draw out your Pafte
into pieces : When they have lain by a little while, they are to
be roll'd out, and cut into fmall round pieces, fo as not to ftick
one to another, and when ready, they may be fried in good
Lard   Having taken them out of the Frying-pan, ftrew fome
Sugar upon them, fprinkling alfo a little Orange-flower-water,
and let them be fpeedily ferv'd up for Out-works.   They may
likewife be us'd for the garnifhing of Cream-tarts.

Inter-

Intermeffes of Blanc-manger-*fritters.*

Take Rice, wafh it in five or fix Waters and dry it well at the Fire · Then pound it in a Mortar, and fift this Flower thro' a Sieve to render it very fine   It would be requifite to ufe a good half ounce of it, according to the bignefs of your Difhes Having put this Flower into a Stew-pan, dilute it well with Milk, afterwards pour in a Quart of Milk, and fet all over the Furnace , but care muft be taken to ftir it continually   You muft alfo put thereto the Breaft of a roafted fat Pullet minc'd fmall and make your Pafte as if it were for Paftry-cream ; neither would it be improper to add a little Sugar, fome candy'd Lemmon-peel and green Lemmon-peel grated, as it is boiling   In the mean while, the Dreffer-board is to be flower'd, and the Pafte being laid upon it, muft be roll'd out with a Rolling-pin   Then having cut it into fmall pieces like thofe of the Water-fritters, flower your Hand, make them up neatly, and fry them in good Lard, as before.   As foon as they are ready to be ferv'd up to Table, ftrew them with Sugar, and fprinkle them with Orange flower-water.   If they are to ferve for a particular Difh, let them be garnifh'd with Water-fritters or others.

Milk-fritters.

They are made after the fame manner as the Water-fritters, but a lefs quantity of Flower muft be us'd, to the end that the Pafte may be fomewhat finer , and if it be not fufficiently fine, fome more Yolks of Eggs may be put into the Stew-pan   Then let the Batter be turn'd into a Plate and well fpread over the bottom of it.   Afterwards having provided fome melted Lard in a Frying-pan and a Spoon, you may make the Fritters with the end of it, which is to be dipt from time to time, in the Lard, to keep the Batter from fticking to it   The Frying-pan muft be gently mov'd without intermiffion, and the Fritters, when well colour'd muft be taken out, in order to be fugar'd hot, and fprinkled with Orange-flower-water   Afterwards being fugar'd again a little, they may be ic'd over, if you pleafe, with the red-hot Fire-fhovel, and ferv'd up hot to Table.

Other

Other forts of Fritters

Fritters may alfo be made with Apples, Apricocks preferv'd dry, Plums, Cherries in Ears, fmooth Piftachoes, red Goofeberries preferv'd, Pomegranate-kernels and Parmefan, fome of them requiring a thin Pafte or Batter, and others thicker But forafmuch as this is rather the Bufinefs of a Confectioner than a Cook, we fhall take no farther notice of thefe Matters in this Place.

F R U I T.

How to make Paftes of feveral forts of Fruit.

As for white Goofeberries, they muft not be too ripe, but for other forts of Fruit, 'tis no great matter. Take thefe Fruits, every one of them a-part, let them be well pickt, and put into a Copper-pan, with a little Water; but if you would have a Jelly made of them, the Liquor of every particular Fruit muft be drawn off feparately When they are fcalded in that little Water, pour all into a Sieve, in order to be well drain'd, and this Liquor will ferve to make your Jelly As foon as the feveral forts of Fruit are fufficiently drain'd in this manner, take a *Spatula* and fqueez every one of them feparately thro' a Sieve into different Silver-difhes; fo as it may become, as it were a kind of Marmelade: Set one of thefe Difhes upon the Furnace, and dry up this Pafte neatly with the *Spatula* till no moifture be left. The fame thing may be done with every fort of Pafte, and they may be left to cool in their proper Difhes In the mean while, you are to provide a large Copper-pan and put into it feven or eight Pounds of Sugar, according to the quantity of your Pafte: Pour in fome Water, with the White of an Egg whipt, and let it be fcumm'd as foon as it boils, for after three or four Walms, a thick Scum will arife, which muft be carefully taken off, to the end that your Syrop may become very clear Then let it boil till it be greatly feather'd, and having fet the Difhes of Marmelade in order, pour fome of this Syrop into them, according to the quantity of your Paftes; fo as every Thing may be well temper'd a-part Afterwards you are to take fome Slates with feveral little Tin-moulds made in the Shape of a Heart, Square, Flower-de-luce, or the like, and of fome other Figures: Set

Set thefe Moulds in order upon the Slates, and by means of a Spoon, fill them up with your Pafte or Marmelade ; taking care not to confound them one with another Laftly, let thefe Slates be put into a Stove, with a little Fire underneath, and fhut up clofe, to the end that the Pafte may be well ic'd over When they are fo order'd, and become firm, the Moulds may be taken away, and they will ferve for a confiderable time, provided that fufficient care be taken of them in the Stove.

For the Jelly of thefe Fruits, take the Liquor that is drain'd from them, that of every fort a-part, and let it boil with Sugar well clarify'd and boil'd till it become pearled. As it is boiling, take off the Scum from time to time, with Paper, and when your Jelly is made, fill up feveral Pots with it, which are to to be fet by to cool. When the Jelly is cold, cover them with Paper, and tye up the Pots all at once, writing on the top of every one, the Name of the Jelly contain'd therein, according to the variety of Fruits, from which the feveral Liquors were extracted.

G.

GALANTINE.

THe Nature of an Intermefs of *Galantine* fhall be hereafter explain'd in the Article of Sucking-Pigs, under the Letter P. and there alfo fhall be fhew'd the Manner of Garnifhing it and Serving it up to Table. We fhall only intimate here, that it may alfo be garnifh'd with its Skin well breaded and brought to a fine colour, by means of the red-hot Fire-fhovel ; for the reft, the Reader is referr'd to the Place even now mentioned.

GALLIMAWFRY.

'Tis no new thing nor very difficult to drefs a Shoulder of Mutton, or fome other Joynt in a Gallimawfry : However in regard that it may ferve to diverfifie the Meffes in thofe Ordinaries, where there is greater ftore of Butchers-meat than Fowl it may not be improper here to fhew the manner of preparing it which is as follows, *viz.*

Let the Skin of a Shoulder of Mutton be flipt off, yet fo as it may continue fticking to the Knuckle ; mince the Flefh fmall and put it into a Frying-pan, with Lard, fine Herbs, whole Chibbols

bols, Pepper, Salt, Nutmeg, Mushrooms, green Lemmon and some
Broth, to be fried or stew'd all together : Then dress it under the
Skin, which may be breaded and colour'd ; adding some Lemmon-juice and good Gravy, when the Dish is ready to be serv'd
up to Table.

GAMMON.

Take small Slices of raw Gammon ; let them be well beaten
and tofs'd up in a Stew-pan, with a little Lard   Then set them
over a Chafing-dish, and by the means of a Spoon, bring them
to a brown colour, with a little Flower   As soon as they are
colour'd put to them good Gravy, a Bunch of Chibbols and fine
Herbs, a few Cloves, a Clove of Garlick, some Slices of Lemmon, a Handful of chopt Mushrooms, *Truffles* likewise minc'd,
some Crusts of Bread and a little Vinegar : When they are all
sufficiently boil'd, strain them thro' a Sieve and put this Liquor
or Gravy into a convenient Place, without suffering it to boil
any longer.   It will be of use for the dressing of all sorts of
Dishes in which Gammon is us'd.

A Gammon-pie.

Having provided a good Gammon, take off the Skin or Sward
with the bad Fat, and cut off the Hock and the Bone in the
middle.   Then covering it with *Bards* or thin Slices of Bacon
and Beef-stakes, also Spice, fine Herbs, pieces of Onion and a
Bay-leaf, set it between two Fires in a Pot, with the Lid close
stopt, so that no steam may evaporate : Stew it thus during
twelve or Sixteen Hours ; taking care that the Fire be not too
quick, and let it cool in the same Pot · In the mean while, prepare a thick Paste, with a little Butter, an Egg, Flower and
Water, and taking the Dish in which you would have it serv'd
up, make a large Border round about it with the same Paste :
This Border ought to be thick, having a Foot to bear some
Weight, because there is no Bottom-crust, and may be wrought
on the out-side with little Flower-de-luces and other fine Pastry-
works : Set it into the Oven, and when it is bak'd, take out
your Gammon, pouring off all the Fat that lies round about,
and put it into a Dish, with its own Gravy.   You may also make
use of the same Stakes or Slices of Beef, to fill up the Intervals,
and some Fat, and compleat the filling them, as if it were done

K   in

in the Pie. 'Tis also requisite to add a little chopt Parsly, to strew
it with Bread-chippings, and to give it a colour with the red-
hot Fire-shovel, in order to be serv'd up cold to Table.

Another Intermeß of Gammon-pie.

Take away the Skin with the bad Fat of your Gammon, cut
off the thin End or Hock, as before : Then, having prepar'd a
thick brown Paste, with Rye-flower and Water, make your
Pie of a round Figure and a considerable heighth ; putting on
the bottom a sufficient quantity of Bacon minc'd and pounded :
Then having well fix'd the Gammon therein, put some Bay-leaves,
four or five Slices of Lemmon and several other *Bards* or thin
Slices of Bacon on the top. Afterwards cover it with a Lid, and
when the Pie is quite finish'd, wash it over with the Yolk of an
Egg   Let it stand in the Oven during six Hours and set it by
cold, before it is brought to Table

Gammon in a Ragoo, with Hypocras.

Take raw Slices of Gammon, and fry them in a Pan ; making
a Sauce with Sugar, Cinnamon, a pounded Macaroon, red Wine
and a little white Pepper beaten   Then put your Slices into this
Sauce, and sprinkle them with Orange-juice, when ready to be
serv'd up to Table
  Gammon is dress'd otherwise among the Salt-meats, with Sausages and dried Tongues.
  For a Gammon-*Omelet* recourse may be had hereafter to the
Letter O. and for Pigeons with Gammon, to the Letter P. in
like manner as Chickens with Gammon and the Gammon-cul-
lis are already set down under C.

Fish-gammon.

Take the Flesh of Tenches, Eels and fresh Salmon, and the
Roes of Carps, which are to be minc'd and pounded in a Mortar, with Pepper, Salt, Nutmeg and Butter.   Mix all these sorts
of Flesh well together, and make of them as it were a kind of
Gammon, upon the Skins of Carps . Then wrap up the whole
Farce in a new Linnen-cloth , which is to be sow'd up very
close, and let it boil in one half Water and the other Wine ; season'd with Cloves, a Bay-leaf and Pepper.   Let it cool in its
own

own Broth, and ferve it up with Bay-leaves, fine Herbs chopt very fmall, and Slices of Lemmon It may alfo be cut into Slices, as the real Gammon

A Leg or fhoulder of Mutton may be imitated after the fame manner, as alfo Chickens and Pigeons or elfe with a fort of Fifh-farce before defcrib'd in the firft Article of the Letter F

G O D I V O E ' S.

We have already taken notice of feveral forts of *Godivoe's* for different Meffes ; fo that it may be fufficient here only to fhew the manner of making the *Godivoe* of a *Poupeton*, which may ferve for many other Things of the like nature.

To make the Godivoe *of a* Poupeton.

Take part of a Leg of Veal , with fome parboil'd Bacon and other Fat, all well minc'd . Then adding to thefe, fome chopt *Truffles* and Mufhrooms, Chibbols, Parfly, the Crum of a Loaf foak'd in good Gravy, four whole Eggs and two Yolks , make the *Poupeton*, as it were a Pie, in the Stew-pan with *Bards* or thin Slices of Bacon underneath. You muft alfo have at Hand, fome Pigeons well drefs'd, with all forts of fine Herbs and good Garnitures, and fome very fmall Slices of Gammon , all well feafon'd : Let your Pigeons be put into the *Poupeton*, and make an end of covering them with the Farce. To keep it from breaking, you may beat up an Egg , and lay it on neatly with your Hand · Then let the *Bards* or Bacon-flices, that are round about be turn'd upon it, and let it be bak'd between two gentle Fires, *viz.* on the top and underneath This is commonly call'd a *Poupeton* farc'd with young Pigeons, and ferves for a Side-difh Quails may alfo be farced with it, or other Fowls of the fame nature.

G O O S E - G I B B L E T S.

There has been occafion to make mention of a Potage of Goofe-gibblets Pag. 26 in order to prepare which, let your Gibblets boil in good Broth feafon'd with a Bunch of fine Herbs and falt Then cut them into pieces and fry them in Lard, with Parfly, Chervil and a little white Pepper . Laftly, having ftew'd all with Yolks of Eggs, a little Verjuice and the Juice of a Lem-

mon

mon, drefs your Potage upon the foaked Crufts. The fame thing may be alfo done with the *Beatils* or Tid-bits of other forts of Fowl.

A Gibblet-pie.

Gibblet-*Tourtes* or Pan-pies may be likewife made in this manner: Let your Gibblets be cut into pieces, fcalded and well cleans'd : Then make your Pie with a fine Pafte, both for the Under and Upper-Cruft; feafoning it with Pepper, Salt, Cloves, fine Herbs, Chibbol and Nutmeg, and adding fome pounded Lard, Artichoke-bottoms *Morilles*, and common Mufh-rooms : Let it be bak'd about two Hours, and ferv'd up with a little white Sauce.

G R A V Y.

Veal-gravy.

Cut a Fillet of Veal into three parts, put it into an earthen Pot, and ftop it up fo clofe with its Lid and fome Pafte, that no Air may come to it : Let it ftand over a gentle Fire about two Hours, and your Gravy will be made; to be us'd for thofe Mef-fes, into which, according to our Directions, fome of it is requi-fite to be put, to render them more fucculent and to heighten their Relifh,

The fame thing may be done, in preparing the Gravy of Mut-ton or Beef, or elfe recourfe may be had to what has been laid down in the firft Article of Cullifes.

Partridge and Capon-gravy.

Let both be roafted, and when they are ready, let them be fqueez'd feparately to get their Gravy. The fame thing may be put in practice for Veal-gravy and others.

Fifh-gravy.

Take Tenches and Carps, cleanfe the former from their Mud, cut them quite thro' the Back, and fcale the Carps Having taken away the Gills from both, put them into a Silver-difh, with a little Butter. Let them be brought to a brown colour, like a
piece

piece of Beef, and when they are drefs'd, put to them a little Flower, which is alfo to be made brown with the reft, and afterwards fome Broth, according to the quantity of Gravy that you would have made · Strain all thro' a Linnen-cloath and let it be very well fqueez'd. Laftly, feafon this Liquor or Gravy, with a Bunch of Herbs, Salt and a green Lemmon ftuck with Cloves, to be us'd, as well for Potages, as for Side-difhes and Intermeffes of Fifh.

GRENADE.

To make a *Grenade*, 'tis requifite to have a fufficient quantity of *Fricandoe's*, or *Scotch*-Collops larded with fmall Slips of Bacon, and a round Stew-pan, that is not of too large a fize. Then put fome thin Slices of Bacon on the bottom, and fet your *Fricandoe's* in Order, with the Bacon on the outfide; fo as they may meet in a Point in the middle, and touch one another   To keep this Order from being confounded in the dreffing of the Meats, they muft be bound together, with the White of a beaten Egg; into which you may dip your Fingers, to moiften them on the Sides, which ought to be thinner than the reft   Into the hollow place made by this means, and alfo round about, you are to put a little of the Farce of *Mirotons*, or of fome other *Godivoe*: referving the middle for fix Pigeons drefs'd in a Ragoo, with Veal-fweet-breads, *Truffles*, Mufhrooms and fmall Slices of Gammon, all well feafon'd. The Ragoo is likewife to be pour'd into it, as if it were a *Poupeton*. Then cover the reft of the Farce on the top, ordering it with your Fingers dipt in a beaten Egg, and join the *Fricandoe's* quite oppofite thereto · Some *Bards* or thin Slices of Bacon are likewife to be laid on the top, and the whole Mefs is to be bak'd *à la Braife* or between two Fires, to give it a fine colour   In order to ferve it up hot, it muft be turn'd upfide down, and when the Fat is all taken away, the Point of the *Fricandoe's* or Collops muft be open'd like that of a *Grenade* or Pomegranate, from whence this fort of Mefs takes its Name.

A GRENADIN,
Of fat Pullets, Chickens, Pigeons, Partridges and all sorts of Fowl

Let a well-season'd *Godivee* be prepar'd, after the same manner as before for the *Poupeton*, remembring to thicken it with
Yolks of Eggs and Bread-crum soak'd in good Gravy, or in a
little Milk-cream : Then take a Baking-pan, according to the
bigness of your Dish, and put into it some *Bards* or very thin
Slices of Bacon · Let your *Godivee* be laid upon these *Bards*,
and with your Fingers dipt in a beaten Egg, make a Hole proportionably to the size of your Dish or Plate, raising up the
sides to the heighth of three Inches, and so as they may be
somewhat firm. Take your fat Pullets or other Fowls as they
are raw, cut them into pieces, and let them be well beaten :
Then fry them in a Pan, with Lard, Parsly, Chibbol and a
little Flower, and afterwards put to them a little Gravy; seasoning them well, and adding *Truffles* cut into Slices, Mushrooms and Veal-sweet-breads When they are almost ready,
so that little Sauce is left, set the Fowls in order in your *Grenadin*, and let it be neatly breaded on the top, to give it a
good colour in the Oven As soon as it is drawn, drain it well
from the Fat, cut off the *Bards* round about, and turn it into
your Dish or Plate A Mushroom-cullis may also be pour'd
upon it, in order to serve it up hot to the Table for a Side-
dish.

A GRILLADE, or
Dish of Meat broil'd upon the Grid-iron.

When any Turkeys, or other sorts of Fowl are left cold, a
Side-dish may be made of them in this manner : Take their
Wings, Legs and Rumps, and broil them upon the Grid-iron,
with Pepper and Salt. Then fry some Flower in Lard, with
Oisters, Anchovies, Capers, Nutmeg, a Bay-leaf and a piece
of green Lemmon, also a little Vinegar and Broth, and let
them all be well soak'd together

GRU-

GRUEL,
An Intermeß of Gruel or Milk-potage.

Let some fine Oat-meal be put into a little Pot, full of Milk, with a Stick of Cinnamon, a piece of green Lemmon-peel, a little Salt, Coriander-seed and a few Cloves: Let it boil till it becomes a fine Cream; then strain it thro' the Hair-sieve, and having pour'd it into a *Cuvet*, Bason, or Dish, put a little Sugar therein: Afterwards bring it to a Furnace, the Fire of which is not too quick; because it ought not to boil any longer. Stir it about gently, from time to time, and when the Sugar is melted, set it upon the hot Embers; covering it close, till a kind of thick Cream over-spread the top: Then take it off, and let it be serv'd up hot in the same Dish.

H.

HASHES.

A Hash of Partridges.

TO make a Hash of Partridges, the same Method is to be obferv'd, as in preparing an ordinary Mutton-hash; only you may add some Gammon, and temper it with good Gravy; garnishing your Dish with small Crufts of fried Bread, and sprinkling it with Lemmon-juice, when ready to be serv'd up to Table.

A Carp-hash.

For a Carp-hash, a few Capers are to be put into it, with Mushrooms, *Truffles* and other proper Garnitures, after all has been well minc'd and season'd

There are also some other sorts of Hashes, which may be found by means of the General Table, in the several Places to which they properly belong, and where they are treated of in particular.

K 4 HARI-

HARICOTS.

The manner of dreſſing an *Haricot* of Mutton, has been already explain'd in the laſt Article of *Cutlets* under the Letter C; and for Fiſh-*Haricots*, they may be prepai'd as a Pike in *Haricot*, under P.

HATLETS.

A Diſh of *Hatlets* is proper for the Intermeſſes, and may be thus made, *viz* Let ſome Veal-ſweet-breads be parboil'd and cut into ſmall Pieces, with Capons livers and young ſtreaked Bacon likewiſe parboil'd: Then let all be well ſeaſon'd and fry'd with a little Parſly, Chibbol and fine Flower When they are almoſt ready, ſo that only a little thick Sauce is left, you are to make ſmall *Hatlets*, and ſpit the pieces of Livers, Sweet-breads and Bacon upon them, according to the bigneſs you would have them to be of Afterwards, having dipt them in the Sauce and well breaded them, they may be broil'd upon a Grid-iron or fried.

Hatlets are alſo often us'd for the garniſhing of Diſhes of Roaſt-meat.

HEADS.

An Intermeſſ of a Boar's Head.

Let a Boar's Head be well ſindg'd at a clear Fire, and rubb'd with a piece of Brick to take off all the Hair, let it alſo be ſcrap'd with a Knife and well cleans'd: After having boned it, cutting out the two Jaw-bones and the Snout; ſlit it underneath, ſo as it may ſtick to its Skin on the top, and take away the Brain and Tongue: Then take up ſome Salt with the Point of your Knife, and cauſe it to penetrate thro' all the Parts of the Fleſh: Afterwards let the whole Head be ſet together again, and well tied up, wrapping it in a Napkin. In the mean while, a great Kettle, almoſt full of Water, is to be hang'd over the Fire, and the Head put into it, with all ſorts of fine Herbs, ſome Leaf-fat out of a Hog's Belly, two Bay-leaves, Coriander and Anis-ſeed, Cloves and Nutmeg beaten, and ſome Salt, if it has not been ſufficiently corned before; adding alſo ſome Onion and Roſemary. When it is half boil'd, pour in a Quart

of

of good Wine, and let it continue boiling for the fpace of twelve Hours; the Tongue may alfo be boil'd in the fame Liquor If time will permit, the Head may be falted before it is drefs'd, and left for a while in its Brine. When it is ready, let it cool in its own Liquor, then having taken it out, let it be neatly put into a Difh and ferved up to Table cold, either whole or in Slices.

Fifh-heads.

The Head of a Pike may be drefs'd in a *Court-bouillon*, as it appears in the Second Article of Pike under the Letter P, and may alfo be ferv'd up in Potage, as well as others; more efpe-cially that of Salmon, for which fee *Joll*.

Lambs-heads in Potage, or for a Side-difh.

Take the Heads, Feet and Livers of Lambs, with young Bacon, and having well fcalded them, let them boil all together in fome Broth in a great Pot · As foon as they are boil'd and well feafon'd, lay your Potage a foaking with good Broth and Gravy, and fet the Lambs-heads in Order in the middle. Then having breaded the Brains, fry them, 'till they become as it were *Croquets*, and put them again into their Place; garnifhing your Potage, with the Livers, Feet and Bacon: To thefe is to be added a White Cullis, made with a piece of Bread-crum fteept in good Broth, a Douzen and half of fweet Almonds, and three Yolks of hard Eggs, all pounded in a Mortar, ftrain'd thro' a Sieve, well foak'd and feafond, with the Juice of a Lemmon, when ready to be ferv d up to Table

A green Cullis may alfo be prepar'd with Chibbol-tops, Spi-nage and Crufts of Bread, which are likewife to be foak'd in a Stew-pan, with good Broth, well feafon'd with Cloves, Thyme and Gravy · Pound your Chibbol-tops and Spinage in a Mortar, and having ftrain'd the reft thro' a Sieve, put them into the Po-tage; ftrewing it with Afparagus-tops, and fprinkling it with the Juice of a Lemmon.

Inftead of this Cullis, a good fort of green Peafe-foop may be pour'd upon the Potage of Lambs-heads, otherwife to diverfi-fie them, a Cullis may be made of the Livers, to be garnifh'd with the Feet and young Bacon At another time, they may be cover'd with green Peafe, and a Cullis of the fame, according

'ding to the Seafon. And at another time, the Lambs-heads may be carefully fcalded in Water that is not too hot; then all the Bones muft be cut out with the Tongue, taking care that the Skin remain quite entire : Thefe Heads are to be ftuff'd with fome good Farce, and neatly tied up, in order to be drefs'd : Then they are to be put into the Potage, and garnifh'd as before; or elfe with Lambs-lungs marinated and fried in Pafte

A fmall Side difh of Lambs-heads may be prepar'd with a good Ragoo pour'd upon it; as alfo a kind of Lamb-potage, with Roman Lettice farced; garnifhing the faid Potage with the Stalks of the Lettice fried in a Pan with Lard and Flower, and afterwards laid a foaking in a Pot with good Broth, which muft be thicken'd before it is drefs'd, with Yolks of Eggs ftrain'd thro' the Hair-fieve.

H I N D.

To know the manner of dreffing a Hind, 'tis only requifite to have recourfe to the Article of a *Stag*; as being of the fame Nature, except that the former is fofter and more infipid. Therefore it ought to be fteept in a Marinade of the fame, after it has been larded, with fmall Slips of Bacon : It muft be well bafted as it is roafting; and when it is ready, Capers and fried Flower are to be put into the Dripping, with a little green Lemmon; it muft alfo be foak'd in its Sauce.

When your Hind is larded, marinated and roafted, cover'd with Paper; a fweet Sauce may likewife be prepared for it, with Vinegar, Pepper, Sugar, Cinnamon and a whole Shalot.

For a Hind-*Civet*, fee the Letter C.

I.

J E L L I E S.

THe manner of making a Jelly of Fruits has been already ex-prefs'd under the Letter F, and in the Article of *Blancman ger* may be found the Jelly which is requifite for that purpofe, as alfo that of Harts-horn, for Fifh-days, fo that we fhall only here produce a fort of Jelly proper for fick Perfons, which neverthelefs will be of a much better Relifh to thofe that are in Health, when ferv'd up among the Intermeffes as the reft.

To make an excellent Jelly.

Take Calves-feet, according to the quantity of Jelly that you would have made, with a good Cock, and having well wash'd all, put them into a Kettle or Pot, filling it with a proportionable quantity of Water. Let them boil together, and be more especially careful to look after the scumming of the Pot When these Meats are almoft reduc'd to Rags, 'tis a fign that the Jelly is fufficiently boil'd, but care muft be taken that it be not too ftrong. Then having provided a good Stew-pan, ftrain the Jelly thro' a Sieve, that is to fay, nothing but the pure Broth; clear it well from the Fat, with two or three Feathers; and put fome Sugar into it proportionably; with a Stick of Cinnamon, two or three Cloves and the Peel of two or three Lemmons, the Juice of which muft be kept Let your Jelly boil thus a little while, and in the mean time, make fome Snow with four or fix Whites of Eggs' Squeez the Juice of your Lemmons into it, and pour all into the Jelly; ftirring them together, a little while over the Furnace: Then leaving them till the Liquor rifes, and is ready to run over the Pan, pour it out into the Straining-bag, and ftrain it two or three times, till you perceive it to be clear Whilft the Jelly is boiling with the Meats, fome think fit to pour in a little white Wine. In order to ferve this Jelly up to Table, it muft be put into a very cold Place, to the end that it may be well coagulated in the Difhes

How to colour Jellies.

Thefe Colours being well order'd, may produce very agreeable Effects in a *Blanc-manger*, or any other Mefs of the like nature. For Example, the Jelly may be left in its natural Colour, or made white with Almonds pounded and ftrain'd after the ufual manner: For yellow, fome Yolks of Eggs may be put into it, for Grey, a little Cochineel, for Red, fome Juice of red Beet or Turnfole of *Portugal*; for Purple, fome purple Turnfole, or Powder of Violets, and for Green, fome Juice of Beet-leaves, which is to be boil'd in a Difh to take away its Crudity.

JOLL.

J O L L.

A Joll of Salmon.

Let your Joll be fcal'd, larded with Slips of Eels-flefh and feafon'd with Pepper · Then fry it with burnt Butter and afterwards ftew it in an Earthen Pan, with clear Peafe-foop, fine Herbs and green Lemmon : Add to thefe, fome Capers, Mufhrooms and Oifters, fry d with burnt Butter and a little Flower ; and drefs all artificially in the Potage, with Lemmon-juice, as they are ferving up to Table.

J U L I A N.

The *Julian* is a very confiderable Potage, and may be made in this manner . Having roafted a Leg of Mutton, let the Fat and Skin be taken away, and let it be put into a Kettle or Pot, of a fufficient bignefs to hold fome Broth for the Potage. Then add a good piece of Beef; another of a Fillet of Veal; a fat Capon ; Carrets, Turneps and Parfneps, two of each; Parfly-roots, Celery and an Onion ftuck with Cloves; and let all boil together a long while, to the end that your Broth may be fufficiently enrich'd In the mean time, another Pot muft be provided, and therein three or four Bundles of Afparagus, as much Sorrel as may be cut with a Knife at two ftrokes and fome Chervil. Let them be well boil'd with fome Broth taken out of the great Pot, and when the Crufts are foak'd, let the Afparagus and Sorrel be laid in order upon them, but nothing round about.

Julian-Potages are alfo made of a Breaft of Veal, Capons, fat Pullets, Pigeons and other forts of Meat: When they are well prepar'd and fcalded, let them be put into a Pot with good Broth and a Bunch of fine Herbs ; afterwards adding the above-mentioned Roots and Pulfe ; which may alfo ferve to garnifh the Potage, with Heaps of Afparagus chopt into pieces, and nothing elfe, but what is green, fuch as green Peafe, &c.

K

K.

K I D S.

Kids may be dress'd after the same manner as Lamb, either in Potage, or for Side-dishes; so that it is only requisite to per-use what is hereafter set down in that Article; and for roasted Kids, to turn to the Letter R.

L.

L A M B.

IT were needless to take notice, That Quarters, or whole Sides of Lamb, often serve for the great Roast, when it is in sea-son; and more especially, for the meaner sort of Ordinaries. And in regard, that there is nothing either difficult or unknown rela-ting to this Article, we shall here only shew the manner of ma-king a Ragoo of Lamb; at the same time, referring the Rea-der, for Lambs-heads, to the third Article of *Heads*, and, for Lambs-feet, to the Letter F

Lamb in a Ragoo.

A Ragoo of Lamb may be prepar'd thus · Cut it into four quarters, and, after having larded it with middle-siz'd Slips of Bacon, and given it somewhat of a colour, let it be boil'd in an Earthen Pot or Stew-pan, with Broth, Pepper, Salt, Cloves, Mushrooms, and a Faggot of fine Herbs. When it is ready, let a Sauce be made for it, of Oisters fried with a little Flower, two Anchovies; and Lemmon-juice, when ready to be serv'd up to Table, and let it be garnish'd with fried Mushrooms.

L A M P R E Y S.

Lampreys may be dress'd two several ways, *viz.* Take some of their Blood and let it be kept a-part · Then cleanse them from their Slime with hot Water and cut them into pieces; which are to be stew'd in an Earthen Pot, with burnt Butter, white Wine, Pepper, Salt, Nutmeg, a Bunch of Herbs and a Bay-leaf. Afterwards let their Blood be put to them, with a little
fried

J O L L.

A Joll of Salmon.

Let your Joll be scal'd, larded with Slips of Eels-flesh and season'd with Pepper: Then fry it with burnt Butter and afterwards stew it in an Earthen Pan, with clear Pease-soop, fine Herbs and green Lemmon · Add to these, some Capers, Mushrooms and Oisters, fry'd with burnt Butter and a little Flower ; and dress all artificially in the Potage, with Lemmon-juice, as they are serving up to Table.

J U L I A N.

The *Julian* is a very considerable Potage, and may be made in this manner   Having roasted a Leg of Mutton, let the Fat and Skin be taken away, and let it be put into a Kettle or Pot, of a sufficient bigness to hold some Broth for the Potage. Then add a good piece of Beef; another of a Fillet of Veal ; a fat Capon ; Carrets, Turneps and Parsneps, two of each ; Parslyroots, Celery and an Onion stuck with Cloves ; and let all boil together a long while, to the end that your Broth may be sufficiently enrich'd   In the mean time, another Pot must be provided, and therein three or four Bundles of Asparagus, as much Sorrel as may be cut with a Knife at two strokes and some Chervil. Let them be well boil'd with some Broth taken out of the great Pot, and when the Crusts are soak'd, let the Asparagus and Sorrel be laid in order upon them, but nothing round about.

Julian-Potages are also made of a Breast of Veal, Capons, fat Pullets, Pigeons and other sorts of Meat: When they are well prepar'd and scalded, let them be put into a Pot with good Broth and a Bunch of fine Herbs ; afterwards adding the above-mentioned Roots and Pulse ; which may also serve to garnish the Potage, with Heaps of Asparagus chopt into pieces, and nothing else, but what is green, such as green Pease, &c.

K

K.

K I D S.

Kids may be drefs'd after the fame manner as Lamb, either in Potage, or for Side-difhes; fo that it is only requifite to per-ufe what is hereafter fet down in that Article, and for roafted Kids, to turn to the Letter R.

L.

L A M B.

IT were needlefs to take notice, That Quarters, or whole Sides of Lamb, often ferve for the great Roaft, when it is in fea-fon; and'more efpecially,for the meaner fort of Ordinaries. And in regard, that there is nothing either difficult or unknown rela-ting to this Article, we fhall here only fhew the manner of ma-king a Ragoo of Lamb, at the fame time, referring the Rea-der, for Lambs-heads, to the third Article of *Heads,* and, for Lambs-feet, to the Letter F

Lamb in a Ragoo.

A Ragoo of Lamb may be prepar'd thus : Cut it into four quarters, and, after having larded it with middle-fiz'd Slips of Bacon, and given it fomewhat of a colour, let it be boil'd in an Earthen Pot or Stew-pan, with Broth, Pepper, Salt, Cloves, Mufhrooms, and a Faggot of fine Herbs. When it is ready, let a Sauce be made for it, of Oifters fried with a little Flower, two Anchovies; and Lemmon-juice, when ready to be ferv'd up to Table, and let it be garnifh'd with fried Mufhrooms.

L A M P R E Y S.

Lampreys may be drefs'd two feveral ways, *viz.* Take fome of their Blood and let it be kept a-part · Then cleanfe them from their Slime with hot Water and cut them into pieces; which are to be ftew'd in an Earthen Pot, with burnt Butter, white Wine, Pepper, Salt, Nutmeg, a Bunch of Herbs and a Bay-leaf. Afterwards let their Blood be put to them, with a little

fried

fried Flower and Capers, and let them be garnish'd with Slices of Lemmon

To dress them with sweet Sauce, when they are clear'd from their Slime, let them be stew'd in red Wine, with burnt Butter, Cinnamon, Sugar, Pepper, Salt and a piece of green Lemmon; adding some Lemmon-juice, when they are set upon the Table

If it be requir'd to make a Potage of Lampreys, cut them into pieces, after having taken away their Slime, and fry them in burnt Butter, with Salt, Flower, fine Herbs chopt small, Mushrooms, strained Pease-soop, and a piece of green Lemmon Then let them be dress'd upon the soak'd Crusts, and sprinkled with Lemmon-juice, as they are serving up to Table.

For Pies of Lampreys, see the Letter P.

LARKS.

Larks may be put into a Ragoo for Side-dishes, as also into a standing Pie, to be serv'd up hot, and into a *Tourte* or Pan-pie, for the two latter, it would be requisite only to observe the Directions given for the dressing of other sorts of Fowl of the like nature, and among others, for young Pigeons; except that Larks are not farced as larger Birds. Only their Ghizzards are usually taken out, and set in order on the bottom of the Pie, which is also to be fill'd with Mushrooms, Capons-livers, *Truffles*, pounded Lard and other seasoning Ingredients. When the Pie is ready to be serv'd up, some good Gravy of Veal or Mutton must be put into it, with the Juice of a Lemmon; and some Capers must be reserv'd for the Pan-pie

As for the Ragoo; after having drawn your Larks, fry them in Lard with a little Flower, and afterwards stew them in an Earthen Pan, in Broth, with white Wine, Dates cut into pieces, candy'd Lemmon-peel, Pistachoes, Cinnamon, Pepper, Salt and Prunelloes; adding Lemmon-juice when ready to be brought to Table They may be garnish'd with the same Things, and serv'd up with short Sauce

It will not be worth the while to observe, that fat Larks are sometimes roasted; it being a very common Dish.

For Potages of Larks, see the Letter P.

LEGS.

L e g s.

Altho' there is nothing more common than a Leg of Mutton or Veal, yet they may be dress'd after several manners, so as to give good satisfaction, and even to grace the most sumptuous Tables.

Legs of Mutton.

A Side-dish of a farced Leg of Mutton.

As soon as your Leg of Mutton is dress'd, take away all the Meat, so as nothing may remain but the Bones sticking together. Then clear this Meat from the Fat, and mince it with parboil'd Bacon, a little Sewer, or Marrow, some fine Herbs, Chibbol, Parsly, a little piece of Calves-udder, the Crum of a Loaf soak'd in good Broth, two whole Eggs and two separate Yolks. Thus, all being well minc'd and season'd, let the Bone be laid in the Dish, that is to be serv'd up, so as the small end of the Leg may appear; one half of this *Godivoe* being put round about. Afterwards, having made a hollow place of the shape of the Leg, and having dipt your Fingers in a beaten Egg, that nothing may stick to them, fill up that place with a Ragoo of all sorts of Garnitures, well boil'd, strain'd and season'd; as also, the rest of the vacancy with the Farce, which may supply the place of a real Leg. Then having breaded the whole Mess, set it into the Oven, to give it a colour, and afterwards, when drawn, take away the Fat, that lyes round about the Dish. Lastly, pour in a small quantity of a well-season'd Cullis, thro' a little hole on the top, and cover it again, to be serv'd up hot to Table.

Another way of dressing a Leg of Mutton.

Another middling Side-dish may be made of a large farced Leg of Mutton with Cream. Having boned it, take the Flesh, with a piece of Veal, another of Bacon, some Leaf-fat out of a Hog's Belly and Beef-sewer, and let all be well minc'd together; adding a little Chibbol and Parsly chopt, with two or three Rocamboles, a little sweet Basil and Thyme, all well season'd, with Pepper, Salt, Spice and a few Coriander-seeds

Then

Then mingle and beat the whole Mass in a Mortar, with Cream, Yolks of Eggs and Bread-crum; stuff the Bone with this Farce in the Shape of a Leg; wash it over with the White of an Egg, covering the top with Bread-crum; and give it its due Form, if you please, with the Back of a Knife. Let it be bak'd in a Silver-dish or in a Baking-pan, with *Bards* or thin Slices of Bacon laid underneath; but your Farce must be made very strong, lest it should break, or fall in the Oven. The Dish may be garnish'd with *Petits-patez* or little Pies, farced Veal-cutlets, marinated Chickens, or any other proper Garniture; taking care, that all be well dress'd and brought to a fine colour.

A middling Side-dish may also be made of a Leg of Mutton farc'd in its Skin, and dress'd in a Ragoo with Artichoke-bottoms, Veal-sweet-breads, *Truffles,* Mushrooms, Capons-livers and Asparagus-tops, all well season'd. It ought to be garnish'd with little Rolls of Fennel and farced *Poupiets,* and sprinkled with Lemmon-juice, when serv'd up to Table.

A Leg of Mutton dress'd à la Royale.

Having taken away the Fat from a good Leg of Mutton, with the Flesh round about the small End, let it be beaten and larded with thick Slips of Bacon; a piece of Buttock-beef or of Veal may also be larded with it at the same time. Let all be well season'd, let the Leg and the other Meat be flower'd, and let them be brought to a colour with some melted Lard: Then being put into a Pot with all sorts of fine Herbs, an Onion stuck with Cloves, some good Broth, or Water, let them be close cover'd, and boil'd for a considerable time. In the mean while, a proper Ragoo is to be made, with Mushrooms, *Truffles,* Artichoke-bottoms, Asparagus-tops, Veal-sweet-breads, all well prepar'd, and enrich'd with a good Cullis. Afterwards having taken your Leg out of the Pot, dress it in a Dish, and cut your pieces of Beef or Veal, very neatly into Slices, to make a Border round about; so as the Bacon may appear on the Slices. Lastly, the Ragoo must be pour'd upon it scalding-hot, but if you would have the Leg take its whole relish, when it is almost ready, let it be stew'd a little while in the said Ragoo, and serv'd up in the same manner. It may also be garnish'd with larded *Fricandoe's* or Scotch-Collops and *Marinade.*

Ano-

Another Side-dish of a Leg of Mutton.

Take a Leg of Mutton, and having cut off the Fat, as before, let it be well larded and feafon'd ; it may alfo be larded with raw Gammon Then provide a Pot with fome *Bards* or thin Slices of Bacon, and Stakes of Beef or Veal and fet them in order therein, as it were for baking or ftewing between two Fires : Let the Leg be put into this Pot, and let a Fire be kindled both underneath and on the top, fo as to bring it to a fine colour Afterwards take out the *Bards* and the other Meat, and dra'n them a little from the Fat, but let the Leg of Mutton be ftill left for fome time, whilft you put as much Flower as may be taken up between your Fingers, round about the Pot, and caufe it to take a colour with the Leg • As foon as it is colour'd, put the Meat in again, that was taken out, with good Gravy and a little Water, keep the Pot clofe cover'd, and make an end, of boiling all together As for the Sauce, it ought to be fomewhat thick, otherwife a Cullis muft be pour'd into it, made of the Meat which lay round about the Leg, pounded, and ftrain'd with good Gravy. To thefe may be added all forts of Garniture, particularly, Afparagus, *Morilles*, and common Mufhrooms, and let all boil together, as alfo fome *Truffles*, Cockscombs and Veal-fweet-breads, if they may be conveniently procur'd. When every thing is ready, drefs the Leg after the ufual manner, let the Ragoo be well clear'd from the Fat, and put a little Verjuice into it. The Difh may be garnifh d with farced Cutlets of Mutton or Veal, as is before fpecified

A Leg of Mutton drefs'd with Succory and Cucumbers

Let a Leg of Mutton be roafted, taking care that it be not done too much, whilft a Ragoo is preparing with Succory, that is fcalded a little and cut into pieces. Take fome Lard, make it fomewhat brown, with Flower and good Gravy, and let all be well feafon'd ; adding a Faggot of fine Herbs and a few drops of Vinegar : Then let your Succory be boil'd, fo as not to turn black, but that it may have a fomewhat ftrong Savour, and let it be put under the Leg The fame Thing may be done with Cucumbers, but they muft be marinated, cut into fmall Slices, and afterwards drefs'd in the fame manner If you would not have the Leg ferv'd up who'e, it may be cut into thin Slices, and

L.   put

put into the same Ragoo ; taking care that they do not boil together, and that the Sauce be not either too thick or too thin. Let all be well clear'd from the Fat and brought hot to Table.

A roasted Leg of Mutton may also be serv'd up with *Robert-Sauce*, Capers and Anchovies, either for Out-works, or even for a Side-dish, when set out with proper Garnitures, and a Shoulder of Mutton may be dress'd after all the manners that have been before-describ'd for a Leg.

Legs of Veal.

Having already shewn how a Leg of Veal may be dress'd in a *Daube*, under the Letter D ; we shall here explain some other Preperations that may be made with that Joint of Meat, *viz.*

A farced Leg of Veal.

The Farce must be made of the same Flesh, with Sewet, Bacon, fine Herbs, Chibbols, Pepper, Salt, Nutmeg, Yolks of raw Eggs and Mushrooms, and when 'tis sow'd up, let it boil in good Broth. Thus a Side-dish may be made of it, or it may be serv'd up in Potage ; adding a Cullis of poach'd Yolks of Eggs and Almonds, strain'd thro' a Sieve, with the same Broth When the Dish is ready to be serv'd up, let some Lemmon-juice and good Gravy be put therein ; garnishing it with Mushrooms farced and ragoo'd, or any Thing else that you have at Hand , as Cutlets, Veal-sweet-breads, &c.

A Leg of Veal à l' Estoufade, or stew'd in a Pan.

Let your Leg of Veal be larded with thick Slips of Bacon, and fried a while in a Frying-pan : Then stew it in an earthen Pan, with Mushrooms, a Spoonful of Broth and a Glass of white Wine ; seasoning it with Pepper, Salt, a Faggot of fine Herbs, Cloves and Nutmeg. When it is ready, let some Flower be fry'd to thicken the Sauce, and garnish it with fry'd Bread, Veal-sweet-breads and Lemmon-juice, as it is serving up to Table.

I. 3 H.

LEMMONS.

To preserve Lemmon-peel dry.

Take Lemmons, and let them be well turn'd with clean Hands, to the end that your Fruit may be always kept white   Then cut them into quarters taking away all the inner Rind, and order them so as their Pulp may be very thin : Let them be steept in fair Water, and afterwards scalded in hot Water ; but care must be taken, that they be not done either too much or too little : Throw them again into fresh Water, and having prepai'd some Syrop with clarified Sugar, let them boil a little therein : Let them lye by a while, and then let them be laid upon a Grate or Hurdle, to dry up their moisture. In the mean time, having boil'd up your Sugar, till it become a little feather'd, put the Lemmon-peels into it with a Table-fork, but be careful that the Liquor be not too thick.   When they are sufficiently boil'd, take them out, leave them again on the Grate to be dried, and let them be well ic'd   There are several other Ways of preserving Lemmon-peels, which we shall pass by at present ; as being the Business of a Confectioner, rather than of a Cook.

LENTILS.

A Cullis of Lentils has been already describ'd under the Letter C, and for Lentil-potage, it may readily be found among the other Potages under P

LETTICE

To farce Lettice à la Dame Simonne.

Let headed or Cabbage-lettice, be only heated a little in scalding Water, and well drain'd : Then taking the Flesh of roasted Capons and Chickens, mince it with some pieces of boil'd Gammon, Mushrooms and fine Herbs · Let all be well season'd, and put into a Stew-pan, with two Handfuls of Bread-crum, and four or five Eggs, according to the nature of the Farce   The Lettice, when stuff'd with it in the middle, must be well tied or sow'd up, and boil'd in good Broth · In the mean while, a good White Sauce being duely prepar'd, with several Yolks of Eggs, so as it may not turn, take your Lettice and after having thoroughly drain'd and untied them, put them into this Sauce, to be kept hot. They are usually serv'd up for Out-works and sometimes among the Side-dishes.

The Soops of farced Fowls are also garnish'd with the same sort of Lettice; and the Lettice, on Fish-days, are commonly stuff'd with a good Fish-farce, or with Herbs and Eggs.

L E V E R E T S.

Leverets or young Hares larded.

Let one Shoulder with one Leg of your Leverets be larded, and the others left in their natural condition Then having roasted them, let them be serv'd up, with Sweet Sauce, or else with Vinegar and Pepper, and garnish'd with *Marinade*.

A Leveret dress'd after the Swiss Mode.

Having cut a Leveret into quarters, and larded them with thick Slips of Bacon, let them boil in some Broth, season'd with Pepper, Salt, Cloves and a little Wine. Then fry the Liver and the Blood with some Flower, and mingle all together; adding a little Vinegar, stoned Olives, Capers and Lemmon-slices for their Garniture

Leveret-potage, after the Italian manner.

Let the Leveret be cut into quarters; larded with thick Slips of Bacon, and fried in Lard : Then let them be stew'd in good Broth, such as is describ'd in the Article of Broth, with Dates, Currans, Lemmon-peel, Cinnamon, Salt and a little white Wine : Lastly, let the whole Mess be dress'd upon the soaked Crusts, and serv'd up to Table, with Lemmon-juice, garnish'd with Pomegranate-slices or Kernels.

For Leveret-pies, see the Letter P. among the other sorts of Pies.

L I Q U O R S, see *Broth.*

LIVERS.

An Intermess of Capons-livers dress'd in a Veal-caul.

Take the largeft and leaneft Capons-livers and having minc'd them, with fome parboil'd Bacon, a little Sewet and Marrow, *Truffles*, Mufhrooms, and Veal-fweet-breads; alfo a little Parfly, Chibbol and boil'd Gammon, let the whole Farce be bound with the Yolk of an Egg Then cut a Veal-caul into pieces, according to the thicknefs of your Livers, fo as they may be conveniently roll'd up in them; and let fome of the Farce be put upon the Caul, then a Liver upon that, and afterwards the Farce again thereupon, and take care that all be well wrapt up in the Caul. Thefe Livers fo drefs'd are to be laid upon a Sheet of Paper in order to be broil'd upon the Grid-iron, with a little Lard, or elfe in a Baking-pan and fet into an Oven When they are ready, let them be taken out, thoroughly drain'd from the Fat, and drefs'd in a Difh, with a little hot Broth pour'd upon them: Afterwards feafon them with Pepper and Salt, and having fqueez'd in the Juice of an Orange, ferve them up hot to Table.

An Intermeß of Capons-livers and Mufhrooms.

After having well cleans'd your Livers from the Gall, take a Baking-pan, lay fome *Bards* or thin Slices of Bacon on the Bottom of it, and the Livers upon them Let them be feafon'd and cover'd with other *Bards* on the top, and then fet into the Oven; taking care that they be not too much dry'd Let fome Mufhrooms well pickt and wafh'd be put into a Difh, with a little Bacon and Verjuice, having before caus'd their moifture to be dry'd up, by fetting them on the Fire, and let fome Slices of Gammon be fried a-part, with a little Lard and Flower, and a Bunch of fine Herbs: Afterwards pour in fome good Veal-gravy, that is not Salt, and ftew it with the Mufhrooms and Livers well drain'd, in the fame Sauce Laftly let it be incorporated with fome good thickening Liquor, if there be occafion, and when the Fat is taken away, add a little Vinegar, and let it be ferv'd up hot to Table The Difh may be garnifh'd with what you pleafe, provided it be fomething that is proper for Intermeffes

Capons-livers dreſs'd otherwiſe for Intermeſſes.

Having provided ſome good Capons-livers with a Baking-pan; for every Liver prepare a thin Slice of Bacon, and ſet them in order ſeparately in the Pan, laying the Livers upon them, when well ſeaſon'd · Let them alſo be cover'd with another Slice of Bacon, and dextrouſly breaded, to the end that they may be well bak'd and brought to a fine colour · When they are drawn out of the Oven, let them be ſufficiently drain'd, and neatly laid in a Diſh : Laſtly ſome good Gravy may be added with the Juice of an Orange, and ſo let it be immediately brought hot to Table

Capons-livers with Gammon.

Let ſome Gammon be cut very ſmall, and fry'd brown, with your Livers, alſo a young Chibbol and a little Parſly well chopt : When they are ſeaſon'd as much as requiſite, let them boil over a gentle Fire, with a piece of Lemmon, and ſerve them up with good Gravy for Out-works and Intermeſſes

Capons-livers dreſs'd between two Fires.

Having ſtrew'd your Livers with Pepper and fine Salt, cover them with a thin Slice of Bacon and a piece of Paper, which muſt be wet a little on the top, to keep them from burning . Then tye up the Livers and putting them between two Fires, let them be ſtew'd by degrees, and ſerv'd up to Table, with Gravy.

Another Intermeſs of Capons-livers.

When the Livers are well clear'd from the Gall, and ſcalded a little, put them into fair Water afterwards with the ſame Water into a Diſh, and let them be well ſeaſon'd. Then chopping a few Muſhrooms, *Truffles,* Parſly and Chibbol, let all boil together. As for the Livers, they are to be wrapt up in thin Slices of Bacon, as before, and ſet into an Oven, till they come to a fine colour ; but if it be not ſufficiently done, it may be brought to perfection, with the red-hot Fire-ſhovel. When it is ready to be ſerv'd up, drain the Fat well off, ſet the Livers in order in a Diſh, and pour a little Gravy upon them, with the Juice of one or two Oranges.　　　　　　　　　　　L O A V E S,

LOAVES, *fee* PAINS.

LOBSTERS.

It were needlefs to infift on the manner of making a Lobfter-hafh, as being common with that of other Hafhes of the like nature: In order to drefs them in a Sallet, it would be requifite only to obferve what has been laid down Pag 41. concerning the other Fifh-fallets ; adding to the Sauce of this fort, the infide of the Lobfter's Body. They are alfo prepar'd in a Ragoo, and in Potages, taking away the Shells, after they are boil'd ; neither is there any difficulty in this Matter, provided the Directions be follow'd, that are given elfewhere in feveral Places, for the ordering of other forts of Fifh.

M.

MACKAREL.

WHen the Mackarel are gutted, flit or cut them a little along the Back, and caufe them to take Salt, with Oil, Pepper, fine Salt and Fennel. They may be alfo wrapt up in the fame green Fennel, in order to be roafted , whilft a Sauce is preparing for them, with burnt Butter, fine Herbs chopt fmall, Nutmeg, Salt, Fennel, fcalded Goofeberries in their Seafon, Capers and a little Vinegar. Then they are to be ferv'd up to Table, and garnifh'd with Slices of Lemmon.

They may alfo be drefs'd in Potage, when they have been well fry'd before in refined Butter, and afterwards laid a foaking in a Stew-pan, with good Fifh-broth or Herbs: Let them be garnifh'd with a Ragoo of Mufhrooms, Capers, Gravy and Slices of Lemmon.

MARINADES.

Several Things are put into a *Marinade* or Pickle, either for the garnifhing of other Meffes, or to make a particular Difh. Fricaffies of Chickens are ufually garnifh'd with other marinated Chickens ; a *Marinade* of Veal ferves to garnifh farced Breafts of Veal, or roafted Loins of Veal, and fo of the reft ;

as

as Pigeons Partridges and others, with which feparate Services may be prepar'd for Side-difhes Let us here give fome Account of what is moft obfervable under this Article

A Marinade *of Chickens.*

Let your Chickens be cut into quarters, and marinated, with Lemmon-juice and Verjuice, or with Vinegar, Pepper, Salt, Cloves, Chibbols and a Bay-leaf or two　Leave them in this *Marinade* for the fpace of three Hours, and having made a fort of clear Pafte or Batter, with Flower, white Wine and the Yolks of Eggs, dip your Chickens into it : Then fry them in Lard, and let them be ferv'd up in form of a Pyramid, with fry'd Parfly and Slices of Lemmon, if you defign to make a particular Difh of them.

A Marinade *of Pigeons.*

Pigeons ought to be marinated in Lemmon-juice, and Verjuice, as before, with the other Ingredients; after having flit them on the Back, or cut them into quarters, to the end that the *Marinade* may penetrate into the Flefh.　Thus they are to be left three or four Hours in Pickle and afterwards dipt into Pafte, or flower'd when all over Wet ; in order to be gently fried They may be ferv'd up with fried Parfly ftrew'd upon them, and round about the Difh, adding a little Rofe-vinegar and white Pepper.

A Marinade *of Partridges.*

Let the Partridges be cut into two pieces and fteept in a *Marinade,* as the preceding Particulars . They muft alfo be fry'd after the fame manner, and ferv'd up to Table with Garlick-vinegar and white Pepper

A Marinade *of Veal.*

This fort of *Marinade* is likewife prepar'd in order to garnifh other Difhes, cutting the Veal into Slices, as it were for *Fricandoes* or Scotch Collops, and fo of the other Things that are to be marinated. For marinated Mutton-cutlets, fee the laft Article *of Cutlets* under the Letter C

A Marinade of Fish

Some forts of Fish are ufually put into a *Marinade* and Tortoifes among others As foon as they are drefs'd, let them be fteept in Vinegar, with Pepper, Salt and Chibbols Then let them be flower'd, fiy'd in refined Butter, and ferv'd up with fry'd Parfly, white Pepper and Orange-juice

Another fort of *Marinade* for Fish, may be made, after they have been fried, in this manner. Let fome Slices of Lemmon or Orange be put into the Frying-pan with Bay-leaves, refined Butter, Chibbols, Pepper, Salt, Nutmeg and Vinegar, and let this Sauce be pour'd upon the Fifh ; fuch as Soles, Congers, Pilchards, Tunnies cut into round Slices, &c Other forts of Fifh-*Marinades* may alfo be found in the Article of Potages, which are fet down in the General Table of the Meffes

M A U V I E T T E S.

Befides that for roafted *Mauviettes,* recourfe may be had to the Article *of Roaft-meats* ; under the Letter R ; a S'de-difh may be prepar'd of farced *Mauviettes* with Muftard, as appears from the Example Pag 28 and a Potage of *Mauviettes,* with brown Broth.

M E N U S - D R O I T S *or* M I N E - D R O I T.

Difhes, or Out-works of *Menus-droits* are made for Intermeffes, of different Things, and among others, of an Ox-palate, cut into thin Slices· Aftei having fry'd them in Lard with Parfly, fmall Chervil, Thyme, a whole Chibbol, Pepper, Salt, Broth and white Wine , they are to be laid a foaking in a Pot oi Difh, and the Sauce is to be thicken'd with Bread-chippings ; adding Mutton-gravy and Lemmon-juice, when ferv'd up to Table.

The *Menus-droits* of a Stag and others are drefs'd after the fame manner.

M E R I N G U E S.

Meringues properly belong only to the Confectioner's Art, but forafmuch as Cooks fometimes have occafion to ufe them, for the garnifhing of feveral Things , it may not be improper here to fhew the manner of making them.   To

To that purpose, take three or four new-laid Eggs, according to the quantity of *Meringues* requir'd to be made; reserve the Whites, and whip them till they form a rocky Snow. Then you are to put to them a little green Lemmon grated, with three or four spoonfuls of fine Sugar pass'd thro' the Sieve, and let all be whipt together; a little prepar'd Amber may also be added: Afterwards take some white Paper, and with a Spoon make your *Meringues* of a round or oval Figure, accordingly as you shall think fit, about the thickness of a Walnut; leaving some Distance between every one of them: In the mean while, let some powder'd Sugar be put into the end of a Napkin, and strew the *Meringues* with it. On the same Table, where they are dress'd, may be laid the cover of a Campain-oven, that has not been put into the Fire, but only has had some Fire upon it, and the *Meringues* may be cover'd with it, to give them a kind of Ash-colour; but no Fire must be put underneath: When they are bak'd and well ic'd, let them be taken off from the Paper. You may also put in a little Fruit, as a Rasberry, Strawberry or Cherry, according to the Season, and joyn other *Meringues* to them, to make Twins.

Pistachoe-Meringues.

Take a handful or two of Pistachoes, and let them be well scalded: After having whipt the Whites of Eggs, as for the preceding *Meringues*, and having beaten all together, with fine Sugar; put in the Pistachoes, the Water being well drain'd from them, and with a little Spoon, make the *Meringues* of what thickness you please; icing them in the same manner If you are not desirous to have them ic'd, their natural colour will be as white as Paper. These *Meringues* may serve to garnish all sorts of Pan-pies for Intermesses, and chiefly those of Marchpane.

MILK-POTAGE, *see* GRUEL.

MIROTONS.

A *Miroton* is usually serv'd up for a Side-dish, and may be made several ways; among others thus: Take a good Fillet of Veal, and cut it into several very thin Slices, which are to be beaten on the Dresser with a Cleaver: Another Fillet of Veal must

muſt alſo be provided, which is to be minc'd with parboil'd
Bacon, ſome Sewet, a little Marrow. Muſhrooms, *Truffles* and
fine Herbs, all well ſeaſon'd · To theſe add two or three Yolks
of Eggs, and, as ſoon as the Farce is made, take a round Stew-
pan, that is not too large : Lay ſome *Bards* or thin Slices of
Bacon in good order on the bottom, then the Veal-ſtakes that
were beaten, and at laſt the Farce, which muſt be cover'd on
the top, with the reſt of the Slices, and all 'muſt be well ſtopt
up. Afterwards let the Bacon-*Bards* be turn'd, and, having well
cover'd the whole Meſs, let it be bak'd or ſtew'd *à la Braiſe*,
that is to ſay, between two gentle Fires, one on the top and the
other underneath · When it is ready, let it be well clear'd from
the Fat, and laid upſide-down in a Diſh ; adding, if you pleaſe,
a little Cullis, before it is ſerv'd up hot to Table.

Mirotons *dreß'd after another manner.*

Some Cooks prepare a well thicken'd *Godivoe* of the ſame
nature as that for a *Poupeton*, and afterwards make a Border
of it, round about the Diſh, made of the Whites of Eggs, as
it were for Milk-potage : Then they waſh it over with beaten
Eggs ; and, having neatly breaded it, bring it to a colour in
the Oven : taking away all the Fat when it is dreſs'd. In the
mean while, an Earthen Pan muſt be fill'd with a Breaſt of Mutton, cut into pieces, the ſcraggy end of a Neck of Mutton,
young ſtreaked Bacon, Pigeons and Quails, as occaſion may
ſerve. All theſe being well bak'd or ſtew'd in the Pan, as it
were *à la Braiſe*, between two Fires, prepare ſome ſtrained
green Peaſe, or Aſparagus-tops, according to the Seaſon ; take
your Meats out of the Pan, let the Liquor be well drain'd
from them, and put them into a Diſh, with the Peaſe on the
top : To theſe may be added ſome Lettice, ſcalded and boil'd
in the ſame Sauce, and then let all be ſerv'd up hot to Table.
Inſtead of the Earthen Pan, when the Border is only left, all
ſorts of good Ragoo's are to be pour'd in the middle. A Mut-
ton-haſh may alſo be put to them, with Mutton-gravy and Lemmon-juice, when ready to be ſet on the Table.

To make another Miroton.

Take *Truffles*, Muſhrooms and boil'd Gammon, and let all
be well minc'd together : Then let them be put into a Stew-

pan,

pan, with two or three Anchovies, according to the bigneſs of your *Miroton*, let a handful of Capers be well chopt and thrown into the ſame *Miroton*   As ſoon as you perceive it to be almoſt ready, put your Haſh into a Stew-pan, with a little Parſly, Chibbol and Lard, all well dreſs'd ; ſoak it with ſome Gravy; pour in a little Cullis, and let it boil , taking care that it be not too thick.   Afterwards, having provided ſome tender and lean Beef, cut it into ſmall Slices, ſomewhat larger than if it were for a *Filet*, with Cucumbers, and put them into the Ragoo: Stir it very little, and let it not boil too much   Before it is ſerv'd up, let ſome Lemmon-juice be ſqueez'd in, and let the Diſh be artificially dreſs'd

To make a Miroton for Fiſh-days.

Take four or ſix Whitings, according to the bigneſs of your Diſh, and let them be ſcrap'd and well waſh'd , they muſt alſo be ſlit all along before, but care muſt be taken that their Backs be not ſpoil d.   Take away the Bones, cut off the Heads, and ſpread them upon a Table or Dreſſer.   Then, having made a good Fiſh-farce, according to the above-ſpecified Directions, put ſome of it upon every Whiting; and roll them up, as it were, *Filets-mignons*.   Afterwards, taking a Stew-pan, or a round Earthen Pan, without a Handle, make an *Omelet* or Pancake with a little Flower, which being entire, may cover the whole bottom of the Pan, and let your farced Fiſh be laid upon it, a little Butter being firſt put under the ſaid Pancake.   When the Fiſh is thus ſet in order with ſome *Truffles* and Muſhrooms well ſeaſon'd, another Pancake muſt be made, to be laid on the top, ſo as it may in like manner take up the whole compaſs of the Pan.   Let the Stew-pan be well cover'd, to the end that the Fiſh may be ſtew'd by degrees, between two gentle Fires, on the top and underneath ; and take care that nothing ſtick to the bottom   The whole Meſs being thus made ready, let the Butter be drain'd off, and the *Miroton* turn'd upſide-down into a Plate or Diſh: Then, cutting a ſmall round piece out of the middle, as if it were a *Poupeton*, pour in a ſmall Muſhroom-cullis, and cover it again with the ſame piece   Laſtly, when the Fat is thoroughly taken away, rub the ſide of the Diſh with a Shalot, and ſerve it up hot to Table.

A Farce may alſo be prepar d in the ſame manner as for the *Poupeton* hereafter deſcrib'd, and a Ring or Border may be
made

made with it round about the Dish, which is to be bak'd in an Oven and fill'd with a good Ragoo of *Mousserons*, *Morilles*, common Mushrooms, *Truffles* and Anchovies, all well chopt together, as also all sorts of Fish-*Filets* and Capers, making a Lay of Ragoo and another of *Filets*, till the whole Space be fill'd up. Then let it be set a soaking over a gentle Fire, and serv'd up, with the Ragoo-sauce and Lemmon-juice.

MORILLES.

Forasmuch as it will be requisite in the following Article of Mushrooms, to shew how they may be preserv'd, and in regard that the Directions there laid down, may also serve for *Morilles* and *Mousserons*, as differing from them only in *specie*; it may be sufficient here only to take notice of the particular Dishes that may be made of them for Out-works or Inter-messes.

Morilles *in a Ragoo.*

Morilles may be fry'd brown with Butter or Lard, after they have been cut long-ways and well wash'd. Then it will be requisite to put to them some Salt, Parsly and Chervil chopt very small, Chibbol, Nutmeg and a little Broth, and to lay them a soaking in a little Pot or Stew-pan: Let them be serv'd up to Table with short Sauce and Lemmon-juice.

They may be also put into Cream and otherwise dres'd, as well as common Mushrooms.

Fried Morilles.

Let your *Morilles* be cut long-ways, as before, and boil'd in a little good Broth, over a gentle Fire When the Broth is somewhat wasted, let them be flower'd and fry'd in Lard. In the mean time, having prepar'd a Sauce, with the rest of the Broth, season'd with Salt and Nutmeg, pour it under your *Morilles*, with Mutton-gravy and Lemmon-juice.

Farced *Morilles* are also used in Potage, and *Tourtes* or Pan-pies may be made of them, which shall be hereafter specify'd among those of common Mushrooms.

MOUS-

MOUSSERONS.

Mousserons *in a Ragoo.*

After having well cleans'd your *Mousserons,* let them be wash'd a little, and shak'd in a Linnen-cloath : Then stew them in a Dish or Stew-pan, with Butter or Lard, a Bunch of Herbs, Salt and Nutmeg, and thicken the Sauce with Yolks of Eggs and Flower or Bread-chippings : When it is ready to be serv'd up, squeez in some Lemmon-juice and garnish it with Slices of the same.

MULLETS.

Let your Mullets be broil'd upon a Grid-iron, after they are scal'd, cut and rubb'd with Butter ; whilst a Sauce is preparing for them with burnt Butter, fry'd Flower, Capers, Lemmon-slices, a Faggot of Herbs, Pepper, Salt, Nutmeg and Verjuice, or Orange-juice

They may be also fried in refined Butter, and then put into a Dish, with Anchovies, Capers, Orange-juice, Nutmeg, and a little of the same Butter in which they were dress'd ; having before rubb'd the Dish, with a Shalot, or a Clove of Garlick

Lastly, Mullets may be put into a *Tourte* or Pan-pie, and more especially into a standing Pie, as well as many other sorts of Fish.

MUSCLES

Muscles are generally put into a Ragoo, either with white or brown Sauce, and a very considerable Potage may be made of them : The Ragoo with white Sauce is prepar'd in this manner, *viz.*

Let the Muscles be taken out of their Shells, and fried in natural Butter, with Thyme and other fine Herbs chopt very small : Afterwards season them with Pepper, Salt and Nutmeg, and when their Liquor is consum'd, put in Yolks of Eggs with Verjuice or Lemmon-juice, garnishing the Dish, with the Shells and fry'd Bread.

The Ragoo with brown Sauce is made after the same manner, except that no Eggs are to be put into it, but only a little fry'd Flower.

Muscle-

Muſcle-potage.

Take good Muſcles ; let them be well cleans'd and waſh'd in four or five Waters : Then put them into a Pot with Water, which may ſerve for the Broth, if there be not other good Fiſh-broth at Hand : Add to your Muſcles, a little Parſly, ſweet Butter, and an Onion ſtuck with Cloves, and ſcald them till the Shells open, which ſignifies, that they are ſufficiently done; but let the Liquor or Broth be pour'd into another Pot a-part : Take the Muſcles out of their Shells and only leave a few to garniſh your Potage ; whilſt the Fleſh of the others is put into a little Pot or Stew-pan   Afterwards you muſt throw in ſome Muſhrooms cut into pieces, *Truffles* in Slices, and Carp-roes, with a whole Artichoke-bottom, if you have no mind to farce a Loaf with a Carp-haſh , that is to ſay, the Artichoke bottom muſt be reſerved entire to be laid in the middle of the Potage, and three or four other Artichoke-bottoms are to be cut into Quar-ters : Having toſs'd up this whole Ragoo in a Stew-pan, with good Butter and a little Flower, let it be ſoak'd in the Muſcle-broth, and boil'd a little while : Let a Faggot of fine Herbs be added, with a Slice or two of Lemmon; all being ſtew'd by degrees and well ſeaſon'd. Then lay your Potage and Cruſts of Bread a ſoak-ing with the ſame Muſcle-broth, which muſt not be too fat : Garniſh your Diſh with the Muſcles that were laid by in their Shells, and if you have a farced Loaf, leave ſome alſo to ſerve for Garniture round about it   When the Potage is thus thorough-ly ſoak'd, and the Ragoo pour'd thereupon, a white Cullis muſt be prepar'd with Almonds, Bread-crum, and ſix or eight Yolks of Eggs, all ſtrain'd thro' the Hair-ſieve, with a little of the ſame Muſcle-broth ; taking care that it do not turn, nor be too much ſeaſon'd with with Salt : Laſtly, having ſprinkled your Potage, with this white Cullis, let it be ſerv'd up hot to Table.

MUSHROOMS.

Muſhrooms are of great uſe in Ragoo's ; ſeparate Diſhes and Potages are alſo made of them for Intermeſſes ; ſo that it is ab-ſolutely neceſſary to be always provided with good Store of them for that purpoſe, and they well deſerve a particular De-ſcription in this Place.

Fried

Fried Mushrooms.

Having tofs'd up your Mushrooms in a Stew-pan, with a little Broth, to take away their bitterness, strew them with fine Salt, a little Pepper and Flower, and fry them in Lard   They may be serv'd up to Table, with Beef-stakes, Parsly and Lemmon-juice, for Intermesses, or else they may be used for the garnishing of some other Dish.

Mushrooms in a Ragoo.

Let the Mushrooms be cut into Slices, and fried in Lard or Butter, seasoning them, with Salt, Nutmeg and a Bunch of Herbs. The Sauce may be thicken'd with a little Flower, Yolks of Eggs and Lemmon-juice.

Mushrooms dress'd in Cream and otherwise.

Having cut your Mushrooms into pieces, and fry'd them in Butter over a quick Fire, let them be season'd with Salt, Nutmeg and a Faggot of Herbs. When they are ready, and very little Sauce is left, pour some natural Cream upon them, and let them be serv'd up to Table

They may also be put into a Baking-pan, with Lard or Butter, Parsly and Thyme chopt very small and whole Chibbols, after they have been season'd with Pepper, Salt and Nutmeg Thus they may be bak'd in the Oven as it were a Pan-pie, till they become very brown, let them also be well breaded; in order to be serv'd up with Slices and Juice of Lemmon, and garnish'd with Parsly.

Potage of farced Mushrooms.

Let a Farce be made with Veal, Beef-marrow and Lard, season'd with Pepper, Salt, Nutmeg and the Crum of a Loaf soak'd in Broth or in Yolks of Eggs. Stuff your Mushrooms with this Farce, and bake or stew them in an Earthen Pan, with Salt, a Bunch of Herbs and some Broth. When they are ready, let them be dress'd upon the soaked Crusts, and garnish'd with Chickens-livers in a Ragoo, fried Mushrooms and Lemmon-juice, as they are serving up to Table.

They

They may alfo be garnifh'd with Veal-fweet-breads, larded *Fricandoe's,* Cocks-combs and *Truffles,* and a *Profitrolle* loaf may be fet in the middle, farced with Mufhrooms, Artichoke-bottoms, and Veal-fweet-breads, all cut into pieces in form of a Die, and drefs'd in a Ragoo A white or brown Cullis may be prepar'd for both, but the latter is moft proper The Beef and Veal, of which you would have the Cullis or Gravy to be made, muft be pounded in a Mortar, with Crufts of Bread, and ftrain'd thro' the Hair-fieve, with fome Broth, and then it may be us'd for the Ragoo

Other Potages are made of Mufhrooms, with different forts of Fowls, as Capons, Quails, *&c.* And on Days of Abftinence, your Mufhrooms may be farced to that purpofe, with the Flefh of Fifh, as for other Difhes

To extract the Juice of Mufhrooms

After having well cleans'd the Mufhrooms, let them be put into a Difh with a piece of Lard, or Butter, if it be a Fifh day; and let them be brought to a brown colour over the Fire, till they ftick to the bottom of the Difh · Then throw in a little Flower, and let that alfo be made brown with the Mufhrooms : Afterwards let fome good Broth be added, and let them be taken off from the Fire, putting that Gravy into a Pot a-part, feafon'd with a piece of Lemmon and Salt. The Mufhrooms may ferve, either whole or chopt fmall, for Potages, Side-difhes, or Intermeffes.

To Preferve Mufhrooms.

Let your Mufhrooms, as foon as they are well pickt and wafh'd be tofs'd up a little in a Stew-pan, with good Butter, and feafon'd with all forts of Spice. Then put them into a Pot with a little Brine and Vinegar, as alfo, a great deal of Butter on the top and let them be well cover'd · Before they are us'd, they muft be thoroughly clear'd from the Salt, and then they will be ferviceable upon all manner of Occafions

A Powder may alfo be made of them, when they are very dry, and the fame thing may be done for the *Mousserons* or white Mufhrooms To preferve the latter entire, let them be dry'd in an Oven, as Artichokes, after they have been fcalded in Water: When they are dry, put them into a Place where there is no

M   Moi-

Moifture, and when you would make ufe of them, let them be fteept in Luke-warm Water

MUTTON.

Among the feveral Meffes that may be prepar'd with Mutton, we have already explain'd the different Manners of Dreffing Legs for Side-difhes, and we have alfo obferv'd what relates to Cutlets and *Filets* of Mutton under the Letters C and F. In like manner, in the Second Article of *Mirotons*, mention is made of an Earthen Pan fill'd with a Breaft of Mutton, the fcraggy end of a Neck of Mutton and fome other forts of Meat; fo that it remains only here, to take notice of fome other Joynts of Mutton that are proper for Side-difhes

A great Side-difh of Mutton.

Take a Crupper of very tender Mutton, let the firft Skin be dextroufly loofen'd on the top to the fmall end, and left hanging: Then having prepar'd fome thin Slices of Gammon, feafon'd with Parfly, Chibbol, and black Pepper, let them be laid upon the Joint of Mutton, with fome *Bards* or thin Slices of fat Bacon, and let the Skin be turn'd over them: Afterwards let it be tied up and roafted on a Spit, cover'd with Paper. When it is ready, let it be neatly breaded, and garnifh'd with Mutton-cutlets. Laftly, having pour'd an exquifite Ragoo thereupon, let it be ferv'd up hot to Table.

The fame thing may be done with a Quarter of Mutton or of Lamb.

Another Side-difh of a Quarter of Mutton.

Let it be farced on the Leg, with a *Salpicon*, or with a Hafh of the fame Meat that was taken out of it, according to the Method before obferv'd in ordering a fhort Rib of Beef in the Article of Beef, or for a *Salpicon* hereafter explain'd under the Letter S. Then let your Quarter of Mutton be breaded, and fet into an Oven to be brought to a good colour: Let it alfo be garnifh'd with fry'd Bread, marinated Cutlets and fried Parfly, and marbled with Lemmon-juice and its own Gravy.

Car-

Carbonado'd Mutton

Let a Joint of Mutton cut into Carbonadoe's be fry'd in a Pan with Lard, before it is ftew'd in Broth, with Pepper, Salt, Cloves a Bunch of Herbs, Chefnuts and Mufhrooms, whilft fome Flower is frying to thicken the Sauce: Then let the Difh be garnifh'd with Mufhrooms and fried Bread, and ferv'd up, with Capers and Lemmon-juice.

A Breaft of Mutton.

In order to drefs a Breaft of Mutton for an Out-work, let it be ftuff'd with Parfly and roafted · Then let it be feafon'd with Bread, white Pepper and Salt; adding the Juice of an Orange and good Gravy, when ready to be ferv'd up to Table

At another time, after the Breaft has been boil'd in a Pot, let it be dipt into a clear Pafte or Batter, and fry'd in Lard · Then adding fome Verjuice with the Grapes entire, and white Pepper, it may be ferv'd up to Table

For Mutton-cutlets, See the Article of *Cutlets* under the Letter C.

A Loin of Mutton à la Sainte Menehout.

To drefs a Loin of Mutton in this manner, fuch a Kettle or Pot muft be provided, as is convenient for that purpofe, covering the Bottom of it with good *Bards* or thin Slices of Bacon, Veal-ftakes, and Slices of Onion. Then let the Loin of Mutton be laid upon them, which likewife muft be cover'd with other Slices of Veal and Bacon; all well feafon'd with fine Herbs and Spice. Afterwards fet your Pot into an Oven, or between two Fires, and let all be well bak'd, but not over-done When they are drawn, or taken out, they muft be well breaded and broil'd upon a Grid-iron; whilft a Sauce call'd *Ramolade* is preparing, with Anchovies, Capers cut fmall, Parfly and Chibbols chopped a-part: Having ftew'd thefe in good Gravy with a little Oil, a Clove of Garlick and other feafoning Ingredients, pour them upon the Loin, in order to be drefs'd in a Difh, and ferv'd up hot to Table. This Sauce may ferve for feveral forts of cold Fowl, which are to be breaded and broil'd, and alfo for many other neceffary ufes.

M 2 'A

A Loin of Mutton dreß'd after other manners.

A Loin of Mutton may be larded with thick Slips of Bacon, and boil'd in a Pot a-part, with Water and a little white Wine, well season'd with Pepper, Salt, Bay-leaves, Cloves, a Bunch of Herbs, and a Slice of Lemmon In the mean while, let some Capers and Anchovies be fried in Lard and a little Sauce in which the Loin was dreß'd, and let it be pour'd upon it when ready to be serv'd up to Table, with Lemmon-juice, or a little Garlick-vinegar

At another time, when the Loin of Mutton is boil'd, take off the Skin, and steep the Flesh in a sort of Batter made with Flower, Yolks of Eggs, Pepper, Salt and Broth, in order to be well fried in a Pan. It may be serv'd up, with white Pepper, Verjuice with the Grapes, and fried Parsly.

Otherwise, after having taken off the Skin, let your Loin be basted with Lard; breaded three several times, to produce a fine Crust upon it in the Oven; and ic'd, by rubbing it with the White of an Egg.

N.

N e a t s - t o n g u e s.

Neats-tongues bak'd between two Fires.

HAving cut off the Roots of your Neats-tongues, broil them a little on the Coals, to the end that the Skin may more easily be peel'd off, and lard them with thick Slips of Bacon and raw Gammon , all well season'd Let some *Bards,* or thin Slices of Bacon be laid in order on the bottom of a Pot, with Beef-stakes beaten, and the Tongues upon them, with Slices of Onions, and all sorts of fine Herbs and Spices, seasoning them also with Pepper and Salt: Then having cover'd the Tongues, with other Beef-stakes and Bacon-*Bards,* in the same manner as they were put underneath, so as they may be well wrapt up on all sides , set the Pot between two Fires, that is to say, one on the top, and the other underneath. Let it continue therein for the space of eight or ten Hours, till the Meats are well bak'd, or stew'd, and in the mean time, prepare a good Cullis of Mushrooms, or some other choice Ragoo, with all sorts of Garnitures,

nitures, *viz.* Mushrooms, *Truffles,* Veal-sweet-breads, *&c.* When the Tongues are taken out, let them be drain'd, thoroughly clear'd from the Fat, and dress'd in a Dish; turning the Ragoo upon them. The Juice of a Lemmon may be squeez'd into the Cullis, and if you would have the Dish garnish'd, one of the Tongues must be cut into Slices, or else you may garnish it with *Fricandoes* or Scotch Collops The same thing may be done in dressing Calves-tongues; but if it be requir'd to farce them without larding, you may make use of the same Ragoo; taking care nevertheless, that both the Neats-tongues and Calves-tongues be always serv'd up hot to Table

Dried Neats-tongues.

Dried Neats-tongues are usually salted after the same manner as dried Hogs-tongues hereafter specify'd, except scalding. However they must be steept in Water, the thick End or Root being cut off, and salted after they have been well wip'd: They must be left three or four Days in the Brine or Pickle, and when they are taken out, if you have any petty Salt-meats to be prepar'd, this Pickle may serve for that purpose; whether it be a wild Boar, Hog or Fawn, so that within the space of five or six Days, some of these Salt-meats may be dress'd, and serv'd up for Out-works, or Side-dishes with good Peas soop As for the Neats-tongues, they must be tied at the small end or tip, and hang'd up in the Chimney to be smoak'd and well dried. They may be kept, as long as you please, and dress'd in the same manner as Hogs-tongues.

A Side-dish of Neats-tongues.

Let your Tongues be boil'd in fair Water with a little Salt, and a Faggot of fine Herbs Then cut the end next the Root, peel off the Skin, and Lard them with somewhat long Slips of Bacon Afterwards they must be roasted, but not too much, and as they are serving up, you may pour upon them a good Ragoo, according to the season, or a rich Cullis, or a *Rimolade*-sauce· The same thing is to be done with Calves-tongues, as well as for the following Dish

Another Side-dish of Neats-tongues.

After having order'd your Tongues, for the peeling off their Skins, as before, and having larded them a-cross with thick Slips

M 3   of of Bacon, let them be well bak'd *à la Braife*, or between two Fires · As they are drefling in the Difh, flit them all along, fo as the Bacon may appear, and make a Ragoo, or a Cullis to be pour'd upon them Let them be well clear'd from the Fat and ferv'd up hot to Table.

O.

O I L S.

THe *Oil* is a very confiderable Potage, which may be ferv'd up as well on Days of Abftinence, as on Flefh-days

An Oil *for Flefh-days.*

Take all forts of good Meats, *viz.* Part of a Buttock of Beef a Fillet of Veal, a piece of a Leg of Mutton, Ducks, Partridges, Pigeons, Chickens, Quails, a piece of raw Gammon, Saufages and a Cervelas, all roafted or fried brown : Let them be put into a Pot, every Thing according to the time that is requifite for boiling it, and let a thickening Liquor be made of the brown Sauce to be mingled together As foon as the fcum is taken off, feafon your Meats, with Pepper, Salt, Cloves, Nutmeg, Coriander-feed and Ginger, all well pounded, with Thyme and fweet Bafil, and wrapt up in a Linnen-cloth Afterwards add all forts of Roots and Herbs well fcalded, accordingly as you fhall think fit, such as Carrets Turneps, Parfnips, Cabbage, Parfly-roots, Onions, Leeks and other Herbs in Bunches. In the mean while, you are to provide *Cuvets*, Silver-pots and other Veffels proper for that purpofe, and when your Potage is fufficiently boil'd, let fome Crufts be broken into pieces, and laid a foaking in the fame Broth, after it has been clear'd from the Fat, and well feafon'd. Before it is ferv'd up, pour in a great deal more Broth, ftill continuing to take away the Fat ; drefs your Fowls and other Meats, and garnifh them with the Roots if you have only one great Difh : Otherwife they may be ferv'd up without Roots ; putting the *Cuvets* on a Silver-difh, with a Silver-ladle in it, with which every one of the Guefts may take out fome Soop, when the *Oil* is fet on the Table

See among the Potages, another fort of *Oil* with young Ringdoves and other Fowl.

An

An Oil *for Fish-days.*

Take some good Broth, Peas-soop, or half Fish-broth ; let all the above-mentioned Roots be put into it, and boil'd as much as is requisite · Then dress your Oil, with a *Profitrolle-* loaf in the middle, and garnish it with Roots.

An *Oil* or Potage of Roots and several sorts of Pulse with *Oil,* may likewise be prepar'd for Good-Friday, as it has been observ'd Pag. 47.

O I S T E R S.

To dress Oisters.

Let your Oisters be put into a Stew-pan, with a little Water and Verjuice, and let them have one Walm or Seething · Then take them out, and reserve the Liquor that is in the Shells, to be put into the Ragoo's, when ready to be serv'd up to Table.

Thus a Side-dish may be made of Chickens farced with Oisters, as it appears in the Second Article of Chickens, under the Letter C. We have also elsewhere explain'd the manner of dressing a Duck with Oisters under the Letter D and that of preparing a Pike with other sorts of Fish with Oisters shall be shewn in its due Place under P.

Oisters in a Daube.

Open your Oisters, and season them with fine Herbs, *viz.* Parsly, Chibbol, Thyme and sweet Basil, putting a very little of each into every Oister ; as also, some Pepper and a little white Wine : Then cover them again with their Shells, lay them upon a Grid-iron, and pass the red-hot Fire-shovel over them from time to time · When they are ready, they may be dress d, and serv'd up uncover'd.

Farced Oisters.

Having open'd your Oisters, let them be scalded and afterwards minc'd small, with Parsly, Chibbols, Thyme, Pepper, Salt, Anchovies and good Butter. Let the Crum of a Loaf be soak'd in the Sauce, with Nutmeg and other Spice, and two or

M 4

three

three Yolks of Eggs, and let all be pounded together Then let the Oifter-fhells be farced, and having breaded,or wafh'd them over, let them be put into an Oven upon a Grid-iron. They may be brought to Table, either dry or with Lemmon-juice.

Oifters marinated and fried.

After the Oifters have been marinated in Lemmon-juice,they may be put into Fritters, and fried till they come to a fine Co.lour.

OLIVES.

Side-difhes may be made of large fat Pullets, Wood-cocks, Partridges, and other forts of wild Fowl with Olives, all which are drefs'd after the fame manner: So that explaining one, a fufficient light will be given as to what relates to the others.

A Side-difh of fat Pullets, with Olives

Take large fat Pullets that are very tender; let them be well trufs'd and roafted with a good Slice of Bacon upon their Breaft. In the mean while, prepare a Ragoo, with Chibbols and Parfly chopt,and fried with a little Lard and Flower Then put into it two Spoonfuls of Gravy, a Glafs of *Champagne*-Wine, minc'd Capers, an Anchovie, bruifed Olives, a little Oil of Olives and a Bunch of fine Herbs : To thicken the Sauce, add a good Cullis, and let all be well feafon'd, and thoroughly clear'd from the Fat: Then take the roafted Pullets, cut off their Legs at the Joints, and tie up their Wings, Legs and Breaft. Let them alfo be bruifed a little, and afterwards put into the Sauce A little before they are ferv'd up hot to Table, they muft be drefs'd in a Difh, pouring in the Ragoo, and fqueezing upon them the Juice of an Orange.

OMELETS.

An Omelet with Sugar.

Having wh'pt as many Eggs as you fhall think fit, put to them a little Milk-cream and Salt, with fome Lemmon-peel cut very fmall: Let all be well beaten together, and make
your

your *Omelet.* Before it is put into the Dish it muſt be ſugar'd in the Frying-pan, and turn'd as it is frying on the ſide that is colour'd, the Plate upon which it is to be laid muſt likewiſe be turn'd downwards: Then ſtrew it with Sugar and ſome candy'd Lemmon-peel minc'd, and Ice it all at once with the red-hot Fire-ſhovel, in order to be ſerv'd up hot to Table.

Omelets *of green Beans and other Things, with Cream.*

Let your Beans be ſhell'd, ſlipt out of their Skins, and fried in good Butter, with a little Parſly and Chibbol: Then, having pour'd in a little Milk-cream, let them be well ſeaſon'd, and ſoak'd over a gentle Fire. Let an *Omelet* be made with new-laid Eggs and Cream, and let ſome Salt be put into it according to diſcretion. When it is ready, dreſs it on a Diſh, bind the Beans with one or two Yolks of Eggs, turn them upon the *Omelet*; ſo as they may ſtick to the ſide of it, and bring it hot to Table.

Omelets of the like nature may be made with *Mouſſerons, Morilles*, common Muſhrooms, green Peaſe, Aſparagus-tops and Artichoke-bottoms, white and black *Truffles*, Spinage, Sorrel, &c all with Cream; but tis requiſite that they be cut into ſmall pieces.

A very great quantity of *Omelets* may be thus diſguiſed, and theſe little Cream-ſauces may ſerve to fill up your Plates or Diſhes, garniſhing them with ſmall Garnitures; ſuch as fried Artichokes, Bread-toſtes, Puffs, *Fleurons, Feuillantins*, Artichoke-bottoms fried in Paſte, and others of the like nature that ſhall be judg'd requiſite, and taking care that all be ſerv'd up hot to Table.

To make a Gammon-Omelet.

Having prepar'd a Haſh of good boil'd Gammon, with a little raw Gammon, let your *Omelet* be made and dreſs'd in a Diſh, ordering it with this Gammon-haſh according to the preceding Method. The ſame thing may be done with boil'd Neats-tongues.

Another

Another farced Omelet.

Take the Breaſt of a roaſted Chicken or other Fowl, cut it into little pieces in the form of a Die, as alſo ſome boil'd Gammon and Muſhrooms likewiſe in little ſquare pieces, with Capons-livers, *Truffles*, and other ſorts of Garniture, all well dreſs'd in a Ragoo. In the mean time, let the *Omelet* be made, but before it is dreſs'd in the Diſh, let ſome Crum or Cruſt of Bread be put therein, and let your Ragoo be turn d into the ſame Frying-pan. When it is ready, let it be moiſten'd with a little Gravy and ſerv'd up hot to Table. Thus *Omelets* may be farc'd with all ſorts of Ragoo's, ſo that it were needleſs to inſiſt on them any longer, particularly, with Calves-kidneys boil'd, Veal-ſweet-breads, Livers of Rabbets, or Leverets, thoſe of Capons, *&c* as well as on Fiſh-days, with a Fiſh-farce, Carp-roes and a good Herb-farce

P.

PAINS.

THere are ſeveral Side-diſhes call'd *Pains, i e.* Loaves, as being made of Bread ſtuff'd with different ſorts of Farces; ſuch are the *Pains* of Gammon, Partridge, Veal, and the Spaniſh *Pain* Let us give ſome Account of theſe in their order.

*To make a Gammon-*Pain,

Let ſome Slices of Gammon be dreſs'd in the ſame manner as for Gammon eſſence, already deſcribed in the firſt Article of *Gammon,*under the Letter G ; except that you muſt not put any Muſhrooms to them, nor ſtrain them thro' a Sieve. If your Slices, when dreſs'd, are not ſufficiently thicken'd, a little Bread-culliſ may be added to bring them to a due Conſiſtence : Then, having provided a Potage-loaf, cut it thro' the middle, ſo as both the upper and under Cruſts may remain entire ; take away the Crum from the inſide, and let the reſt of the Loaf be toaſted and brought to a colour at the Fire, or in an Oven, till it become brown. When it is ready, joyn the two Cruſts together, in a little Diſh, after having ſoak'd them a little in the Sauce ; and put your Ragoo into it with the Sauce. It may be
gar-

garnifh'd with Capons-livers drefs'd in a Veal-caul, and ferv'd up among the Intermeffes.

A Side-difh of Partridge-Pains.

Take roafted Partridges, with the Flefh of a Capon or Pullet, parboil'd Bacon, tried Sewet, *Morilles* and common Mufhrooms chopped, alfo *Truffles*, Artichoke-bottoms, fine Herbs, and a Clove of Garliek, all well feafon'd and cut fmall, and, to bind them, add the Crum of a Loaf foak'd in good Gravy and fome Yolks of Eggs: Then let your *Pains* be made upon Paper, of a round Figure, and of the thicknefs of an Egg, at a convenient diftance one from another. The Point of your Knife muft be dipt in a beaten Egg, in order to fhape them, and bread them neatly. They may alfo ferve to garnifh other Side-difhes of a larger fize, and of more confiderable Meats.

To make a Veal-Pain.

Having cut a Fillet of Veal into thin Slices, beat them with the Back of a Knife, and take as great a quantity of them, as will be requifite, proportionably to the bignefs of your Difh Then let another Fillet of Veal be well minc'd, with parboil'd Bacon, drefs'd Gammon, tried Sewet, all forts of fine Herbs, the Breaft of a Capon and Partridge, a few *Truffles, Moufferons,* and common Mufhrooms chopped, all well feafon'd with all forts of fine Spice, and mixt with a little Milk-cream. Afterwards let fome *Bards* or thin Slices of Bacon be laid in order in a round Stew-pan, as alfo one half of the beaten Veal-ftakes, and then the Farce; continuing to cover it on the top, in the fame manner as underneath; fo as the whole Farce may be enclos'd on all fides: Laftly, let it be well cover'd and bak'd *à la Braife*, between two Fires A little piece of Garlick may be put into the Farce, which muft be brought hot to Table, after it has been well clear'd from the Fat, and neatly drefs'd in a Difh

This Veal-*Pain* may alfo be ferv'd up with green Peafe and Afparagus, when they are in feafon.

To make a Spanish Pain.

Take the Breasts of roasted Partridges, mince them small, with a Handful of scalded Pistachoes and a little beaten Coriander-seed, and let all be well pounded in a Mortar; adding three or four Yolks of Eggs, according to the bigness of your Dish, a little Lemmon-peel and some good Veal-gravy. Let the whole Mixture be well temper'd in a Mortar, and strain'd thro' the Sieve, as if it were Cream made after the Italian Mode: Then let the Dish be set into the Oven, and let all be turn'd into it, keeping a Fire on the top and underneath, till it be thoroughly coagulated. But it must be set on the Table by a neat-handed Servitor, left it should be broken, as it is serving up.

Another Side-dish of a farced Pain.

Another Side-dish may be made of a *Pain* or Loaf farced with Veal-sweet-breads, Artichoke-bottoms, *Truffles* and Gammon dress'd in a Ragoo, with a white thickening Liquor of roasted Veal and Lemmon-juice: Let your Loaf be well soak'd for a quarter of an Hour in good Broth, and serv'd up with Mutton-gravy, a little thickening Liquor and Lemmon-juice.

You may hereafter observe among the Potages, the manner of preparing *Profitrolle*-loaves, and several sorts of farced Crusts, as well for Flesh-days, as those of Abstinence, of which also may be made as many Side-dishes, for the meaner sort of Ordinaries.

PAN-PIES, *see* TOURTES.

PARTRIDGES.

Having a little before explain'd the manner of making Partridge-*Pains*, as also Partridge-Hashes in the first Article of *Hashes*, under the Letter H; we shall here produce some other Side-dishes of the same sort of Fowl

Partridges, with Spanish Sauce.

After having roasted some Partridges, let one of them be well pounded in a Mortar, and soak'd in good Gravy : The Li-

vers of the Partridges muſt likewiſe be pounded with ſome pieces of *Truffles,* and let all be well moiſten'd with Gravy, ſo as
the Cullis may become ſomewhat thick; ſetting it aſide for a
while in a Diſh. Then pour two Glaſſes of *Burgundy*-wine into
a Stew-pan, with a Clove or two of Garlick, two or three Slices
of Onion, a few Cloves, and two Glaſſes of the Sauce; ſo that
only one may be left; but if the Diſh be large, the Quantity of
the Wine and Cullis may be augmented. When your Sauce is
ready, ſtrain it thro' a Sieve into a Stew-pan, pour the Cullis
upon it, and let all be well ſeaſon'd · To theſe add a little Gammon-eſſence, and let all boil together for ſome time Laſtly,
cut your Partridges into pieces, put them into the Sauce, and
let them be kept hot; ſqueezing in the Juice of two or three
Oranges, before it is ſerv'd up to Table.

*A Partridge-*Biberot.

Take the Breaſts of roaſted Partridges, and if they are not
ſufficient, ſome of fat Pullets likewiſe roaſted, and let them be
minc'd upon a Dreſſer that is well flower'd · Let the Carcaſſes
be pounded in a Mortar, and ſtew'd in a Pan with good Gravy: Then, having ſtrain'd them thro' a Sieve, put them into a
little Pot, with your *Biberot* or minc'd Meat Let it boil over
a gentle Fire, taking care that it do not ſtick to the bottom,
and adding a Spoonful of Gammon-eſſence; but it muſt be ſo
order'd, as not to be too thin or too fat When it is ready, it
may be diſpoſed of in a Plate or two, and ſerv'd up hot to
Table. Some are content to make uſe of it in this manner; and
others, after having dreſs'd the whole Meſs in a Plate or Diſh,
ſtrew it with Bread-chippings grated very fine, and give it a colour with the red-hot Fire-ſhovel. When ſo order'd it may be
eaten with a Fork, and otherwiſe with a Spoon.

*Partridge-*Filets, *with Gammon.*

When your Partridges are roaſted, let them be cut into *Filets,* and ſtew'd with Gammon, an Anchovie, Capers, Chibbol and Parſly chopt very ſmall. Thus they are to be ſerv'd
up among the Out-works, and may alſo be dreſs'd with Wood-
cock or Pike-ſauce.

Ano-

Another Way of dreſſing Partridges.

Partridges may likewiſe be bak'd between two Fires, or roaſted in *Sur-tout*, according to the Method hereafter laid down for
Pigeons ; or elſe dreſs'd with Olives, as it has been already obſerv'd under the Article of *Olives*.

For Partridge-pies, ſee the firſt Article of Pies, as alſo Partridge-potages under that of Potages, or rather, look for them
in the General Table of the Meſſes.

P A S T E S.

It would be needleſs here to inſiſt on the different ſorts of
Paſtes, which are uſually made ; that is to ſay, ſome thin as it
were Batter, and others of a more firm Conſiſtence ; the latter
to be us'd for Pies and Pan-pies, and the other for Fritters, or
to cover ſeveral Things in order to be fried. It may well be
preſum'd, that the Reader is ſufficiently inſtructed in this Matter, and ſome particular kinds of Paſtes have been already produc'd, as thoſe of Almonds and Fruit, under thoſe Articles ; ſo
that we ſhall only add one or two that are no leſs curious and
remarkable.

Paſte for crackling Cruſt.

Take Sugar beaten to Powder, with as much fine Flower,
Whites of Eggs, according to the quantity of your Paſte, and
a little Orange-flower-water.   Then having caus'd the Paſte to
be well made upon the Dreſſer-board, ſo as it be not too ſoft,
roll out a piece for the Bottom-cruſt, as thin as Paper, if it be
poſſible, and flower it continually underneath, working it in
with your Hands : And indeed, it will be ready almoſt to ſpread
of it ſelf, after it has been beaten a little with the Rolling-pin.
Then rub a Plate or Baking-pan with a little Butter, put your
piece of Paſte into it, and pare it round about ; afterwards it
muſt be prickt with the Point of a Knife, that it may not puff
in the Oven. When it is ſufficiently bak'd, let it be dreſs'd on
a Diſh or Plate, laying thereon, before it is ſerv'd up, ſome
Marmalade, with Apricocks, Peaches, Plums, and other ſorts
of preſerv'd Fruit.

With

With this Pafte, you may roll out feveral very thin pieces, which may be neatly cut and dried in an Oven, always remembring to butter the Plate or Pie-pan, left they fhould ftick to it. Afterwards they may be ic'd, if you fhall think fit, and laid upon the *Tourtes* or Pan-pies, which are to be fet out with *Savoy*-Biskets, or other fmall Garnitures

Syringed Pafte.

Take Almond-pafte, prepared according to the Method defcrib'd in the firft Article of Almords, pound it in a Mortar, with a little natural Cream boil'd, and having pafs'd it thro' the Syringe, let it be fried in a Pan, adding fome muskèd Sugar and fweet Water, when ready to be ferv'd up to Table. This Pafte may be prepar'd after many other manners, at pleafure, as has been before obferv'd in the fame place.

PASTIES.

Pafties made of Stags-flefh or other forts of Venifon.

Having caus'd your Venifon to be mortified, or marinated, let it be larded with thick Slips of Bacon, and feafon'd with Pepper, Salt, Nutmeg and Cloves, all well beaten together. Then let a brown Pafte be made with Rie-flower, as being more proper to preferve Meats, and more portable, adding fome Salt and a little Butter. After having drefs'd the Pafty with pounded Lard, *Bards* or thin Slices of Bacon, Bay-leaves, and the above-mention'd feafoning Ingredients, let it be wafh'd over with the Whites of Eggs, and bak'd for the fpace of three or four Hours. A Hole muft be made in the middle, left it fhould burft, or the Liquor fhould run out; but it may be ftopt up when taken out of the Oven, and the Pafty fet upon a Hurdle or Pie-plate. It may be ferv'd up to Table either entire, or cut into flices.

A Pafty may be made after the fame manner, with the Flefh of a wild Boar, or Roe-buck, but it is not neceffary to bake it fo long, or to feafon it fo high

PERCHES.

A Side-difh may be made of Perches in a Sauce of *Mouffetons*, fried in natural Butter with Cream. They may also be
ferv'd

ferv'd up in *Filets*, with Cucumbers, as well as Soles, hereafter mentioned; cutting them into pieces, after they have been fcal'd, and boil'd in Broth Laftly, Perches may be drefs'd with green Sauce, or otherwife thus :

Perches in Filets, *with white Sauce.*

Let Mufhrooms be tofs'd up in a Pan, with natural Butter, and afterwards boil'd in a little Cream, without any thing to thicken them   Then let your Perch-*Filets*, ready cut, be put to them, and thicken'd with three Yolks of Eggs, chopt Parfly, grated Nutmeg, and the Juice of a Lemmon : Let all be ftirr'd together very gently, for fear of breaking the *Filets*, and drefs'd with Slices of Lemmon, or fome other fort of Garniture.

PETITS OEUFS, *fee* EGGS.

PETITS PATES, *fee* PIES.

PHEASANTS.

Two particular Side-difhes may be made with Pheafants, *viz* one a hot Pie and the other with Carp-fauce.

A Side-difh of Pheafants, with Carp-fauce.

Let your Pheafants be well trufs'd, barded with a good Slice of Bacon, and roafted, taking care that they be not dry'd   To prepare the Sauce, let fome tender Veal-ftakes be laid in order on the bottom of a Stew-pan, as if it were to make Gravy, with feveral Slices of Gammon and Onions, Parfly-roots and a Faggot of fine Herbs   In the mean while, having gutted a Carp, wafh it only in one Water, without fcaling it, cut it into pieces, in the fame manner as for ftewing, and put it into the fame Pan . Then fet it over the Furnace to give it a fine Colour, as is ufually done in making Gravy, and foak it with good Veal-gravy and a Quart of *Champagne*-wine, adding a Clove of Garlick, fome chopt Mufhrooms, *Truffles*, and fmall Crufts of Bread   Let the whole Mefs be boil'd, taking care that it be not too much falted, ftrain it well thro' the Hair-fieve, and order the Sauce fo as it may be fomewhat thick Otherwife, fome Partridge-cullis may be added, and put with it into a Stew-pan

After-

Afterwards having tied up the Pheasants let them be laid in this Sauce, and kept hot, till it be requisite to serve them up to Table · Then dress them in a Dish , and pour the Sauce upon them. They may be garnish'd with Partridge-*Pains*, which have been already describ'd in the second Article of *Pains*.

A Side-dish of a hot Pheasant-pie.

Take the Flesh of a Pheasant, with that of a large fat Pullet and a tender piece of a Leg of Veal, and let all be well minc'd together, with Parsly, Chibbol, *Mousserons*, common Mushrooms, Veal-sweet-breads, boil'd Gammon and raw Bacon   Then having season'd them with fine Herbs, Spice, Pepper and Salt, make a good *Godivoe* of them, as also, a somewhat strong Paste, and let your Pie be rais'd either with double, or single Crusts, accordingly as you shall think fit   As soon as it is bak'd, take away the Fat, pour in a Mushroom-cullis, and serve it up hot to Table.

PICKLES, *see* MARINADES.

PIES.

Pies are brought to Table, either hot or cold , that is to say, the former for Side-dishes, and the other for Intermesses.

A hot Pie of Partridges, Wood-cocks, &c.

Take two Partridges and as many Wood-cocks, and let them be well drawn, reserving the Livers   Let them also be neatly truss'd, and beaten on the Breast, with a Rolling-pin . Then having larded them with thick Slips of Bacon and Gammon, season them with Pepper and Salt, and slit them thro' the Back   In the mean time, let a Farce be made of a tender piece of Veal, as thick as an Egg, with raw Bacon, a little Marrow, Parsly and fine Herbs, a few *Truffles* and Mushrooms chopped, and a little Veal-sewet: When the whole Farce is thus duely prepar'd, let it be bound with the Yolk of an Egg, and let the four Fowls be stufft with it on the Back. It will also be requisite to mince and pound some Bacon, with the two Partridge-livers, and to season all with beaten Spice. Afterwards having made some Paste, with an Egg, fresh Butter, Flower and a little Salt, roll out

N   two

two pieces of it; lay one of them on butter'd Paper, and let some Lard pounded in a Mortar be neatly spread upon it. Let your Partridges and Wood-cocks be seafon'd, and set in order round about, after all their Bones have been broken; adding some *Truffles* and Mushrooms, with a Bay-leaf, and covering all with *Bards*, or thin Slices of Bacon: After having laid on your other piece of Paste for the Lid, close up the Sides round about, wash over the whole Pie, and set it into the Oven; taking care of the Fire. When it is bak'd, let the Paper be taken away from underneath, preparing at the same time a good Cullis of Partridges, Veal-sweet-breads, Mushrooms and *Truffles* Then cutting off the Lid of the Pie, remove all the Bacon-*Bards*, clear it well from the Fat, and squeez in the Juice of a Lemmon. Let the whole Cullis be likewise pour'd into the Pie very hot, and having cover'd it again with the Lid, let it be immediately serv'd up to Table for a Side-dish.

Hot Pies of Chickens, Pigeons, Larks, Quails, Thrushes and others of the like nature, are usually made after the same manner, and we have already shewn in the preceding Article, how to prepare a hot Pheasant-pie, which is a kind of *Godivoe.*

A Pie of large Pigeons, or young Turkeys.

Having provided large Pigeons, let them be drawn, truss'd and beaten on the Breast, to Break the Bones: Then let them be larded with thick Slips of Bacon, and well seafon'd. Take the Livers, with raw Bacon, Parsly, Chibbol, fine Herbs, all well chopt and seafon'd; as also, some *Truffles,* Mushrooms and Marrow, and pound all together in the Mortar: Stuff the Bodies of your Pigeons, or young Turkeys with this Farce, and reserve a little of it to be put underneath. In the mean while, the Pie being made of good Paste, some of the Farce must be put on the Bottom, and afterwards the Pigeons in due order, and well seafon'd; adding also a Bay-leaf Then all must be cover'd with thin Slices of Bacon, and with a Lid on the top When the Pie is bak'd, let it be clear'd from the Fat, and at the same time, let a good Ragoo be pour'd into it, ready prepar'd with Veal-sweet-breads, Mushrooms, Cocks-combs, &c. accordingly as occasion may serve, or the Season will admit. But let it be set on the Table hot among the Side-dishes.

A

A Chicken-pie, with Cream.

- As foon as the Pie is made, let your Chickens be put into it in Quarters, feafon'd with Pepper, Salt, Nutmeg, Cinnamon, melted or pounded Lard and fine Herbs; and let it be cover'd with a Lid of the fame Pafte When it is bak'd, pour in fome Cream, and let it ftand a little while longer in the Oven Laftly, add fome Mufhroom-juice, and ferve it up hot to Table.

A Pie of a boned Capon.

The Capon is to be ftuff'd with a Farce made of its own Flefh, part of a Fillet of Veal, Beef-marrow, or Sewet and Bacon; feafon'd with Pepper, Salt, Nutmeg, Cloves, Veal-fweet-breads, *Truffles*, Mufhrooms and fine Herbs : Then it muft be cover'd with *Bards*, or thin Slices of Bacon, and put into a Pie made of fine Pafte, which is to be wafh'd over, and bak'd about two Hours Some Lemmon-juice muft alfo be fqueez'd upon it, when ready to be brought to Table

A Duck-pie.

After having beaten the Breafts of the Ducks, let them be larded with middle-fiz'd Slips of Bacon, and drefs'd as the above-mentioned forts of Fowl; covering them with Mufh-rooms, Capons-livers, *Truffles*, and the neceffary feafoning Ingredients When the Pie has been bak'd during two Hours, let fome Juice of Shalots or of Garlick, with that of Orange be put therein, as it is ferving up to Table.

A Pie after the German Mode.

Take Lamb cut into Quarters, which is to be larded with middle-fiz'd Slips of Bacon, and put into a Pie made of indifferent fine Pafte ; feafon'd with Pepper, Salt, Nutmeg, Cloves, a Bay-leaf or two, pounded Lard, fine Herbs and Chibbol: Let it be cover'd with a Lid of the fame Pafte, and bak'd three Hours. Laftly, let fome Oifters be fried in Lard, with Flower, Capers, ftoned Olives, Mufhrooms, Mutton gravy and Lemmon-juice, and let all be turn'd into the Pie with the Oifter-liquor

A

A Godivoe-*Pie.*

Let a good *Godivoe* be prepar'd, with a Fillet of Veal, some Marrow or Beef-sewet, and a little Lard; season'd with Pepper, Salt, Cloves, Nutmeg, fine Herbs and Chibbols, and let your Pie be made of fine Paste, of the height of three or four Inches, and of a round or oval Figure, accordingly as you shall think fit, garnishing it with *Morilles,* common Mushrooms, Veal-sweet-breads, Artichoke-bottoms and *Andouillets,* round about the opening in the middle, and pouring in a white Sauce, when ready to be brought to Table

The Plate-pies, of a round Figure, are made in the same manner, when they are entirely cover'd, and a little Coronet is usually set on the middle. They are to be wash'd over, and scarce require an Hour for Baking.

A Pie made of a Fillet of Veal.

The Fillet is to be cut into pieces larded with thick Slips of Bacon · Afterwards, being dress'd in a good *Godivoe,* it must be fill'd with Asparagus-tops, Mushrooms, Veal-sweet-breads and Artichoke-bottoms · When it is ready to be serv'd up, it would be requisite to pour into it a little thickening Liquor, with some Lemmon-juice, and to garnish it with its own Crust, as well as the other sorts of Pies.

A Blood-pie for a Side-dish.

On those Days that young Turkeys, fat Pullets and other sorts of Fowl are kill'd, some of their·Blood may be preserv'd, to the quantity only of a large Glass full. It must be put into an Earthen Pan, with some *Filets* of a Hare and of Veal: Let these *Filets* be larded with Gammon and thick Slips of Bacon, and steept in the Blood; seasoning them a little. To make the *Godivoe,* you are to provide some Flesh of Chickens and Partridges, a good piece of a Leg of Veal, some Bacon, Marrow and a little Sewet; with Parsly, Chibbol, a Clove of Garlick and *Truffles,* all well season'd, enrich'd and chopt small: Let the Blood be put into this Farce and temper'd with it. In the mean time, let two sorts of Paste be prepar'd, *viz.* one ordinary, of a greater quantity, and the other less, consisting of Eggs,

But-

Butter, Flower and Salt, all well workt, without any Water. Thus two large pieces are to be roll'd out of the common Paſte, and two leſſer ones of the finer ſort · Let the great piece for the Bottom-cruſt be put upon Paper, and the leſſer on the top of it: Take one half of your *Godivoe*, and ſpread it neatly upon thoſe two pieces of Paſte ; then ſet your *Pulets* in order, and the reſt of the Farce upon them; covering all with *Bards* or thin Slices of Bacon, and afterwards with a ſmall piece of the fine Paſte ; wetting the greater round about . At laſt, the other large piece being put on the top, to compleat the Lid or upper Cruſt ; the whole Pie is to be waſh'd over with an Egg, and bak'd in the Evening, for the ſpace of eight or ten Hours : For it muſt be left all Night till the ſame Hour next Morning, taking care that the Oven be not over-heated It muſt be ſerv'd up hot to Table, after having pour'd a Partridge-cullis into it, and both the Meat and Cruſt ought to be eaten with a Fork.

A Chibbol-pie.

For the Farce, or *Godivoe*, 'tis requiſite to provide a piece of Beef, or of very tender Veal, with Beef-ſewet, raw and tried, Parſly and a great deal of young Chibbol: Let it be chopt together, ſufficiently enrich'd, and well ſeaſon'd with all ſorts of beaten Spice; adding a little Beef-marrow, Bread-crum ſteept in Gravy, ſome pieces of *Truffles* and Muſhrooms cut ſmall: Then let two pieces of good Paſte be roll'd out, *viz.* one for the Lid very thin, and the other for the Bottom-cruſt ſomewhat thicker; let the Pie be rais'd upon Paper, three or four Inches high; and let the Farce be put into it, all well ſeaſon'd and diſpos'd of in good order . Laſtly, let it be cover'd with Bacon-Bards and Slices of Lemmon, and when the Lid is laid on over all, let it be ſet into the Oven As ſoon as it is drawn, a good white Cullis, or one of Partridges, may be pour'd into it, in order to be ſet hot on the Table.

A Pie after the Engliſh Way.

Take the Fleſh of a Hare, and of a tender Leg of Veal, according to the ſize of your Pie: Let all be chopt upon the Dreſſer, with good raw Bacon, Marrow, a little Veal-ſewet, candy'd Lemmon-peel, Sugar, beaten Cinnamon, and Coriander-ſeed; all well order'd and ſeaſon'd with all ſorts of ſweet Spices,

N 3   and

and bound with four or five Yolks of Eggs In the mean while, a Paste being duly prepar'd, raise it of a convenient height, put your Farce into it, with some Slices of Lemmon and Bacon-*Birds*, and cover it with a Lid When the Pie is bak'd, let a Sauce be made for it, of two good Glasses of Vinegar, with a little Sugar, some Cloves and a Stick of Cinnamon ∙ Let all boil together, till the Sauce be almost ready, and if the Pie be large, a proportionable quantity will be requisite : Afterwards, the Pie being open'd, clean it thoroughly from the Fat, and pour in the Sauce. It may, if you please,-be adorned with fine cut Pastry-works, and ought to be serv'd up hot for a Side-dish.

A Fish-pie.

For a Fish-pie to be serv'd up on Days of Abstinence, let a *Godivoe* be made in the same manner as the Fish-farce describ'd in the Article of *Farce* ; except the Yolks of Eggs and the *Omelet*, which may be omitted : For the rest, the Mushrooms and *Truffles* must be chopt, as before, and this *Godivoe* may serve as it were instead of a *Godivoe*-pie on Flesh-days. After having made the Paste and rais'd the Pie, one half of this *Godivoe* is to be put into it, as also at the same time, all sorts of Garniture for Fish-days ; such as *Truffles*, Mushrooms, *Andouillets*, Artichoke-bottoms, and raw Fish-*Filets* cut into small pieces ∙ Then having put the rest of the *Godivoe* well season'd on the top, let your Pie be cover'd and bak'd ∙ Lastly, you may prepare for it a white Sauce or Cullis of Mushrooms, or some other sort of Ragoo, but more especially take care, that it be serv'd up hot to Table.

The General Table at the end of this Volume, shews some other particular Fish-pies, that are occasionally describ'd upon account of the same Fishes: Those that remain are as follows, *viz.*

A Carp-pie.

The Carp must be scal'd and larded with Eels-flesh, season'd with good Butter, Pepper, Salt, Cloves, Nutmeg, a Bay-leaf and Oisters: Then the Pie being made of fine Paste, according to the length of the Carp, must be cover'd, and set into an Oven moderately heated ; so as half a Glass of white Wine may be pour'd in, when it is half bak'd.   The

The Carp may also be farc'd, according to the Method explain'd in the fifth Article *of Carps,* with Roes of the same, Oisters, Mushrooms and Artichoke-bottoms, in order to be serv'd up, with Lemmon-juice: Or else it may be cut into *Filets,* of the same nature as those for the above-mentioned Pies, as well as the following sorts of Fish and others

A Turbot-pie.

A Turbot may be bak'd in a round or oval Dish, or in a standing Pie, after the usual manner: When it is well scal'd and wash'd, let the Tail be cut off, with the end of the Head and the Gills: Season your Pie with Pepper, Salt, Cloves, Nutmeg, young Chibbols, fine Herbs, *Morilles,* or common Mushrooms and sweet Butter, and cover it with a Lid. As soon as it is half bak'd, pour in a Glass of white Wine, and serve it up with Lemmon-juice or Verjuice with the entire Grapes.

A Roach-pie.

A Roach-pie may be made, as that of a Tunny, and set out with the same sort of Garniture; only adding some Cray-fish-claws, if you have any at hand When it is half bak'd, let the Livers be first fried in a Pan with burnt Butter, then pounded in a Mortar, and strain'd thro' the Hair-sieve, with half a Glass of white Wine: Let all be put into the Pie, with some Lemmon-juice, when ready to be brought to Table.

A Trout-pie.

The Trout being well scal'd and cut, may be larded with Eels-flesh, and afterwards put into a Pie, made in the usual manner; season'd with Pepper, Salt, Cloves, Nutmeg, a Bay-leaf, Butter and fine Herbs, and enrich'd with Mushrooms, Artichoke-bottoms, Capers, Oisters and Fish-roes; squeezing in some Lemmon juice before it is serv'd up to Table.

A Sole-pie.

When your Soles are scal'd and wash'd, let them be put into a Pie made of Paste, and season'd with Pepper, Salt, Nutmeg, fine Herbs chopt very small, Chibbols, *Truffles, Morilles* or *Mouf-*

N 4 *ferons,*

ferons, common Mushrooms, fresh Oisters, and a great deal of Butter: As soon as it is bak'd, let it be serv'd up with Lemmon-juice

A Tunny-pie.

Let the Tunny be cut into round Slices, and dress'd, as it is usually done, with Oisters, Artichoke-bottoms, and other seasoning Ingredients; as also, one or two Slices of green Lemmon: Let it be bak'd in an Oven moderately heated, and put in some Lemmon-juice, or a little Vinegar, as it is serving up to Table.

A Lamprey-pie after the English manner.

Let your Lampreys be well cleans'd from their Slime, reserving their Blood, and afterwards put into a Pie of fine Paste, season'd with Pepper, Salt, beaten Cinnamon, Sugar, candy'd Lemmon-peel, Dates and Currans: When it is half bak'd in an Oven moderately heated, pour in the Blood, and half a Glass of white Wine; adding also some Lemmon-juice, before you serve it up to Table

Petits Patez, or little Pies of Fish.

Take the Flesh of Carps, Eels and Tenches; let all be half stew'd in a Pan with Mushrooms, and afterwards chopt small, with Parsly, Chibbol, Thyme, Pepper, Salt, Cloves and Nutmeg· Then put in as great a quantity of Butter as of Meat, and let your Pies be made of Puff-paste.

Petits Patez after the Spanish way

With this Article we shall conclude what relates to hot Pies for Side-dishes, as well on Flesh-days, as those of Abstinence. To make this sort of Pies, take only a Slice of Bacon, a little piece of Veal and the Breast of a Chicken· Let all be parboil'd in a Pot, minc'd very small, and season'd with beaten Spice. They must also be pounded in a Mortar, adding a little Garlick and Rocambole; whilst your *Petits Patez,* or little Pies are made with fine Paste, which will serve for garnishing other Dishes, or instead of an Out-work.

Cold

Cold Pies for Intermeſſes.

Having already given Directions for making a Gammon-pie in the third Article *of Gammon,* let us now take a View of ſome other ſorts of Pies that are likewiſe ſerv'd up among the Inter-meſſes, *viz.*

Pies of Beef-ſtakes and other ſorts of Butchers-meat.

Take ſome Buttock-beef cut out into Stakes ; let them be well beaten, larded with thick Slips of Bacon and ſeaſon'd as before : Let them alſo be dreſs'd and bak'd in the ſame man-ner.

According to the bigneſs, you would have your Pie to be of, a Leg of Mutton may likewiſe be added , or elſe a particular Pie may be made of it : To that purpoſe, having taken away the Skin and Fat from the Leg, let it be boned, well beaten and larded with middle-ſiz'd Slips of Bacon ; ſeaſoning it at the ſame time, with fine Herbs, Parſly, Chibbol and Spice.   In the mean while, let a piece of ordinary Paſte for a ſtrong Under-cruſt, be roll'd out and laid upon thick Paper well butter'd ; and let the Joynt of Mutton be dreſs'd upon the ſame Paſte, with thin Slices of Bacon, Bay-leaves and the neceſſary ſeaſoning In-gredients · Then cover your Pie with a Lid, and having ſhap'd it neatly, let it be bak'd as the former, about three Hours. When it is drawn out of the Oven, let a Clove of Ga-lick, or a Shalot bruiſed be put in thro' the Breathing-hole, and let it lye by, in order to be ſerv'd up cold to Table.

To make a Pie of a Fillet of Veal, it muſt be larded in like manner, after it has been marinated for a while, with well ſea-ſon'd Vinegar ; and for the reſt, you need only obſerve the Di-rections even now laid down for the Mutton-pie.

A Hare or Leveret-pie.

If you would have your Hares and Leverets entire, with the Bones, let them be larded with middle-ſiz'd Slips of Bacon, and ſeaſon'd with Pepper, Salt, Nutmeg, Cloves and a Bay-leaf : Neither muſt you be ſparing of your pounded Lard or Bacon-*Bards,* in making the Pie, either of courſe or fine Paſte. When it is bak'd, let it be ſet a-ſide in a dry place and ſtopt up cloſe.

If

If the Hares or Leverets are to be boned, endeavours muſt be us'd to keep the Fleſh, as entire, as is poſſible, and they muſt be larded with thick Slips of Bacon Then having feaſon'd them, they may be put into a Pie and bak'd as the others.

A Pullet-pie and others.

Having neatly trufs'd your large fat Pullers, and broken their Bones, let them be larded with thick Slips of Bacon, alſo feaſon'd with fine Herbs, Parſly, Chibbol and Spice · Then let them be laid in order in a Pie made of ordinary Paſte, with freſh Butter, *Bards*, or thin Slices of Bacon, a Bay-leaf or two, and other feaſoning Ingredients · Laſtly, let the Pies when well order'd, be bak'd during two or three Hours according to the Heat of the Oven.

PIGEONS.

Pies of young Turkeys, Ducks, Partridges, Pheaſants, Wood-cocks, large Rabbets, young Rabbets, green Geeſe, Teals and others are uſually made after the ſame manner.

Pigeons afford a great Variety of Ragoo's and ſome of them have been already produced ; particularly, a *Bisk* of Pigeons, in the firſt Article of *Bisks*; a *Godivoe* farced with young Pigeons, in that of *Godivoe*; and a Pie of large Pigeons, a little before, in the ſecond Article of Pies : There ſtill remain many other ſorts, ſo that it would be expedient here, to give ſome account of them in their Order.

To dreß Pigeons, with ſweet Baſil.

Let your Pigeons be well ſcalded, and ſlit a little on the Back, to let in a ſmall Farce, made of raw Bacon well minc'd, with Parſly, ſweet Baſil and Chibbol, all well feaſon'd Then having ſtew'd them in a Pot, with ſome Broth, an Onion ſtuck with Cloves, a little Verjuice and Salt, let them be roll'd in beaten Eggs, and at the ſame time wrapt up in Bread-crum, to the end that they may be well breaded. Every one of the Pigeons being thus order'd a-part, they muſt be fried in hot Lard, till they come to a fine colour, and afterwards fried again all at once with Parſly ; which is to garniſh them when they are ready to be ſerv'd up among the Side-diſhes.

A

A Side-dish of Pigeons, with Fennel.

Having provided Pigeons of the beft fort, let them be well truſs'd and only findg'd at the Fire Then taking the Livers, with fome Lard, Chibbol, Parſly, and a little green Fennel ; let all be chopt and well feaſon'd, in order to ſtuff the Bodies of the Pigeons Afterwards let them be roaſted, and let a good Ragoo be turn'd upon them, when ready to be brought to Table.

A Side-dish of Pigeons bak'd between two Fires.

Take large Pigeons, that are well truſs'd , and, if you pleaſe, prepare a ſomewhat thick Farce to ſtuff their Bodies Then let them be bak'd, or ſtew'd between two Fires, as many other Things are uſually dreſs'd : Afterwards they muſt be laid in order in a Diſh , and well clear'd from the Fat , pouring upon them at the ſame time, a Ragoo of *Truffles,* and Veal-ſweetbreads.

Pigeons ſtewed in Compote.

The Pigeons muſt firſt be larded with thick Slips of Bacon, and fried for ſome time in melted Lard · Then they are to be ſtew'd in Broth, with a Glaſs of white Wine, Pepper, Salt, Nutmeg, green Lemmon, Cloves, Muſhrooms and *Truffles* , whilſt a white or brown Cullis is preparing, as it were for a Fricaſſy of Pigeons cut into pieces · The Diſh may be garniſh'd with little Rolls cut into halves, or any thing elſe at pleaſure, and ſome Lemmon-juice muſt be ſqueez'd in, as it is ſerving up to Table.

A Side-dish of Pigeons, with Gammon.

This Diſh is uſually prepar'd after the ſame manner, as that of Chickens, with Gammon, already ſpecified in the firſt Article of Chickens, under the Letter C. If the Pigeons are very large, they muſt be larded with thick Slips of Bacon and others of Gammon, and bak'd between two Fires Then let them be put into a Gammon-ragoo, prepared for that purpoſe, and let all be well clear'd from the Fat ; ſprinkling them with a little Verjuice, or Vinegar Take care that they be not too high ſeaſon'd with Salt and let them be brought hot to Table

Ano-

Another *Side-dish of Pigeons*, with Truffles.

Another Side-dish may be made of larded or farced Pigeons, in a Ragoo, with *Truffles* and Radishes, or dress'd in a well sea-son'd Ragoo of a fine colour, with Artichoke-bottoms and A-sparagus-tops   They may be garnish'd with Veal-sweet-breads in white Sauce, and fried Parsly; adding some Lemmon-juice, before they are serv'd up to Table.

A Side-dish of Pigeons broil'd or fried, à la Sainte Menehout.

Take large Pigeons, that are well truss'd, let them be cut into two parts and broil'd upon the Coals: Then let them be neatly breaded, taking care that they be not spoil'd.   If you would have them fried; before they are breaded, they must be roll'd in beaten Eggs, to the end that the Bread may more easily stick to them.   When they are dress'd either way, they may serve for garnishing; but if a separate Dish be made of them, a *Ramolade*-sauce must be put underneath, ready prepared, with Anchovies, Parsly, chopt Capers, a little Chibbol, Vinegar and Gravy, and then all may be set hot on the Table.

All other sorts of Fowl, may be dress'd in the same manner Pigeons may also be larded, if you shall think fit, with thick Slips of Bacon and Gammon, to heighten their Savour, and some call Fowls so dress'd *Pieces à la Sainte Menehout.*

Moreover Pigeons, after they have been well season'd, may be stew'd in a *Court-bouillon*, that is duly order'd and made very Savoury : Then they must be well breaded, so as no part of the Meat may be any longer seen, and brought to a colour, with the red-hot Fire-shovel.

Pigeons in Sur-tout, *roasted, and bak'd between two Fires.*

Having caus'd large Pigeons to be well order'd and truss'd, let a Farce be made of raw Bacon, boil'd Gammon and Veal-sweet-breads, with *Truffles* and Mushrooms, chopt with the Li-vers, also Parsly, Chibbol and a Clove of Garlick; all cut small, well season'd, and bound with one or two Yolks of Eggs Let the Pigeons be stuff'd with this Farce between the Skin and the Flesh, as also in the Body, and afterwards well tied up, pro viding at the same time a large *Fricandoe,* or *Scotch* Collop larded,

ed, for every Pigeon, which is to be laid upon the Breaft. Then all the Pigeons being neatly tied and fpitted, are to be co-ver'd with Paper, and roafted in this manner; whilft a good Ragoo is preparing for them   Before they are ferv'd up, 'twill be requifite to drefs them in a Difh, taking away the Collops, and pouring on them the Ragoo or Cullis, of whatfoever Nature it be, provided it be well boil'd and feafon'd   Laftly, let the Collops be laid again upon the Breafts of all the Pigeons, and let them be brought hot to Table

The fame thing may be done for Pigeons in *Sur-tout* bak'd be-tween two Fires : All the difference between them, and other forts of Fowl drefs'd in this manner, is, That no Bacon-*Bards*, nor Meat are to be put upon the Collops, to the end that they may take a fine colour.   As foon as the Pigeons are ready, let the Fat be taken away, and a Ragoo prepar'd with *Truffles*, ac-cordingly, as occafion may require.

Other Side-difhes of the like nature, may be made of Par-tridges, Wood-cocks and other forts of Fowl, and to diverfifie them, a Ragoo may be drefs'd with Oifters, or *a la Saingaraz*, or a Partridge-cullis, according to the Expences allotted to be laid out : But all muft be well clear'd from the Fat, and ferv'd up hot to Table.

*A Pigeon-*Tourte, *or Pan-pie.*

After having provided good tame Pigeons, let them be well fcalded and trufs'd : Then taking melted Lard, Marrow, Veal-fweet-breads cut into halves, Artichoke-bottoms in quarters, and a whole one to be fet in the middle, with Capons-livers, Cocks-combs well pickt, Mufhrooms cut into fmall fquare pie-ces, and *Truffles* in Slices ; let all be well ftew'd in a Pan, with a little Flower, and well feafon'd.   In the mean while, let your Pafte be made (according to the bignefs of the Pie-pan) of an Egg, Butter, Salt and Water ; as alfo, a piece of Puff-pafte : let a good piece of the former be roll'd out for the Bottom-Cruft, which is to be put into a Pie-pan of a fize proportionable to that of your Difh : Then having pour'd in fome melted Lard, that is moderately hot, let the Pigeons be well moiften'd and laid in order, with the Artichoke-bottom in the middle, the Sli-ces of *Truffles*, Mufhrooms and Veal-fweet-breads in the Inter-vals.   Afterwards let the reft of the Sauce be infus'd, and ta-king another piece of Pafte, that was roll'd out of a round Fi-gure,

gure, let it be clapp'd with your Hand, spreading it upon the dresser-board; to the end, that the Puff-paste may be put upon it, and that the Lid may be neatly spread on the top. But too great a quantity of Puff-paste must not be made, that the other Piece may be thicker. Having thus cover'd your Pie with this Lid, make a neat Border or Side-crust round about, and when 'tis ready to be serv'd up, remove the Bacon-*Bards*, drain off the Fat, and pour in a Cullis of Pigeons-carcasses, or some other white thickening Sauce

Other ways of dressing Pigeons.

Pigeons may be otherwise dress'd *au Pere Douillet*; and to that purpose, after they have been well order'd, let them be stew'd in a little Pot, well seasoned and enrich'd, with Salt, Cloves, Thyme, Onion, and a little white Wine. They may be garnish'd with Parsly and Lemmon-slices; squeezing in some of the Juice, when ready to be brought to Table.

At another time, your Pigeons, after they have been roasted, barded and brought to a fine colour, may be serv'd up in Veal-gravy, without any other Garniture, or with white Sauce; or lastly, in a *Marinade*, as it appears from the second Article of *Marinades*.

P I G S.

A Side-dish of a young sucking Pig.

After a young sucking Pig has been well scalded and drawn; let the Liver be minc'd a-part, with parboil'd Bacon, *Truffles*, Mushrooms, an Anchovie, half a Clove of Garlick, a few fine Herbs and a little Sage. The whole Farce being thus dress'd in a Stew-pan and well season'd, stuff the Body of your Pig with the same, tye it up neatly, and let it be roasted; basting it with good Oil of Olives. It must be serv'd up hot to Table, and may be garnish'd with fried Bread

To scald a sucking Pig well, it must be rubb'd with Rosin, and put into Water moderately heated.

A sucking Pig dress'd after the German Fashion.

The Pig must be first cut into quarters, and fried in a Pan with Lard: Then let it be stew'd in Broth, with a little white
Wine,

Wine, a Faggot of Herbs, Pepper, Salt and Nutmeg Afterwards having toſs'd up in a Stew-pan with Lard, ſome Oiſters and Flower, a piece of Lemmon, Capers and ſtoned Olives, let them be added to the reſt, with Slices and Juice of Lemmon, as they are ſerving up to Table.

For a ſucking Pig roaſted, ſee the Letter R.

An Intermeß of a ſucking Pig in Galantine.

After having cauſ'd your Pig to be well ſcalded and drawn, cut off the Head and the four Legs. Then let the Skin be ſlipt off, beginning at the Belly ; but care muſt be taken that it be not cut, eſpecially on the Back · Let this Skin be neatly ſpread upon the Dreſſer, whilſt a Farce is preparing, with the Fleſh of the Pig, a piece of very tender Veal, a little raw Gammon, and Bacon, alſo, a little Parſly, chopt Chibbol, and all ſorts of fine Herbs, except Roſemary and Sage In the mean while, a Strong Liquor is to be made, with a Quart of Water, two Bay-leaves, ſome Thyme, ſweet Baſil, Savoury, three Cloves of Garlick, and two or three Shalots , this Liquor when half boil'd away, will ſerve to moiſten your Farce Let ſome Piſtachoes and Almonds be alſo ſcalded, according to diſcretion, and let ſix Eggs be harden'd to get their Yolks · Afterwards let ſome of your Bacon and Gammon be cut into thick Slices, taking only the lean part of the Gammon : When they are all well ſeaſon'd, let a Slice of Gammon, another of Bacon ; as alſo, a Lay of Almonds, another of Piſtachoes, and a third of hard Yolks be ſet in order. Beſides, you muſt put into the Farce, ſome *Truffles* and Muſhrooms cut ſmall, with a little Milk-cream, and ſoak them in your ſtrong Liquor ; adding afterwards the Yolk of one Egg. The Bacon and other Things being thus order'd, this Farce is to be ſpread over them, beginning at one of the ends of the Skin, and then roll'd up ; drawing the two Swards on both Sides cloſe together, ſo as the Farce may not fall out : When it is well roll'd up of a convenient length, let it be tied, or ſow'd up on all Sides, and put into a Napkin ; which muſt be bound at both end Ends and in the middle, to keep it very firm and compact. At laſt, it muſt be bak'd in a Stew-pan between two Fires, *viz.* one upon the Lid and the other underneath, for the ſpace of ten or twelve Hours, with ſome Slices of Bacon and Beef-ſtakes, both on the Bottom and Top of the Pan : Let your farced Pig cool in the ſame Pan, and as ſoon as it is
taken

taken out of the Napkin, let it be untied, and cut into Slices, which are to be laid in a Dish, upon a clean Napkin, and so ferv'd up cold, with Slices of Lemmon and Flowers

A Pig dreſs'd au Pere Doüillet.

When the Pig is well scalded in Water, and order'd as before, it muſt be larded with middle-siz'd Slips of Bacon, and seafon'd high, with Pepper, Salt, Cloves, Nutmeg, Bay-leaves, young Chibbols and green Lemmon · Then let it be wrapt up in a Linnen-cloth, and boil'd in a Pot, with Broth and a little white Wine. Afterwards it may be fet by, till it be half cool'd, and so ferv'd up for a Side dish.

Pigs-pettitoes à la Sainte Menehout

Take Pettitoes that are well drefs'd, cut them into halves, and let every Pettitoe be tied up together : Then having provided a Pot, put into it a Lay of *Bards*, or thin Slices of Bacon, another of Pettitoes and fine Herbs, and a third of Pettitoes and *Bards*; and so on, till all your Pettitoes are difpofed of, as alfo, afterwards a Glaſs of Spirit of Wine, and a Quart of white Wine, with Anis, Coriander, a Bay-leaf or two, and a little Quick-filver : Let all be cover'd with Bacon-*Bards*, and let the Edges of the Pot be lin'd with ftrong Paper, fo as the Lid may be exactly fitted, and kept clofe ftopt. Then let the Pot be fet between two Fires, which muft not be too quick, that the Pettitoes may be leifurely ftew'd, during ten or twelve Hours, more or lefs. When they are taken out and cool'd, they are to be neatly breaded, and broil'd upon the Grid-iron, in order to be ferv'd up hot among the Intermeffes. They may be drefs'd with lefs charge, only with Water and white Wine mingled together, feafoning them well, and putting in fome Leaf-fat out of a Hog's Belly ; as it may alfo be done, in the other Way of drefsing them.

The Denomination of *à la Sainte Menehout* is likewife attributed to Pigeons, Chickens, or other forts of Fowl, drefs'd in that manner, which fome call *à la Mazarine*, and which has been elfewhere explain'd in the third Article of Chickens, under the Letter C.

P I K E S.

PIKES.

Pike with Oifters

Let the Pike be cut into pieces and put into a Stew pan, with white Wine, Parfly, Chibbol, Mufhrooms, chopt *Truffles*, Pepper, Salt and good Butter In the mean while, let your Oifters be fcalded a little in Water, with a few Drops of Verjuice, and thrown in among the reft, with their Liquor, when the Pike is ready to be ferv'd up to Table Afterwards let all be drefs'd in a Difh, and garnifh'd with what you fhall think fit.

The fame thing may be done for other forts of Fifh that are drefs'd with Oifters.

A Side-difh of a large Pike.

After having cut your Pike into four Quarters, let the Head be drefs'd in a *Court-bouillon*, one of the middle-pieces with white Sauce, the other in a Hafh, or in a Ragoo, and the Tail-piece fried with Caper-fauce The Hafh is to be garnifh'd with fmall Crufts of fried Bread, and all drefs'd in a large Difh. To thefe may be added a fmall Ragoo of Pike-livers, Roes and Capers; garnifhing the Difh with Flowers, or green Herbs

A Pike with Sauce, after the German Way.

When the Pike is well cleans'd and gutted, let it be cut into two parts and boil'd in Water, but not outright: Having taken it out, let it be fcal'd till it become very white, and put into a Stew-pan, with white Wine, chopt Capers, Anchovies, Thyme, fine Herbs and Mufhrooms cut fmall, as alfo *Truffles*, and *Morilles* Then let all boil together gently, left the Fifh fhould break, and throw in a Lump of good Butter, to thicken the Sauce, with a little Parmefan. When it is ready, you may drefs your Difh, and garnifh it with what you pleafe.

Pike-Filets fried and otherwife.

As foon as your Pike is gutted and fcal'd, cut it into pieces, and make *Filets* of it, which are to be marinated for fome time: Then let them be fried, after having dipt them into a thin Pafte

O or

or Batter, or otherwife, and let them be ferv'd up to Table, garnifh'd with Parfly and Slices of Lemmon.

Pike-*Filets* may alfo be put into white Sauce, which is a kind of thickening Liquor proper for that fort of Fifh, made of a little Bread-crum pounded and ftrain'd thro' the Sieve, after having boil'd two or three Walms in a Stew-pan, with a little Broth, or Fifh-cullis. Let your *Filets* be foak'd in this Sauce, that is well feafon'd, and if you pleafe, fome *Truffles* may be added, with *Moufferons* and common Mufhrooms, as alfo fome Lemmon-juice, as they are ferving up to Table.

Laftly, they may be drefs'd with Cucumbers, as many other Things, and fprinkled likewife with Lemmon-juice.

A Pike-pie.

The Pike may be cut into *Filets* or fmall pieces of the length of your Finger, which are to be fcalded, well feafon'd, and tofs'd up in a Stew-pan with fweet Butter, Mufhrooms, *Truffles*, Afparagus-tops and Carp-roes, alfo a piece of Lemmon thrown in as they are Stewing. Then a fmall *Godivoe* is to be made of the Flefh of Carps or Eels, feafon'd according to the ufual manner, and bound with Bread-crum foak'd in Broth. The bottom of your Pie muft be fill'd with this Farce, and a thickening Liquor with Lemmon-juice muft be pour'd in, before it is brought to Table

A Pie may likewife be made of a boned Pike, and farced in the mannner hereafter exprefs'd in the eighth Article. The Pafte for this Pie out to be fine, and it muft be fhap'd according to the fize of your Pike. Both thefe forts of Pies muft be bak'd in an Oven moderately heated, and ferv'd up hot for Side-difhes

A Pike in Haricot with Turneps.

Let the Pike be cut into fmall pieces about the length of half your Finger, and then fcalded : When they are drain'd, let them be fried brown, and one half of the Turneps likewife fried brown. Afterwards they muft be ftew'd together, over a gentle Fire, adding a good thickening Liquor and Lemmon-juice, when they are ferv'd up to Table.

Pike in a Court-bouillon *or* au Bleu.

The Pike being cut into quarters, and put into a Dish, let Vinegar and Salt be pour'd upon it boiling hot Then having caus'd white Wine, Verjuice, Pepper, Salt, Cloves, Nutmeg, a Bay-leaf, or two, Onions and green Lemmon, or Orange, to boil together, over a quick Fire ; let your Pike be put in, and afterwards ferv'd up dry among the Intermeffes.

Forced Pike.

Let the Pikes be fcal'd, and let the Bones be taken out at the Back, yet fo as the Heads and Tails may be left fticking , whilft a Farce is preparing with fome of the fame Flefh and that of Eels, feafon'd with Pepper, Salt, Nutmeg, Cloves, Chibbol, Butter, Mufhrooms and fine Herbs. Let the Skins be ftuff'd with this Farce and fow'd up, in order to be ftew'd in a Dish, with burnt Butter, fried Flower, white Wine, Verjuice, a little Broth and a piece of green Lemmon. Then a Ragoo of Oifters, Carp-roes and Mufhrooms is to be added ; garnifhing the Dish, with fried Bread, Lemmon-flices and Capers.

Pike in Cafferole

Scale your Pikes, Lard them with Eel-flefh, and let them be ftew'd with burnt Butter, white Wine, Verjuice, Pepper, Salt, Nutmeg, Cloves, a Bunch of Herbs, Bay-leaves and green Lemmon In the mean while, let a Ragoo be made for them, with Mufhrooms, Oifters, Capers, fried Flower and fome of the fame Sauce in which they were ftew'd. They may be garnifh'd with Lemmon-flices, Carp-roes and fried Mufhrooms.

Pikes fried with Anchovie-fauce.

Let the Pikes be cut open in the Belly, and marinated in Vinegar, with Pepper, Salt, Chibbols and Bay-leaves , let them alfo be flower'd before they are fried. For the Sauce, let Anchovies be diffolv'd in burnt Butter, and having ftrain'd them thro' the Sieve, add fome Juice of Orange, Capers and white Pepper The Dish is to be garnifh'd with fried Parfly and Slices of Lemmon, before it is brought to Table.

Roafted

Roasted Pike.

The Pike must be scal'd, cut lightly and larded with middle-siz'd Slips of Eels-flesh, season'd with Pepper, Salt, Nutmeg, Chibbols and fine Herbs : It must be Spitted at its whole length, and basted with Butter, white Wine, Vinegar and green Lemmon Then having dissolv'd Anchovies in the Sauce, strain them thro' the Hair-sieve, with a little fried Flower, and add some Oisters mortified in the Sauce, with Capers and white Pepper. The Dish may be garnish'd with fried Mushrooms, Carp-roes and Lemmon-slices.

Pike on Flesh-days, for an Intermeß.

After having scal'd your Pike, and drawn out the Guts at the upper part of the Belly, it must be scalded in luke-warm Water, and larded with thin Slips of Bacon : Then it must be roasted on a Spit, and basted as before ; the same sort of Sauce being also prepared for it. The Dish is to be garnish'd with larded Veal-sweet-breads, farced Mushrooms and Lemmon-slices.

It may also be dress'd according to the Directions laid down in the first Article of *Trouts* under the Letter T.

Pike-potage.

This sort of Potage may be made with Oisters, Turneps, or Cabbage ; cutting the Pike into several pieces, which are to be first fried in a Pan with Butter, and afterwards stew'd in an earthen Pot, with some Fish-broth, or strained Pease-soop, season'd with Pepper, Salt, and a Bunch of Herbs : Then having added Oisters, the Potage is to be laid a soaking with the Broth, in which the Fish was stew'd ; the Pike must be dress'd in the same Potage, as also the Oisters ; and the whole Mess must be garnish'd with Bread and Mushrooms fried, squeezing in some Lemmon-juice, as it is serving up to Table.

When Turneps are us'd, they must be fried with burnt Butter, and Flower and then stew'd with Pepper and Salt. Afterwards they are to be laid in good order upon the soaked Crusts, with the Pike.

The same thing may be done with the Cabbage, after it has been scalded and chopt small, and as for the Pike, it may be larded with Eels-flesh.   A

A Potage may alfo be made of farced Pike, and to that purpofe, it would only be requifite, to look a little backwards upon the Inftructions contain'd in the preceding Article of *farced Pike* Pag. 195. and for the Potage of *Pike-Filets* and Crufts farced with Pike, fee the following Articles of Potages.

PLAICE.

After having roafted and flafh'd your Plaice on the Back, in form of a Crofs, cutting off the Nofe and Tail, they are to be put into a Stew-pan, with white Wine, Fifh-roes, *Morilles*, common Mufhrooms, *Truffles*, Parfly, Chibbol, Thyme, and a Slice of good Butter, all well thicken'd; but care muft be taken to ftir them gently leaft they fhould break When they are ready, let them be neatly drefs'd and made very white; pouring fome good Sauce upon them, and garnifhing them with any thing that is at Hand.

As for thofe that are fried, they muft be firft ftrew'd with Salt and Flower, and when drefs'd, they may be ferv'd up, with Salt and Orange-juice.

POTAGES.

Altho' mention has been already made of feveral Potages, as well for Flefh-days, as thofe of Abftinence, particularly, the *Bisk*, *Cafferole*, *Oil* and *Julian*, as alfo Potage of Lambs-heads, Pike, Cray-fifh, Sea-ducks, Mufcles and fome others, according to the refpective Meffes that were treated of Neverthelefs this Subject is very copious, and capable of furnifhing matter for a large Article A general Account has likewife been given of the peculiar Broths, that ought to conftitute the Body of all thofe Potages, and of all others, as alfo of the Cullifes that are ufually made. Let us now proceed to a more particular Enumeration of them; beginning with the Potages of Pulfe, that may be proper for feveral forts of Fowls, to avoid the unprofitable Repetition of the fame Thing, for every one of them.

POTAGES FOR FLESH-DAYS.

Potage with Peafe.

Take green Peafe, and having fhell'd them, let the Peafe be fet by a-part, which will ferve to make green Peafe-foop To that purpofe, taking the Cods with the Peafe, let them be fcalded a little, with the green top of a Chibbol and a little Parfly, and drain'd from their Liquor: Then they muft be pounded with a little Bread-crum foak'd in good Broth, and well ftrain d thro' a Sieve; fo as your Soop may be fomewhat thick Afterwards your Peafe muft be put into a Stew-pan, with a little Lard; having before fried in it, a little chopt Parfly and Savoury: Let all be ftew'd together, and moiften'd with good Broth; adding a Faggot of fine Herbs · When the whole Mefs is put into a Pot, and almoft ready, the Soop may be pour'd in, and fome Cabbage-lettice, cut into fmall Slices, may alfo be ftew'd before the green Peafe are put in, all being well feafon'd. Let your Potage be laid a foaking with good clear Broth, and having pour d in a little Peafe-foop, let your Fowls be laid in order upon the Potage. They may be garnifh'd either with farced, or unfarced Lettice, or with Cucumbers, or elfe with lean Bacon, accordingly as you fhall think fit. Laftly, let your Potage be foak'd with the Soop and green Peafe, and let all be ferv'd up at once

Many Potages of the like nature are ufually made with green Peafe in their Seafon, particularly for Lambs-heads, Ducks, green Geefe, farced Chickens, young Turkeys and others, which ought to be boil'd feparately in a Pot, with good Broth. They are to be garnifh'd with Afparagus-tops, farced Lettice, or Cucumbers. When green Peafe are out of Seafon, the Soop may be made with old ones; and this fort is more efpecially proper for Ducks, *Andouilles*, &c.

'Tis an eafie Matter to take Meafures in reference to this Article, for Peafe-potage on Fifh-days; for then the Peafe are to be ftew'd with natural Butter, and the Crufts laid a foaking, with good Herb-broth, according to the Directions laid down in the laft Article of *Broths*, under the Letter B.

For the Fowls that are farced, the Method is explain'd in the refpective Articles, where mention is made of thofe Fowls; and for the reft, fee what is obferv'd in the following Potages.

Potage,

Potage, with Turneps.

After having well scrap'd your Turneps, cut them into round pieces, or long-ways, and fry them with Lard and a little Flower: You may make use of the same Lard, in which your Fowls were fried brown, whether they were Ducks, Teals, green Geese, or others; at least if you would not have them roasted a little on the Spit. So that either Way, all may be put into a Pot together, with good Broth, season'd with Pepper, Salt, and a Faggot of Herbs, adding a brown thickening Liquor, as they are stewing · Thus, having laid your Potage a soaking with the same Broth, let the Fowls and Turneps be neatly dress'd, and garnish'd, sometimes with fried Bread, and sometimes with Sausages, *Andouillets*, or young Bacon boil'd together · Afterwards let some Lemmon-juice and good Gravy be put to them, before they are serv'd up to Table. Some cause the Turneps to be boil'd separately.

Large Geese, green Geese, Ducks and other Fowls of the like nature, that are usually dress'd with Turneps, ought to be larded with thick Slips of Bacon, before they are fried, and the lighter Fowls may be farced, more especially Chickens

The Houghs of a Stag, and of a wild Boar, may also be serv'd up in the same sort of Potage

A Potage with Turneps may likewise be prepar'd for a Shoulder of Mutton; which being well mortified, you are to lard with thick Slips of Bacon, and cause it to be half roasted; as well as for a farced Leg of Mutton, which must be fried as the above-mentioned Fowls

Cabbage-potage.

Take large Pigeons, Partridges and other sorts of Fowl well truss'd; lard them with three or four Rows of Bacon, and let them be roasted only till they come to a colour · In the mean time, having provided Cabbages that are well headed, let them be cut into quarters and scalded · Then they must be drain'd and put into a Pot, as also the Fowls, with young Bacon parboil'd, a little sweet Basil, an Onion stuck with Cloves, and one or two Cloves of Garlick · They must also be season'd, pouring in some good Gravy and Broth, and afterwards all boil'd together. When they are half boil'd, a brown thickening Liquor

O 4

must

muft be prepar'd with Lard and Flower, as if it were to make
a good *Robert*-Sauce   As foon as the Flower has taken colour,
moiften your thickening Ingredients with good Gravy, or with
the fame Cabbage-broth, and when it is ready, turn all upon the
Cabbage.   Let your Potage be laid a foaking with good Gravy and the Cabbage-broth, when you perceive them to be favoury, and that they are well boil'd.   Afterwards let the Fowls
be laid in order upon the Potage ; let a fine Border be made
round about the Difh, or in the Intervals, with young ftreaked
Bacon cut into Slices, let all be foak'd with good Broth, and
ferv'd up hot to Table.

As for *Milan* Cabbages and others, after having fcalded them,
they may be chopt fmall and fried, before they are put into a
Pot, in the above-mentioned manner ; except fome of the In-
fides, which are to be preferv'd for garnifhing   See alfo what
has been already deliver'd upon this Subject in the firft Article
of Cabbage, under the Letter C.

Root-potages.

After having made good Broth, pour it into a Pot, and put
in at the fame time a fat Capon, with Parfly-roots, Parfnips,
and fmall Chibbols, entire.   Then, all being boil'd together, let
your Potage be laid a foaking, with the Capon on the top, garnifhing it with Parfnips and young Chibbols, and foaking it with
good Veal-gravy, before it is ferv'd up to Table.

Potages may alfo be made of Quails, young Ring-doves, fat
Pullets and others, with Roots, after the fame manner.

Potages, with Lentils.

Having provided Partridges, Pigeons, Ducks, or other Fowls ;
let them be larded with feveral Rows of Bacon and fpitted.
When they are half roafted, let them be put into a Pot and
boil'd with good Broth, a Faggot of fine Herbs, and other feafoning Ingredients.   Then taking fome Lentils ready boil'd,
pound them with Onions, Carrets and Parfly-roots, and ftrain
them thro' the Hair-fieve, in order to make the Cullis.   In the
mean while, having caus'd other Lentils to be ftew'd in a Pan,
with a little Parfly, Chibbol and Savoury chopt fmall, pour in
fome of the Broth, in which your Fowls were boil'd, as alfo
the Cullis, and let all be put into a Pot, till you have laid them

a

a foaking and drefs'd your Potage. 'Twill be requifite to provide fome young ftreaked Bacon, Cervelas, or Saufages for the Garniture; and, if the Expences are not grudged, a Border may be made round about the Difh, with Cocks-combs and Veal-fweet-breads in a Ragoo; all well drefs'd and clear'd from the Fat. The Potage may alfo be enrich'd with a Beefcullis, Partridge-carcaffes, Crufts of Bread, and a piece of green Lemmon, all pounded in a Mortar, ftrain'd thro' a Sieve, and well feafon'd See the Lentil-cullis, in the laft Article of *Cullifes,* under the Letter C.

Another fort of Lentil-potage is fometimes made, and garnifh'd with a farced Loaf in the middle, as well on Flefh-days, as thofe of Abftinence: For the latter, it may be ferv'd up with Oil, and more efpecially for the Entertainments with Roots, or on other Days of Lent, when a particular Plate, or Difh may be made of them, drefs'd in a Ragoo, with fine Herbs.

Potage of young Ring-doves, in form of an Oil

After having neatly trufs'd your Ring-doves, let them be fcalded in Water, and put into a Pot with good Gravy; throwing in at the fame time, a Bunch of Leeks cut into pieces, another of Celery, a third of Turneps, a fourth of other forts of Roots, a few Chibbols, and a Faggot of fine Herbs. All being well boil'd, you muft lay your Potage a foaking with the fame Broth; fetting the Ring-doves in order in it, and garnifhing the whole Difh with your Roots Let them alfo be foak'd with good favoury Gravy, and ferv'd up hot to Table The Garnitures ought only to take up the fides of the Difh, fo as the Soop may be left free: And the fame thing may be done for Quails, and all other forts of Fowl.

At another time, young Ring-doves may be drefs'd in Potage, with Cabbage, Mufhrooms, or otherwife at pleafure.

Potage à la Reyne, *with Partridges, Quails, or other forts of Fowl.*

Let frefh Partridges, after they have been fcalded and well trufs'd, be boil'd in good Broth, with a good Faggot of fine Herbs, fome thin flices of Bacon and pieces of Lemmon, whilft a Cullis is making of the Breaft of a roafted fat Pullet, or Capon; minc'd and pounded in a Mortar, with the Crum of a

Loaf

Loaf foak'd in Broth, and ftrain'd thro' the Hair-fieve. Let this Cullis be put into a little Pot, well cover'd, and let your Potage, that ought to be made of Bread-crufts, be laid a foaking with ftrained Broth. Afterwards fet your Fowls in the fame Potage, fprinkle all with good Gravy, and before they are ferved up, fqueez the Juice of a Lemmon into the Cullis: A farced Loaf muft alfo be put in the middle of the Potage, with the Fowls round about; the Cullis muft be pour'd upon them, and a Border is to be made about the Difh, with farced Cocks-combs, Sweet-breads of Veal larded and roafted, other Slices of Veal-fweet-breads in a Ragoo, and Artichoke-bottoms: Laftly, the Breafts of the Partridges, or other Fowls, muft be cover'd with Slices of black *Truffles*, and all difpos'd of in good order As for the farced Loaf, it muft be ftuff'd with a good Hafh of a roafted Fowl, pieces of *Truffles* and Mufhrooms, and fmall Afparagus-tops, according to the Seafon.

A leffer quantity of Potage, may be made of a fingle Partridge, without a farced Loaf, obferving all the reft of the Circumftances, as much as Convenience, or the allotted Expences will admit of.

A Potage of farced Partridges, may be alfo prepar'd, which ought to be garnifh'd with larded *Fricandoes* drefs'd in a Ragoo, alfo Veal-fweet-breads, Mufhrooms, Artichoke-bottoms, Cocks-combs, and *Truffles*, adding the Juice of a Lemmon, when brought to Table.

Another white *Potage* à la Reyne.

This fort of Potage does not require any Fowl, only the Breaft of a Capon, and a piece of a Neck of Veal, fome Almonds, two or three Yolks of hard Eggs, and the Crum of a Loaf fteept in good Broth. All thefe Ingredients are to be pounded in a Mortar, and afterwards laid a foaking in a Sauce pan, with good Gravy and Broth, till they have acquir'd an exquifite Relifh · Then they muft be ftrain'd thro' a Sieve, and fpread over the Potage, when it is fufficiently foak'd; which may alfo be marbled with well feafon'd Gravy.

Potages of farced *Quails and young Partridges.*

Having caus'd your Quails to be farced, with Capons-breafts, Beef-marrow, Pepper, Salt, Nutmeg, and the Yolks of raw

Eggs,

Eggs, let them be ſtew'd in good Broth, with a Bunch of Herbs, as in the preceding Potage. For the Cullis, ſtrain thro' the Sieve, two Bottoms of boil'd Artichokes, and ſix Yolks of Eggs, with the ſame Quail-broth, and let them be gently ſtew'd over the hot Embers Then dreſs your Quails upon the ſoaked Cruſts, and garniſh them with ſmall Artichoke-bottoms; pouring in the Cullis, with Muſhroom-juice and Mutton-gravy, as they are ſerving up to Table. A Ragoo of Turkeys may alſo be made, for that purpoſe, or elſe the Quails may be ſtuff'd with Sweet Baſil.

As for large Partridges and young Partridges, that are farced, after they have been boil'd in good Broth, a white Cullis may be prepar'd for them, with Almonds and green Lemmon. They may be garniſh'd with Cocks combs and Muſhrooms, adding ſome Mutton-gravy and Lemmon-juice, when ready to be brought to Table

Potage, without Water.

Take a good piece of Beef, another of Mutton, part of a Fillet of Veal, a Capon, four Pigeons and two Partridges; all the Fowls being well truſs'd, and the Butchers-meat ſufficiently beaten. Then put them into a Pot that is well tinn'd over, with Slices of Onions, Parſnips and Parſly-roots, and ſeaſon them with all ſorts of fine Herbs and a little Salt In the mean while, having provided ſome Paſte and ſtrong Paper, let the Edges of your Pot be ſtopt up cloſe; ſo as all the Steam may be kept in, and that the leaſt Air may not either be let in or out Afterwards let this Pot be ſet into another of a larger ſize, the void ſpace being fill'd with hot Water and ſtuff'd with Hay, to the end that the leſſer Pot may remain ſteady in its proper place, without moving on either ſide · Thus the Water in the greater Pot muſt be kept continually boiling, and cloſe ſtopt up, for the ſpace of five or ſix Hours When that time is expir'd, it muſt be uncover'd, ſo as all the Gravy of the Meat may be pour'd off, and well clear'd from the Fat Let the Fowls that were ſtew'd, be minc'd, in order to farce a Loaf, with good Garnitures; then let the Soop, as well as the Loaf, be ſoak'd with the ſame Gravy; and let a Ragoo be made of all ſorts of Garnitures, fried in Lard, to be pour'd thereupon. Laſtly, let the whole Meſs be neatly dreſs'd, and garniſh'd with farced Cocks-combs, Veal-ſweet-breads, or ſomething elſe of the like nature, in order to be ſerv'd up to Table. Po-

Potage de Santé.

After having caus'd some good Broth of Buttock-beef, a Knuckle of Veal and Mutton, to be put into a Pot, with Capons, fat Pullets, or other Fowls proper for the Potage *de Santé*, and having made the same Broth very savoury; let the Crusts be soak'd with it, whilst some fine Herbs are boiling in another Pot, such as Sorrel, Purslain, Chervil, &c. all cut very small. These Herbs may serve to garnish your Potage and Fowls; or they may be strain'd, so as nothing be put into the Dish, but the Broth and good Gravy, when served up to Table.

Another sort of Potage *de Sante*, is made quite clear, of a Chicken or Pullet, and a piece of a Fillet of Veal, without any Garniture; only it may be brought to a colour, by passing the red-hot Fire-shovel over it.

Potage of farced Chickens.

The Chickens must be farced with a good *Godivoe*, between the Skin and the Flesh; the Breasts may be also taken away. When they are well order'd and scalded, they must be put into a Pot, with good Broth, and may be garnish'd with Veal-sweet-breads and Cocks-combs, as a *Brk*, or with Pulse; a Cullis and some Gravy being added, before they are set on the Table. See hereafter, different sorts of farced Chickens.

Potage of Barn-door-chickens.

After they have been farced with a delicious *Godivoe*, soak'd in Cream, let them be well boil'd in a Pot, and garnish'd with fried Paste or Pulse; squeezing in some Lemmon-juice, before they are brought to Table.

Potage of farced Chickens, with Onions.

Let a white Cullis be made of Capons-breasts, or of Veal, and three or four Yolks of hard Eggs, all well pounded in a Mortar, with some Bread-crum soak'd in good Broth After this Mixture has been season'd, let it have five or six Seethings in a Stew-pan. Then, having strain'd it thro' the Hair-sieve, squeez in the Juice of a Lemmon, and sprinkle all your Potage with it, when ready to be serv'd up to Table.   The

The Potage of Pigeons with a white Cullis, garnish'd with white Onions, or Cardoons, is usually prepar'd after the same manner.

Potage of farced Chickens, garnish'd with Chesnuts.

Let your Chickens be boil'd in the ordinary Pot, and the Chesnuts in a little Pot a-part (after their second Skin has been peel'd off) with savoury Broth; but so as they be not broken. With these a Border is to be made round about the Dish and the Chickens, which are to be sprinkled with a good Cullis, as they lye a soaking, and with Lemmon-juice, as they are serving up to Table.

Another Potage of farced Chickens.

A Potage of Chickens is also sometimes made, with a green Cullis, Asparagus, and a Border of young streaked Bacon

A Potage of Chickens and other sorts of Fowl, with Cucumbers.

Let your Chickens, Pullets, or Capons, be boil'd, in well-season'd Broth, according to the usual manner. As for the Cucumbers; after having taken out the Seeds and scalded them in Water, let them be stuff'd with a good Farce, and stew'd in Broth, with Salt and a Bunch of Herbs: In the mean while, let some Yolks of poach'd Eggs be strain'd thro' the Hair-sieve, with Beef-juice and good Broth, and let them be boil'd and soak'd a-part. Then dress your Potage with the Crusts, the Chickens in the middle, the farced Cucumbers for Garnitures, and the Cullis pour'd upon all, with Lemmon-juice The same thing ought to be observ'd in dressing Turkey-powts, and other Fowls of the like nature.

Other Potages may be prepar'd with Cucumbers, without farcing, only frying them in Lard, and dressing them, as before.

Potage, with Crusts farced with Partridge-breasts.

As soon as the Partridges are roasted, take their Breasts and cut them into small pieces, in form of a Die, and some Arti-
choke-

choke-bottoms in like manner: Let thefe be ftew'd together, and made very favoury, in order to farce your Crufts, and let a Cullis be made of a piece of Beef roafted brown, which you muft pound in a Mortar, with the Partridge-carcaffes, and let all boil in a Sauce-pan; feafoning them as much as is requifite Afterwards they are to be ftrain'd thro' the Sieve, with good Gravy and a piece of Lemmon, and the Crufts are to be foak'd with them Laftly, let a fmall Mutton-hafh be made, which is to be ftrew'd on the top, whilft a Border of Crufts is fet round about the Difh

Another Potage is fometimes made of Crufts farced with Lentils, with a Cullis of the fame, as for Pigeons, and other forts of Fowl, before-mention'd in the fifth Article, and 'tis an eafie thing to order others, conformably to the Model of the former, according to the Variety of Meats that are to be drefs'd, or elfe the Loaf may be ftuff'd with a good Ragoo

Another Potage, with Crufts farced with Gammon.

The Crufts are to be farced with Gammon, Veal-fweet-breads, Capons-breafts, *Moufferons* and Artichoke-bottoms, all cut into little fquare pieces, and ftew'd in a Ragoo with a Veal-cullis Let thefe Crufts be enclos'd in others, and neatly tied up, that they may not be broken, as they are foaking. When they are ready, let them be drefs'd in the Potage, and garnifh'd in a Difh, fprinkling them with the Juice of a Lemmon

Potage of Profitrolle.

Having provided a little round Loaf, of the fame fort as thofe for Soop, with Crufts, let it be farc'd, and foak'd with Veal-gravy and good Broth Let it alfo be drefs'd upon the other foaked Crufts, with a little of a Partridge or Capon-hafh Then having prepar'd a Cullis, with the Meats of which the Gravy was made, and having ftrain'd it, let it be pour'd upon the Potage. When you would have it ferv'd up, a fine Artichoke-bottom may be laid upon the Loaf, with fome Mufhrooms on the infide, and it may be garnifh'd with *Fricandoe's*, or Veal-fweet-breads

A

A Potage of Profitrolle, *garnish'd with* Poupiets.

Let the *Poupiets*, the manner of ordering which you'll find in its proper place, be put into a Dish or Sauce-pan; and let a Cullis be made of a piece of roasted Veal, pounded in a Mortar, well season'd and strain'd thro' the Hair-sieve, for the soaking of your *Poupiets*. Then a Ragoo is to be made of Veal-sweet-breads, Cocks-combs, *Truffles*, *Morilles*, *Mousserons*, common Mushrooms and Artichoke-bottoms, all dress'd with white Sauce, and well season'd, with which the Potage is to be garnish'd, the *Profitrolle*-loaf being laid in the middle, and the Juice of a Lemmon squeez'd in, as it is serving up to Table.

Another Potage of Profitrolle.

This Potage is to be set out with six small Loaves and one great one in the middle, that is to say, three farced with Gammon; three others with Capons, and the large one, with a Hash of Gammon and Capon; as also, Veal-sweet-breads, *Truffles*, *Mousserons*, common Mushrooms, and Artichoke-bottoms cut into pieces in form of a die The whole Mess is to be garnish'd with larded *Fricandoes*, or Scotch Collops fried brown, a Border of Cocks-combs, and a Ragoo of *Mousserons*, or common Mushrooms, with Artichoke-bottoms and Asparagus-tops, all dress'd with white Sauce, squeezing in the Juice of a Lemmon, when ready to be brought to Table.

See afterwards the Potages of *Profitrolles* for Fish-days.

Potage of a Capon, or of a Fat Pullet, with Rice.

Let the Rice be boil'd in good Broth, and then serve to garnish your Capon or fat Pullet; upon the soaked Crusts Afterwards you must strew some rasped Parmesan and grated Cinnamon on the top, and give it a colour, with the red-hot Fire-shovel. The Side of the Dish may be garnish'd with Bread-crusts made very brown with Lard, in order to be serv'd up with Mutton-gravy and Lemmon-juice.

The Potage of *Vermicelli* is made after the same manner.

Potage of Teals and other Fowls, with Mushrooms.

Lard your Teals with middle-siz'd Slips of Bacon, and after having fried them in Lard, let them be stew'd in good Broth, according to the usual manner, with Salt, and a Bunch of Herbs: In the mean time, let some Mushrooms and Flower be toss'd up in the same Lard, and put to the Teals, when they are half-stew'd. Lastly, let them be neatly dress'd, and serv'd up in Slices, with Mutton-gravy and Lemmon-juice

The Mushroom-potages have been already explain'd in the fourth Article of Mushrooms.

Potage, with Truffles.

The *Truffles* must be boil'd in good Broth and Gravy in a little Pot, with a Faggot of Herbs and a thickening Liquor, that is well enrich'd. When the Potage is sufficiently soak'd, and the *Truffles* dress'd, they must be laid in order therein, adding some Lemmon-juice, when the Dish is serv'd up to Table. A *Profitrolle*-loaf may also be set in the middle.

For the Potages of young Pheasants, Quails and other sorts of Fowl, which you would have dress'd with *Truffles*, let them be put into a Pot in the usual manner, and well season'd. But your *Truffles* must be cut into little pieces and not into Slices, and after having fried them in a little Lard, they must be stewed, as before. To make the Potage brown, let a good Cullis of Beef or Mutton be pour'd in, and some Lemmon-juice, before the Dish is brought to Table.

Potage, with Truffles *and* Mousserons.

Let a Cullis of Veal or Capons-breasts be well season'd, and let a Loaf farced with every thing that you shall think fit, be set in the middle of the Potage. Then dress your *Truffles* and *Mousserons* in a good Ragoo, and garnish the Potage with them; squeezing in the Juice of a Lemmon, when ready to be set on the Table.

Potages of farced Pigeons, with a brown Cullis.

Let Onions be fried brown to make the Border; whilſt a
Cullis is preparing with a piece of Beef roaſted very brown,
and pounded in the Mortar with Cruſts of Bread. Then let all
be ſtew'd in a Sauce-pan and well ſeaſon'd, and afterwards
ſtrain'd thro' a Hair-ſieve, with the Juice of a Lemmon, to ſoak
the Potage, when ready to be ſerv'd up. It ought alſo to be
enrich'd with Muſhrooms, Artichoke-bottoms, and other ſorts of
Garnitures.

Potage of Pigeons, with Radiſhes.

Having larded your Pigeons, with thick Slips of Bacon, and
having fried them till they come to a fine brown colour, let them
be gently ſtew'd in good Broth, with a Bunch of Herbs · Let
a thickening Liquor be alſo prepai'd with fine Herbs and pour'd
upon them. When the Cruſts are ſoak'd in good Broth, garniſh
your Potage with the Radiſhes that are very white and neatly
dreſs'd; one part of them being cut into little ſquare pieces, and
the other remaining entire.

A Potage of farced Pigeons, likewiſe fried brown, may be
made after the ſame manner; ſo as a thickening Liquor may be
added as they are ſtewing, and the Diſh garniſh'd in the ſame
manner, with Radiſhes.

Potage of Pigeons, with a white Cullis.

This Potage may be garniſh'd with *Poupiets,* and the Limbs
of Barn-door-chickens marinated and fried   A white Cullis is
to be pour'd upon the Pigeons, and a Loaf ſet in the middle, or
elſe a Border may be made of Aſparagus, with a *Profitrolle-*loaf,
ſqueezing ſome Lemmon-juice upon it, when ſerved up to
Table.

See the white Potage of Pigeons with Onions, before deſcribed
in the fourteenth Article.

Parmeſan-potage.

This Potage may be garniſh'd with little *Profitrolle*-loaves,
very neatly chipt, which are to be ſoak d in melted Lard, and
P   after-

afterwards ftrew'd with rafped Parmefan, to be brought to a
colour in the Oven   When the Potage is laid a foaking in a
Difh, a Lay muft be made of Parmefan, another of fome good
Meat-hafh, and a third of Cinnamon : This is to be done twice,
and all may be colour'd by means of the red-hot Fire-fhovel.
Then let your Potage be garnifh'd on the Sides, with Crufts of
Bread made very brown, the Middle with your Loaves, and
the Intervals with Veal-fweet-breads, larded *Fricandoes*, *Truffles*
and Cocks-combs ; fqueezing in the Juice of a Lemmon, when
ferv'd up to Table.

For another Parmefan-potage, let the Flefh of a Chicken be
minc'd very fmall, which muft be ftrew'd upon the Crufts, and
afterwards fome rafped Parmefan on the top   A Loaf may be
laid in the middle, and the whole Mefs may be fet out with Artichoke-bottoms, and other ufual Garnitures , or elfe it may be
left without garnifhing, only giving it a fine colour with the red-
hot Fire-fhovel

For a *Cafferole*, with Parmefan, fee the fecond Article of
Cafferole, under the Letter C.

Potage of *Quails*, with a Blanç-manger.

Having ftew'd your Quails in good Broth, with Salt and a
Bunch of Herbs, pound fome Almonds, which are to be ftrain'd
thro' a Sieve into the fame Broth, and let them boil, with a
little Cinnamon and Sugar : Then cover the Bottom of your
Difh of Potage, with Macaroons, Biskets and March-panes, and
when the Quails are drefs'd, pour the white Broth upon them ;
garnifhing all with Slices of Lemmon, as alfo with the Juice and
Kernels of Pomegranate, when ready to be ferv'd up to Table.

The other Potages of Quails fhall be hereafter explain'd ,
either in particular in the Article of Quails, under the Letter Q,
or elfewhere, with refpect to other Fowls.

Potage of *Partridges*, with brown Broth.

Lard your Partridges with middle-fiz'd Slips of Bacon, fry
them in Lard with a little Flower, and afterwards put all into
a Pot, with good Broth, a Faggot of Herbs, and as much Salt
as is needful.   In the mean while, the Cullis is to be made of a
piece of roafted Beef, ftew'd in the fame Partridge-broth, and
kept hot ; Then let fome boil'd Artichoke-bottoms be cut into
                                                              pieces

pieces and thrown into the Cullis, with Slices of Lemmon and Cocks-combs ftew'd, and put into a Ragoo. When the Potage is fufficiently foak'd, drefs your Partridges and Garnitures, pour the Cullis upon them, with fome Slices and Juice of Lemmon, as they are ferving up to Table.

A Potage may alfo be made with Cray-fifh, obferving the Directions given for the making of that fort of Potage on Fifh-days, in the fecond Article of Cray-fifh. It may be garnifh'd with Veal-fweet-breads, Capons-livers, *Fricandoes*, Partridge-*Pains*, and other Things that are at hand.

See above, the Partridge-potages that are made with Cabbage, Lentils, and other forts of Pulfe.

Potage of a Breaſt of Veal and Capon, with a Loaf in the Middle.

The Loaf muft be farc'd with the Breafts of Capons and Partridges and fome Mutton minc'd together, as alfo Artichoke-bottoms and Veal-fweet-breads cut into little fquare pieces, *Truffles*, Cocks-combs and Mufhrooms in a Ragoo, and a Veal-cullis. This Loaf ought to be open on the Top, fo as the Ragoo may be feen, and marbled with Veal-gravy and Lemmon-juice. After having drefs'd the Potage, it muft be garnifh'd round about the Veal-fweet-breads and Cocks-combs, all ftew'd with white Sauce, adding fome Lemmon-juice when ferv'd up to Table.

Potage of young Turkeys, with Succory.

Take young Turkeys, large fat Pullets, Chickens and other Fowls, and boil them in a Pot after the ufual manner, with Broth, Salt and a Bunch of Herbs· Let your Succory be fcald-ed in Water, and boil'd with the reft: Then let the Potage be drefs'd and laid a foaking, garnifhing it with Succory, and ferving it up, with natural Broth, Mutton-gravy and Mufhrooms.

Potage of fat Pullets.

Let a large fat Pullet be cut into pieces, and marinated in Lemmon-juice or Verjuice, with the other feafoning Ingredients: Then let a Pafte be made with Verjuice to fry them in, till they come to a fine colour, in order to garnifh the Potage

round

round about another fat Pullet, that has been well boil'd in good Broth In the mean while, prepare a Cullis with the Bones of the marinated Pullet, Crusts of Bread and good Broth, and sprinkle your Potage with it, as it lies a soaking, as also with the Juice of a Lemmon, before it is brought to Table.

Potage after the Italian Mode.

This Potage is a kind of *Oil* dress'd in a large Dish, after having made a Partition in it, in form of a Cross, with Paste baked in the Oven. In one of the Squares, a *Bisk* is to be put; in the second a Potage, of young Chickens; in the third, a Potage *à la Reyne*, with a *Profitrolle*-loaf; and in the fourth, a Potage of farced Partridges; all in their peculiar Broths, and with different Garnitures, as rich as they possibly can be.

Potage of farced green Geese.

Let a Farce be made with the Livers and Hearts of Geese, fine Herbs, and an Omelet of four Eggs, which are to be pounded together in a Mortar, and well season'd, in order to stuff your Geese between the Skin and the Flesh. Then boil them in good Broth, and prepare some green Pease-soop to be pour'd upon the Potage. For want of new Pease, old ones may be taken, to make the green Cullis; and the whole Mess may be garnish'd with farced Lettice.

White Potage.

The Potage *à la Reyne*, described in the seventh Article, may be so call'd, as well as these that follow

Having caus'd the Breasts of Chickens or Capons to be minc'd very small, strew them upon your soaked Potage; marbling it with very brown Veal-gravy, and squeezing in some Lemmon-juice, when serv'd up to Table.

Otherwise pound the Flesh of a Pullet or some Capons-breasts in a Mortar, with a piece of very white Bread-crum, strain all thro' the Hair-sieve, and when the Crusts are soak'd, pour this Cullis upon them, without any Garniture.

Potage of boned Capons, with Oisters.

After having taken out the Bones of your Capons, referving the Skins entire, ftuff the Skins with the fame Flefh, Beef-few-et or Marrow, pounded Lard, fine Herbs, Pepper, Salt, Nut-meg and Yolks of Eggs, and let them boil in good Broth · Af-terwards fry Oisters, Mufhrooms and Flower in a Pan, and put all to the Capons, when they are almoft ready · Let them be drefs'd and orderly ferv'd up, with Lemmon-juice and Mufh-rooms

For the other Potages that are made of Fifh on Flefh-days, fee here after that of Soles.

POTAGES FOR FISH-DAYS.

Potage de Santé.

Let Purflain, Lettice, Sorrel, Beets and other good Herbs be cut and ftew'd a little with Butter in an earthen Pot, to take away their Crudity : Then put fome boiling Water to them, with Salt, a Bunch of fine Herbs, and a Loaf, or Cruft which is to be fet in the middle of the Potage   The Herbs may be ftrain'd, if you fhall think fit; or they may be ferv'd up to Table and garnifh'd, with young Lettice, Mufhroom-juice, and a Spoonful of Peafe-foop.

The Potage without Butter, and the *Julian,* come fo near to this, that it would be needlefs to give a particular Defcription of them.

Potage of Moufferons *and* Morilles, *with Cream.*

The *Moufferons* and *Morilles* muft be ftew'd, or fried in good Butter with fine Herbs, after the fame manner as in Oil, for other forts of Potages   When the Crufts are fufficiently foak'd, the Cream muft be put with the *Moufferons* into the Stew-pan in which they are drefs'd, with a Faggot of Herbs, and all muft be well thicken'd   At the fame time, the Potage is to be drefs'd, with a *Profitrolle* loaf in the middle, and Lemmon-juice, before it is ferved up   The fide of the Difh may be fet out with *Moufferons* fried in Fritters, or fome other convenient Garnitures

Po-

Potage of Onions, with a white Cullis.

This Potage may be dress'd, if you please, with a Loaf in the middle; whilst a Cullis is preparing, with white Almonds, Parsly-roots and Bread-crum soak'd in Pease-soop, all strain'd thro' a Hair-sive. The same Cullis is proper not only for the Onions; but also for Cardoons, Goats-bread, Skirrets, &c.

Another Potage may be made of Onions, cut into square pieces, and fried brown, to be garnish'd with other Onions cut into round pieces, and fried as Fritters, or else whole: As also a Potage of Onions, with sweet Basil.

Potage, with Hops.

The Hops are to be well scalded, tied up in Bunches, and stew'd in good Pease-soop, or in some other sort of Broth proper for Fish-days: Then the Potage may be garnish'd, with a Loaf in the middle.

Potage of Purslain.

The Purslain, if it be small, must be laid at its whole length into a little Pot, and boil'd in Broth, or Pease-soop, with an Onion stuck with Cloves, a Carret, a few Parsnips, and a thickening Liquor: When it is ready, and the Crusts are well soaked, the Potage may be garnish'd in the usual manner.

Potage, with young Sprouts.

Let some Sprouts be well pickt and thrown into fair Water: Then after they have been scalded, let them be put into a Pot, pouring in a small Cullis, as for the Purslain; and let them be garnish'd with other Sprouts.

Potage of Radishes.

After they have been well scrap'd, leave a small Bunch of the Greens at the end: Then let them be scalded and boil'd in good Broth, with some thickening Liquor. This Potage must be dress'd after the same manner as that of Purslain.

Potage, with Cucumbers.

Let your Cucumbers be fcalded, and ftew'd in good Peafe-foop, with an Onion ftuck with Cloves, and fome Roots of Herbs chopt fmall : Then a thickening Liquor muft be made, as for other Potages, on Flefh-days, and the Difh fet out with Cucumbers and Capers. They may alfo be farced with Herbs, or Fifh, and garnifh'd with Afparagus-tops, according to the Seafon.

Afparagus-potage.

For want of Peafe, pounded Afparagus may be ftrain'd thro' the Hair-fieve, with Herb-broth, to make the green Cullis; whilft other Afparagus are fried in Butter, with fine Herbs, and afterwards laid a foaking, feafon'd with Salt and Nutmeg. The Potage muft be cover'd, with the Cullis pour'd into it, and you may add fome natural Cream, or Yolks of Eggs, if the time will allow it.

Potage, of farced Lettice.

Obferve the preceding Directions for farced Lettice, laid down in that Article, under the Letter L, except, that they ought now to be ftuff'd with a good Fifh-farce, fuch as is before defcribed in the Article of *Farces*; and, if the Entertainment be provided for Days of greater Abftinence, or if Fifh be wanting, let them be ftuff'd with a good Farce of fine Herbs, feafon'd with Pepper, Salt, Nutmeg and Yolks of Eggs, or Cream For the reft, they muft be boil'd in ftrained Peafe-foop, or Herb-broth, and drefs'd upon the Crufts, foak'd, with the fame Broth; adding a white Cullis and Mufhroom-juice, when ready to be ferv'd up. The whole Mefs may be fet out with fried Bread, or fome other convenient Garniture.

Marbled Potage.

This is a Potage of Almond-milk, to which are added, Yolks of Eggs, Sugar, Cinnamon and a little Salt It muft be drefs'd upon Bread, or Biskets, and marbled with the Juice, or Jelly of Currans, Beet-juice boil'd with Sugar and Orange-flowers The Difh is to be garnifh'd with Pomegranate-kernels and fmall Sugar-plums, P 4 *Po-*

Potage, with Fennel.

Let Fennel be chopt very fmall, and put into a little Pot, obferving, for the reft, the fame Directions as for the following Potage.

Potage, with Spinage.

Take only the Heart or foundeft part of the Spinage, which muft be chopt fmall and ftew'd in a little Pot with Peafe-foop, a Carret, an Onion ftuck with Cloves, and the other feafoning Ingredients As the Crufts are foaking, fcrape in fome Parmefan, and drefs your Potage; garnifhing it with fticks of Cinnamon, round about, and one in the middle, or elfe with Onions, or fried Bread.

Potage of Vine-buds.

Cut off the largeft Leaves of your Buds, and take care that none of the Wood be left : Then having fcalded 'em in boiling Water and tied them up in Bunches, let them be ftew'd in a little Pot, with a Carret, a Parfnip, Parfly-roots, an Onion ftuck with Cloves, a few Turneps cut into quarters, and a Clove of Garlick.   Add to thefe as they are dreffing, a little thickening Liquor, and garnifh your Potage, with other Buds and a Loaf in the middle.

Green Peafe-potage.

See the Peafe-potage for Flefh-days, and obferve the fame Method; except, that your Peafe muft now be drefs'd with fweet Butter, and ferv'd up in good Broth.   For fimple Peafefoop, the Difh may be fet out with Cucumbers, Artichoke-bottoms, Afparagus-tops, and other things of the like nature.

Cabbage-potage.

See likewife the Cabbage-potage for Flefh-days, in the third Article, where the manner of preparing it is fully explain'd; retrenching the Lard, and making ufe only of Butter and Broth that is proper for Fifh-days, or ftrained Peafe-foop. This Potage

tage muft be garnifh'd with the infide of fome Cabbage, Artichoke-bottoms and fried Bread.

Potage of Citrulls, with Milk.

Cut your Citrulls into very fmall fquare pieces; and fry them
in natural Butter, with Salt, Parfly, Chervil and fine Herbs.
Then let them be put into an Earthen Pot, with boiling Milk,
and drefs them upon the foak'd Crufts Garnifh the Difh with
with fried Bread, and ftrew it with white Pepper, as it is ferving up to Table.

Melon-potage.

Let the Melons be cut as the Citruls, and fried likewife with
Butter . Then let them be ftewed, feafon d with Pepper, Salt
and a Bunch of Herbs, and ftrain'd thro' the Hair-fieve, with
the fame Broth ; with which the Crufts are alfo to be foak'd.
Afterwards having drefs'd the Potage, ferve it up, garnifh'd
with fried Melons and Pomegranate-kernels.

Potage, with Mufcadine-grapes.

Let good Almond-milk be prepar'd, according to the Method laid down in the fecond Article of *Almonds*, under the
Letter A. and when you have a mind to drefs your Soop, let
fome Mufcadine-grapes be put into it, after they have been
ftoned. Inftead of Crufts, or other pieces of Bread, let the Potage be drefs'd with Macaroons, or Biskets, and garnifh'd with
Mufcadine-grapes, preferv'd with Sugar; marbling it with the
Juice of a Lemmon and that of Currans, when ferv'd up to
Table.

Potage of Artichoke-cardoons.

The Cardoons muft be cut very fhort, fcalded and boil'd in
Water, with Butter, Salt, and a Cruft of Bread : Then they
are to be put into melted Butter , whilft the Potage is foaking
with good Herb-broth : Let the Cruft of a fmall Loaf be laid
entire in the middle , let the Cardoons be drefs'd in form of a
Dome or Coronet, upon the Bread , and let fome fcraped Parmefan be added. You may alfo prepare a white Cullis, ftrewing
the

the whole Mefs again with fcrap'd Cheefe, and garnifhing it
with Capers and Lemmon-flices.

Potage of white Cabbage and young Chibbols, with Milk.

After the Cabbage has been fcalded in Water, let it be chopt
and fried in natural Butter : Then let it be put into hot Milk,
feafon'd with Pepper, Salt and a Faggot of fine Herbs, and
drefs'd upon Slices of Bread.

The fame thing is to be done with young Chibbols cut very
fmall.

Potage of Artichoke-bottoms.

Cut your Bottoms into halves, and fry them in burnt Butter,
with Flower, or in natural Butter , referving one entire, for the
middle of the Potage : Then put them into an earthen Pot, with
clear Peafe-foop, Salt and fine Herbs, and when they are ready,
drefs them upon the foaked Crufts ; in order to be ferv'd up,
with Capers and Mufhroom-juice

Thefe Potages are more than fufficient, as to what relates to
Herbs and Pulfe ; either for Good Friday, or for the other
Fifh-days throughout the whole Year : Let us now proceed to
the Fifh-potages, of which we have not as yet given a particular Account.

FISH-POTAGES.

Sturgeon-potage.

When the Sturgeon is well cleans'd , let it be ftew'd for a
while in Water, with Butter, Salt and a Bunch of fine Herbs
As foon as it is half done, take away this Liquor or Broth, and
put the Fifh again into a Stew-pan, or earthen Pan, with white
Wine, Pepper, Salt, beaten Cloves, Verjuice, Onions, and a
Bay-leaf or two, with which you muft make an end of boiling
it : In the mean while, fry fome Mufhrooms and Flower in Butter, which are to be put into the firft Broth for your Potage, with
a Spoonful of Peafe-foop Then let the Crufts of Bread be
foak'd with it, in a round or Oval Difh, and the Sturgeon drefs'd
therein , after having been well drain'd. You may garnifh
the whole Mefs, with Oifters, Mufhrooms and Capers; adding
fome Juice and Slices of Lemmon, when ready to be ferv'd up
to Table.   *Tur-*

Turbot-potage.

Let the Turbot be fcal'd, wrapt up in a Linnen-cloth and boil'd in one half white Wine and the other Water, with Ver-juice, Pepper, Salt, Nutmeg, Cloves and Bay-leaves Then let the Crufts be foak'd in good Fifh-broth, and when the Tur-bot is drain'd, let it be drefs'd and garnifh'd, with Mufhrooms, upon the Body of the Fifh, but the fides of the Difh muft be fet out, with farced Mufhrooms, Roes, Oifters, Capers and Slices of Lemmon, with Juice of the fame.

Potage of frefh Salmon.

The Salmon muft be fcal'd, cut into pieces, and parboil'd as the Sturgeon, to get the Broth Afterwards it muft be feafon'd with Salt, fine Herbs chopt fmall, and ftrained Peafe-foop; and whilft the Crufts are foaking, your Salmon when well feafon'd, muft be boil'd outright over a gentle Fire. When 'tis requifite to ferve it up, let it be drefs'd, and garnifh'd with farced Mufh-rooms, Carp-roes, ftew'd Mufhrooms, Capers, the Juice and Sli-ces of Lemmon and Mufhroom-juice

Sole-potage for Fifh-days.

To prepare a Potage of Soles, having provided fome of the beft fort, that are very frefh, let them be fcrap'd and well wafh'd : If they are fmall, take two of them to be farced, but if large, only one, to be fet in the middle of your Potage The Sole that you would have farced, muft be neatly taken by the Head, and fqueez'd on the top, to get out the Bone entire. Then ta-king a little of this Flefh and of that of a Carp, to make a Farce of it, with Chibbol, Parfly and Bread-crum, fet it together a-gain in the fame manner as when it was whole. It muft be farc'd all at once, and other Soles muft be fried, in order to get the *Filets* for the garnifhing of the Potage In the mean while, a good Ragoo ought to be made, in the fame manner as for the Cray-fifh-potage, and alfo a Cullis of the like nature. Afterwards let the Potage be laid a foaking with good Fifh-broth, whilft the farced Sole is frying, which muft be laid in the Po-tage, when it is fufficiently foak'd, and ready to be ferv'd up. Laftly, let the *Filets* of the other fried Soles be garnifh'd with

Carp-

Carp-roes and Artichoke-bottoms , let the Ragoo be pour'd round about, and let the Sole remain uncover'd, so as it may appear of a fine colour, when the whole Mess is brought hot to Table

If it be not the time of Lent, an *Omelet* may be made to be mingled with the Farce, and instead of frying the Soles, they may also be put into a Baking-pan rubb'd with Butter: They must be breaded to give them a colour, and bak'd in an Oven moderately heated.

A Potage may likewise be made only of Sole-*Filets*, with a Loaf in the middle, garnish'd with Onions fried brown ; also a Potage of Sole-*Filets*, with sweet Basil.

Potage of Soles on Flesh-days.

The Broth and Gravy are the same as for other Potages that are proper for Flesh-days.   For the rest, having provided Soles, take the raw *Filets* of some of them, and stuff them neatly with larded Veal-sweet-breads, which may serve for the Garniture of your Potage : For the farced Sole in the middle of the Potage; let it be scrap'd, and a Hole made in the Head, to get out the Bone, so as the Skin may remain altogether entire : Take some of the Flesh of the same Sole, with a little parboil'd Bacon, a few pieces of Veal-sweet-breads, *Truffles* and Mushrooms, all well minc'd, and to make the Farce more delicious, 'twould be requisite to put into it some Bread-crum soak'd in a little Milk, binding it with two Yolks of Eggs, and adding a little chopt Parsly and Chibbol.   Then the Sole must be stuff'd with this Farce, and when ready to be serv'd up, it must be flower'd and fried in Lard, till it come to a fine colour.   With the rest of the Farce, some small *Andouillets* are to be made and fried, flowering and breading them, after they have been dipt in beaten Eggs, to the end that the Bread may stick to them.   As for the *Filets* ; when they are larded with the Veal-sweet-breads, they must be flower'd a little, and fried in the same Lard   The Potage being well soak'd, let it be garnish'd with these *Filets*, as also with Veal-sweet-breads and *Andouillets*; let the Sole be set in the middle of the Potage, with a Ragoo of Lamb-sweet-breads and *Truffles*, according to the Season ; let all be well garnish'd , let the Potage-loaf be soak'd in good Gravy ; and let the whole Mess be serv'd up hot to Table.

At another time, the Sole in the middle may be larded, and

to

to that purpofe, after it has been fcrap'd, wafh'd and well wip'd, the red-hot Fire-fhovel muft be lightly pafs'd over the Back, to the end that the Larding-pin may have a freer Paffage : Then it may be fried as the other Sole ; it may alfo be put into a Baking-pan with Bacon underneath, and be brought to a colour upon the Spit, or in the Oven.

For Side-difhes, they may be made of Soles, with the above-mention'd Ragoo; garnifhing them with *Filets*, *Andouillets* and other Things, all brought hot to Table.

Potage of Tortoifes on Fifh-days.

Having cùt off the Heads and Legs of your Tortoifes, the Day before, fteep them in Water, to take away the Blood, and then let them be well boil'd in a little Pot of a proportionable fize, in Water, with a little Salt and Parfly, frefh Butter, a Chibbol ftuck with Cloves, and a few fine Herbs If you would have the Broth of a more exquifite relifh, add the Bones of Carps or other Fifh, the Flefh of which was taken to make Farces. Then take out the Tortoifes, and ftrain the Broth, which will ferve both for the Potage and for the Ragoo : The Shell on the top of the Tortoifes muft be taken away, as alfo the Skin, referving the Flefh, which muft not be too much boil'd : But you muft be fure to clear it from the Gall, and keep the Shell to make a thin Pafte or Batter for the frying of it, as if it were marinated Meat in Pafte ; this will ferve to be put in the middle of the Potage. Having likewife taken fome of the Flefh of the Tortoife, ftew it in a Sauce-pan with a little Butter, Chibbol and Parfly, and moiften the Ragoo with the fame Broth. Afterwards turn in the Roes, *Truffles*, Mufhrooms and other Garnitures, if you have any, with a little Cullis of Cray-fifh, or fome other fort of Fifh, and let your Crufts be well foak d · Let fome fried Fifh-*Filets* be alfo ready at hand, as being very proper to garnifh the Potage. Moreover, it will be requifite to provide a fmall white Cullis of Pikes-flefh, to fprinkle the Potage, that it may be marbled with the Ragoo , and alfo, fome Cray-fifh Cullis. At laft, you may drefs your Potage with the Ragoo pour'd on the top, the *Filets* round about marbled with both the Cullifes, and the Shell that was fried, in the middle.

Potage of Tortoises, on Flesh-days.

For this Potage, the Tortoises must be order'd as before, to get their Flesh, which is to be fried in Lard with fine Herbs; whilst a Cullis is preparing, with a piece of Veal roasted very brown, which is to be pounded in a Mortar, with the Breast of a Capon or Pullet, five or six Almonds, and a piece of Bread-crum soak'd in good Broth: Let all be boil'd in a Stew-pan well season'd, and afterwards strain'd thro' the Hair-sieve, with a piece of green Lemmon. This Cullis will serve to enrich the Potage as it lies a soaking: Then you may garnish the sides of the Dish, with Veal-sweet-breads cut into pieces, Artichoke-bottoms, and larded *Poupiets* fried brown a-part; and the Middle with the Shells fried till they come to a fine colour; squeezing in some Lemmon-juice, when serv'd up to Table.

A Potage, with Crusts farced with Quavivers and Perches, with a white Cullis.

Let your Quavivers, or Perches be boil'd in Water with Salt, and having taken away the Skin, let the Flesh be minc'd very small: Then let a Cullis be made with some of the same Flesh, and a douzen of Almonds; pounding them with three or four Yolks of Eggs, if the time will permit. Lastly, let the Hash be dress'd with good Butter and fine Herbs, and make use of it to strew upon the soaked Crusts; adding some Lemmon-juice, before it is brought to Table.

Potage, with Crusts farced with Soles.

The Hash must be made as before, after having fried the Soles, with Lentils dress'd in the Cullis; or else a green Cullis may be prepar'd with Asparagus-tops.

Potage, with Crusts farced with Pike.

This Potage must be order'd as the former, with a green Cullis and Asparagus-tops, in their Season, or else with a white Cullis.

§ *Perch-potage, with a white Cullis.*

After having well wash'd the Perches, let them be boil'd in Water, with Pepper, Salt, Cloves, an Onion and Thyme, and afterwards neatly pickt: But one of them must be taken to make a Cullis, with a few pounded Almonds and some Yolks of Eggs, according to the Season: Let all be pounded together in a Mortar, well season'd and strain'd thro' the Hair-sieve. Then some Carp-hash must be put upon the Crusts, with the Cullis, and the whole Mess must be garnish'd with fried Bread.

Frog-potage.

Let the Legs of your Frogs be cut off, and the Thigh-bones broken, after the Flesh has been taken away; reserving the thickest to be fried: These being marinated with Verjuice, Pepper and Salt, and dipt into a thin Paste or Batter, must be fried till they come to a fine colour, to make a Border round about the Potage. The rest are to be dress'd in a Ragoo, with Roes, Mushrooms and other Garnitures, all dress'd with a white Sauce. Lastly, the Potage must be garnish'd, after it has been well soak'd, pouring a Cullis upon it, and squeezing in the Juice of a Lemmon.

Potage, with a Profitrolle-*loaf.*

Having prepar'd a Carp-hash dress'd in Broth, with Butter, fine Herbs and a piece of green Lemmon, let it be stew'd and season'd till it has acquir'd a good relish. Then cut some Pike, or Quavivers into Collops, which are to be marinated in Verjuice, with Pepper, Salt and Onion; and, when flower'd, must be fried till they come to a fine colour; these will serve to garnish the Potage. Afterwards turn your Hash upon the soaked Bread, set the *Profitrolle*-loaf in the middle, and squeez in some Lemmon-juice, as the Dish is serving up to Table.

Tortoise-potage, with a Profitrolle-*loaf.*

This Potage may be garnish'd with Cray-fish, and fried Shells in the Intervals. Let a brown Cullis be made, as for Cray-fish, and let the Tortoises be cut into *Fricandoes* or Collops, as

it

it were Chickens ; with a white Cullis, and a piece of green
Lemmon.   As the Crufts are foaking, let fome Fifh-hafh be laid
upon them, and Roes fried brown, with fine Herbs. Afterwards
your Tortoifes may be drefs'd, with a Loaf in the middle, and
Lemmon-juice.

Potage à la Royale.

Take Eels-flefh, with the like quantity of Mufhrooms, which
are to be fried in natural Butter, chopt all together, and put
into a Pot, with good Fifh-broth, feafoned with Salt and a
Faggot of Herbs.   In the mean time, the Crufts being foaked
with the fame Fifh-broth, cover them with your minc'd Meat,
and garnifh them with Carp-roes, Pike-livers, and farced Mufhrooms; adding fome Slices and Juice of Lemmon, with the Juice
of Mufhrooms and Capers, when ferved up to Table.

Oifter-potage.

It would be requifite to fry the Oifters in burnt Butter, and
to referve their Liquor, as it has been elfewhere obferv'd · At
the fame time, you muft alfo fry with your Oifters, fome Mufhrooms cut into pieces, and a little Flower, and afterwards let
all boil in ftrained Peafe-foop, with Salt and a piece of green
Lemmon · Then the Bread being foak'd in good Fifh-broth, and
the Oifters and Mufhrooms drefs'd, they may be garnifh'd with
Capers and Lemmon-flices, and fo ferv'd up, after having
pour'd the Oifter-liquor into the Potage, with the Juices of
Mufhrooms and Lemmons.

Potage of farced Tenches, with brown Broth.

The Tenches muft be firft cleans'd from their Slime in hot
Water, and their Skins entirely taken away, as the fame thing
may be done with Soles   Then prepare a Farce with the Flefh,
alfo Mufhrooms, fine Herbs, Yolks of Eggs, Salt and Nutmeg, and
having ftuff'd them with it, as if they were whole; let them
boil in ftrained Peafe-foop, or in fome other Broth, with Butter.
In the mean while, let Mufhrooms be fried in Butter, with
Flower, and ftew'd in other Broth, or Liquor, feafon'd with Salt,
Cloves, and a Bunch of Herbs.   This Broth will ferve to foak
the Crufts, upon which the Tenches are to be drefs'd ; garnifhing

ing the Dish with Mushrooms, Capers, Carp-roes; as also with Lemmon-juice and Slices of the fame, as it is ferving up to Table.

Farced Crabs, and other Fish of the like nature, may also be drefs'd in the fame fort of Potage

A P O T - P O U R R I, *or* Hotch-potch.

This Way of dreffing is proper for feveral forts of Meat, particularly, Ducks, young Turkeys, Leverets, &c. They muft firft be larded with thick Slips of Bacon, and fried in Lard to give them a colour : Afterwards, they are to be boil'd or ftew'd in Broth, with white Wine, a Faggot of Herbs, Pepper and Salt When they are half done, let fome Mufhrooms be fried in the fame Lard, with a little Flower, and let all be mingled together, with Gravy, or an Artichoke cullis, *Andouillets*, Veal-fweet-breads, Oifters (if you fhall think fit) and Cucumbers marinated, according to the Seafon. This Hotch-potch, when neatly drefs'd with Mutton-gravy and Lemmon-juice, muft be ferv'd up hot to Table for a Side-dish

P O U P E T O N S.

In giving Directions for making the *Godivoe* of a *Poupeton* in the Article of *Godivoe*, under the Letter G, we have alfo explain'd, what is moft remarkable, with refpect to all the reft; particularly, for a *Poupeton* farced with young Pigeons and other forts of Fowl So that it only remains here to fhew the manner of diverfifying them, when green Peafe are in feafon.

A Poupeton, *with green Peafe.*

The *Poupeton* being made after the ufual manner, let two or three Handfuls of ftrained Peafe be thrown into it, before it is cover'd with its Farce, and let all be enclos'd with the *Godivoe* Then it muft be bak'd *à la Braife*, that is to fay, between two Fires, one on the top and the other underneath, and afterwards put into a Dish Some Spoonfuls of Peafe may alfo be added, before it is brought hot to Table.

A Poupeton *for Fiſh-days.*

Take the Fleſh of Carps and Pike, and let a well ſeaſon'd *Godivoe* be made of it, with Bread-crum or Flower; all being well chopt together : To theſe you may add an Egg or two, if it be not in Lent; ſhaping your *Poupeton,* as the former, and laying ſome Sole-*Filets,* or others in the middle, which are to be dreſs'd with ſweet Butter and all ſorts of good Garnitures. A fine Artichoke-bottom muſt likewiſe be ſet in the middle, after the Ragoo and Fiſh-*Filets,* and the *Poupeton* is to be quite fill'd up with the Ragoo-ſauce. Afterwards, let all be cover'd with your *Godivoe* or Farce, and bak'd or ſtew'd between two gentle Fires. When it is ready, it muſt be turn'd into a Diſh upſide downwards, and ſerv'd up with Lemmon-juice.

P O U P I E T S.

To make *Poupiets* it will be requiſite to provide ſome *Bards,* or thin Slices of Bacon that are ſomewhat long, but not too broad, according to the thickneſs you would have the *Poupiets* to be of, with as many Veal-ſtakes ; which, when well beaten, muſt be laid upon every *Bard* In the mean while, having prepar'd a good Farce ſeaſon'd with a Clove of Garlick and other Ingredients, let as much of it as you ſhall think fit, be put upon the Stakes or Slices, and then let them be cloſe roll'd up. Afterwards they muſt be pierc'd with a ſmall Iron-Spit, and roaſted wrapt up in Paper When they are almoſt ready, the Paper is to be taken away, in order to bread them, and give them a fine colour Theſe *Poupiets* may ſerve either for a particular Diſh, or for Out-works, or only to garniſh other Meſſes. They are alſo ſometimes dreſs'd in a Ragoo, as *Fricandoes,* with a piece of Lemmon, as they are ſtewing, and ſome Juice of the ſame, as they are ſerving up to Table

Larded Poupiets.

Larded *Poupiets* are likewiſe prepar'd upon occaſion, and fried brown, with pieces of *Truffles, Morilles,* and good Gravy, or a little Cullis to enrich them ; ſqueezing in ſome Lemmon-juice, when ready to be brought to Table.

P U D

PUDDINGS.

There are two forts of Hogs-puddings, *viz.* white and black, and both are ufually ferv'd up among the Side-difhes. The formei is moft delicious, and may be made thus.

To make white Puddings.

Having roafted a young Turkey, and alfo a Capon (if a great quantity of Pudding be required) take the Breafts of thofe Fowls, and let them be well minc'd Then cut fome Leaf-fat taken out of a Hog's Belly, very fmall, and put all into a Stew-pan, with a litle chopt Onion, that was fried in it before, and a few fine Herbs of all forts, except Parfly · Seafon thefe Ingredients with the ordinary Spices, and pour in as much Milk, as you fhall judge needfull Let them alfo boil together, for a while, and then having drawn back the Stew-pan, add two or three Whites of Eggs wh'pt, taking care that the Farce be not too liquid, Afterwards, the Puddings may be made with the prepared Guts, and as they are filling, they muft be prickt a little, to let out the Wind : They muft alfo be fcalded in a little Water and Milk, with fome Slices of Onion, and when taken out, left to cool upon a clean Napkin. In order to ferve them up, they muft be broil d upon Paper, ovei a gentle Fire, left they fhould break, putting to them a little Lard or other Fat ; and, when ready, they muft be brought hot to Table.

To make black Puddings.

Let fome Hogs blood that is not coagulated be put into a Stew-pan, with a little Milk, and a Spoonful of fat Broth, to render it more delicious, and let fome Leaf-fat out of the Hog's Belly be cut into fmall pieces, and mingled with chopt Parfly, Chibbol, and all forts of fine Herbs, which are to be fried in fome of the fame Fat · Then let them all be turn'd into the fame Sauce-pan, and feafon'd with beaten Spices. In the mean time, a Pot or Kettle is to be hang'd over the Fire, with boiling Water, and the Stew-pan containing the Blood muft be fer in it, to be kept hot ; ftiri ng it neverthelefs, continually, to hinder it from fticking to the bottom. As foon as you percieve all to have acquir'd a good Relifh, the Puddings may be made

Q 2

of what thicknefs, or length, you fhall think fit, and fcalded in Water, but as they are fcalding, let them be prickt with a Pin: If nothing comes out but Fat, 'tis a Sign that they are fufficiently parboil'd; fo that they may be neatly taken out, and when cold, they muft be broil'd upon a Grid-iron, as occafion requires, in order to be ferv'd up hot, as before

Other forts of Puddings.

Puddings may be alfo made of the Livers of Capons and Calves: For the former, let a quarter of a Pound of Hogsleaf-fat be chopt fmall, with a Pound of the Livers, and as much of the Flefh of Capons, and let all be well feafon'd with fine Herbs, Chibbols, Pepper, Salt, Nutmeg, beaten Cloves, Cinnamon, fix Yolks of raw Eggs, and two Quarts of Cream. Then fill up the Guts of a Hog, Sheep, or Lamb, and boil your Puddings in Milk, with Salt, green Lemmon and Bay-leaves: They muft be broil'd in the fame manner as the former, and ferv'd up with Orange-juice. For the other fort of Pudding, you are to mince a Calves-liver, and pound it in a Mortar, with Hogs fat, to the quantity of one third part, which muft likewife be cut into fmall fquare pieces: Let this Mixture be feafon'd, as before, and ftuff'd into Hogs or Calves-guts. Thefe Puddings muft be fcalded in white Wine, with Salt and a few Bay-leaves, over a gentle Fire, and left to cool in their own Liquor, to be broil'd and order'd as the others

PULLETS.

We have already produc'd a Side-difh of fat Pullets drefs'd with Olives, which may alfo be made in like manner, with other forts of Fowls, and fhall here fubjoyn fome other particular Difhes of Pullets, no lefs remarkable and delicious.

Large fat Pullets drefs'd after the Englifh Way.

A Farce is to be firft prepar'd, with Bacon, Calves-udder, Veal-fweet-breads, and a little Marrow, as alfo, *Truffles*, Mufhrooms, Artichoke-bottoms, Capers, and a little Garlick; all fcalded, minc'd and well feafon'd The Pullets, being ftuff'd in the Body with this Farce, and well tied up, with a good Slice of Bacon on their Breafts, muft be roafted, wrapt up in Paper: Then
they

they may be dreſs'd with a little Sauce, made of *Truffles*, Muſh-rooms, Anchovies, a few Capers and Veal-gravy; all chopt ſmall, ſtew'd and well ſoak'd   A little Cullis muſt alſo be ad-ded, and the Juice of an Orange ſqueez'd in, when the Diſh is ready to be ſerv'd up to Table.

Fat Pullets farced upon the Bones, with Cream.

After having roaſted large fat Pullets, let the Fleſh of their Breaſts be well minc'd, with boil'd Bacon, a piece of dreſs'd Gammon, a few Muſhrooms, *Truffles*, Chibbols, Parſly, and the Crum of a Loaf ſteept in Cream, after it has been ſoak'd a little at the Fire; to all theſe, when chopt very ſmall, ſome Yolks of Eggs are alſo to be added.   Afterwards, having ſtuff'd your Pullets upon the Bones with this Farce, ſet them in order in a Diſh or Baking-pan, and bread them neatly on the top   Then let ſome whipt Whites of Eggs be put to them, and let them be brought to a colour in the Oven.   If you have ſome of this Farce to ſpare, and if any Legs or Wings of Pullets, or Chickens are at hand, they may be ſtuff'd with it, and theſe will ſerve to garniſh your Diſh   A ſmall Ragoo (if you pleaſe) may alſo be made for the Pullets, of Muſhrooms, and Capons-livers dreſs'd in Cream, to be put underneath.

Fat Pullets dreſſ'd à la Sainte Menehout.

Let your Pullets be truſs'd for boiling, and ſlit in the hinder part: Then ſpread them upon the Table, or Dreſſer; break their Bones, and take away thoſe of the Legs·   Then they muſt be ſtew'd in a Sauce pan, with a great deal of good Lard, a little Parſly, Chibbol, and other ſeaſoning Ingredients   Afterwards, leaving them in the ſame Pan, let them be cover'd with ſome *Bards*, or thin Slices of Bacon, and ſet between two Fires, *viz.* one on the Lid, and the other underneath; taking care that they be not too quick.   Some Slices of Onions muſt alſo be put to them; and, as ſoon as they are ready, they may be neatly bread-ed, put into an Oven for a while, to give them a colour, and ſerv'd up hot, with a *Ramolade* Sauce underneath; if you ſhall think fit

Another Side-dish of fat Pullets in Filets.

Having caus'd large fat Pullets to be roasted, let the *Filets* and all the Flesh be neatly taken away : Then let those *Filets* be clear'd from the Fat, and laid in the bottom of a Dish ; whilst the following Sauce is preparing for them : Let some Parsly be chopt, with a little Chibbol, Capers and Garlick ; and let all, when well season'd, be put into a Stew-pan, with a little Oil and Vinegar: They must be well temper'd together, squeezing in the Juice of a Lemmon ; but the Sauce must not be set upon the Fire. When it is ready, it may be pour'd into the Dish, that contains the Pullet-*Filets*, which are to be serv'd up cold to Table.

A fat Pullet accompanied with a delicious Farce.

Take a large fat Pullet or Capon, or some other Fowl of the like nature, as a Pheasant or Wood-cock · Slit it along the Back, and cut out all the Bones that you can come at in the inside. Then let a Farce be made of delicious Meats, *viz.* the Flesh of young Pigeons, small Chickens, Snipes, *Mauviettes*, &c and a little well season'd Ragoo incorporated with it   The Pullets, when stuff'd with this Farce, must be neatly sow'd up again, and leasurely stew'd between two gentle Fires, in a Pot that is well stopt, with thin Slices of Bacon, Beef-stakes, a piece of green Lemmon, a Bunch of Herbs, and all sorts of Spice.   When it is ready, it must be dress'd upon the Back, and put into a Ra- goo of Mushrooms, Veal-sweet-breads, *Truffles* and Artichoke- bottoms, all well season'd   The Dish may be set out, with marinated Pigeons, or some other convenient Garnitures.

Large fat Pullets dress'd with Gammon-sauce, or otherwise.

When your Pullets are roasted, let a Gammon-sauce be made for them, with Capers and a thickening Liquor ; adding some Lemmon-juice, before they are set on the Table.   At another time, they may be dress'd in a Ragoo with *Truffles*, or *à la Sain- garaz*, or with a Cray-fish Cullis, or else they may be bak'd, or stew'd between two Fires, as many other Things.

Q.

Q.

QUAILS.

QUails may be bak'd *à la Braife*, that is to fay, between two Fires, and drefs'd in a Ragoo. Otherwife they may be ferv'd up in a hot Pie, fuch as that of Partridges, defcrib'd in the firft Article of *Pies* under the Letter P They may alfo be order'd feveral Ways in a Potage, and a *Bisk* of Quails has been elfewhere explain'd in the Article of *Bisks* Let us now produce fome other Methods of dreffing this fort of Fowls.

A Side-difh of Quails drefs'd à la Braife *and in a Ragoo.*

For Quails bak'd or ftew'd *à la Braife*, or between two Fires, 'tis requifite only to follow the Directions fpecified in the third Article of *Pigeons*, and to prepare a Ragoo for them, of Lambs-fweet-breads drefs'd in white Sauce, with Mufhrooms, *Truffles* and Cocks-combs. The Quails being put into this Ragoo, a little before they are ferv'd up, the Yolk of an Egg, or two, and fome Milk-cream, may be temper'd with it

The other fort of Ragoo is made, by flitting the Quails into halves, without feparating them, and frying them in Lard, fea-fon'd with a Faggot of Herbs, Pepper, Salt, Nutmeg, three or four Mufhrooms and a little Flower, adding fome Mutton-gra-vy and Lemmon-juice, at the Inftant of ferving them up to Table.

Quail-potages.

If you would have your Quails ftuff'd, a Farce may be made for that purpofe, with Capons-breafts and Beef-marrow, fea-fon'd with a little Pepper, Salt, Nutmeg, and the Yolks of raw Eggs Let them boil in an Earthen Pot or otherwife, with a Bunch of Herbs and good Broth, fuch as is defcrib'd in the firft Article of Broth : Then ftrain two boil'd Artichoke-bot-toms thro' the Hair-fieve, with fix Yolks of Eggs and fome of the Quail-broth, and let all be ftew'd upon the hot Embers. When the Crufts are fufficiently foak'd, drefs your Quails, and pour the Cullis upon them ; they may alfo be farc'd with *Truf-fles*. The Difh muft be garnifh'd with Artichoke-bottoms, Mut-ton-gravy and Mufhroom-juice

Ano-

Another fort of Quail-potage is made with a brown Cullis, without farcing, only stewing them in a proper Broth with a piece of Veal, and preparing the Cullis, with a piece of a Beef-Filet pounded with Bread-chippings This Potage is to be garnish'd with Mushrooms and *Truffles*, and some Lemmon-juice must be fqueez'd in, when brought to Table.

A Potage of Quails may likewife be ferv'd up with Roots and *à la Reine*, as it appears from the feventh and eighth Articles of Potages and elfewhere · Alfo a Quail-potage in form of an *Oil*, another fort with fweet Bafil, as that of Pigeons, others with Mushrooms and otherwife · So that due meafures may be taken, upon occafion, from the like *Species*, which may be eafily found by means of the General Table

QUAVIVERS.

Quavivers may be fried, and put into a Ragoo made of *Morilles*, *Moufferons*, common Mushrooms and Artichoke-bottoms, and garnish'd with what you shall think fit   They may alfo be broil'd upon the Grid-iron, and dref's'd with a Sauce of Capers and Anchovies

As for Quavivers in *Filets*, with Cucumbers and *Moufferons*, let them be boil'd in a *Court-bouillon*, and cut as the Perches and Soles that are fo dref's'd, according to the Inftructions given in the third Article of *Soles*. See alfo that of *Perches*, for Quaviver-*Filets*, with white Sauce, which are prepar'd after the fame manner, and may be otherwife ferv'd up, with Capers

Quavivers are likewife put into a Fricaffy of Chickens, or a Hash may be made of them, with chopt Anchovies and whole Capers, all well feafon'd, garnish'd with Crufts of fried Bread, and fprinkled with Lemmon-juice, as they are ferving up to Table.

R.

RABBETS.

RAbbets may be put into a ftanding Pie, in order to be ferv'd up cold among the Intermeffes, as it has been already intimated in the laft Article of Pies; or a hot Pie may be made of them for a Side-dish, in this manner.

A Rabbet-pie to be served up hot.

Let the Rabbets be larded, and put into a Pie made of beaten Paſte, ſeaſon'd with Pepper, Salt, Nutmeg, Cloves, pounded Lard, a Bay-leaf or two, and a Shalot After having waſh'd the Pie over, let it be bak'd for the ſpace of two Hours, and let ſome Orange or Lemmon-juice be ſqueez'd in, when brought to Table.

Rabbets and young Rabbets in Caſſerole.

Cut your Rabbets into quarters, lard them with thick Slips of Bacon; and, after they have been fried, ſtew them in an earthen Pan with Broth, a Glaſs of white Wine, a Bunch of Herbs, Pepper, Salt, fried Flower and Orange.

Rabbets dreſs'd with white and brown Sauce.

After having cut the Rabbets into quarters, ſlit their Heads, and fried them in Lard, as before; let them be ſtew'd in an earthen Pot, with Broth, white Wine, Pepper, Salt, Nutmeg and green Lemmon Let a little fried Flower be put to thoſe that are to be dreſs'd with brown Sauce, and for the others, let white Sauce be made, with the Yolks of Eggs, as upon other occaſions.

Rabbets in a Tourte, *or Pan-pie, and otherwiſe.*

Large fat Rabbets and young Rabbets may likewiſe be put into a *Tourte,* or Pan-pie; cutting them into pieces, which are to be fried in Lard, with a little Flower, fine Herbs, young Chibbols, Pepper, Salt, Nutmeg, and a little Broth When they are cold, let your Pie be made of them, with fine Paſte; adding ſome *Morilles, Truffles* and pounded Lard, and covering all with a Lid of the ſame Paſte Let it be bak'd an Hour and half, and, when it is half done, pour in the Sauce in which the Rabbets were dreſs'd, as alſo, ſome Orange-juice, as it is ſerving up to Table

At another time, when the Rabbets are roaſted, they may be cut into halves, and dreſs'd with a good Gammon-ſauce.

Young

Young Rabbets dreß'd à la Saingaraz.

The Rabbets being neatly larded and roasted, some beaten Slices of Gammon are to be fried in Lard, with a little Flower, a Faggot of fine Herbs, and some good Gravy that is not Salt: A few Drops of Vinegar are also to be added, and the Sauce may be thicken'd with a little Bread-cullis. Then let the Rabbets be cut into quarters, and dress'd in a Dish or Plate; pouring the Sauce upon them, with Slices of Gammon, in order to be serv'd up hot, after they have been well clear'd from the Fat.

Large fat Pullets may be likewise dress'd, *à la Saingaraz;* as also, Chickens and Pigeons, except that they must not be cut into quarters.

R A M E Q U I N S.

To make Cheese-*Ramequins;* a Farce is to be prepar'd of the same sort as that before describ'd for Cheese-cakes, only adding a little pounded Parsly, and, if you please, some Yest to render them lighter. Then let some Bread-crum be cut into small square pieces, with the point of a Knife, and let a little of this Farce be put upon every one of those Slices: But it would be requisite to dip your Knife into a whipt Egg, to hinder the Farce from sticking to it; so as the *Ramequins* may be made of a round or square Figure: They are to be bak'd in a Pie-pan, with a little Butter underneath; and care must be taken, that they be not too much colour'd. These *Ramequins* will serve to garnish Pease in Cream, or any thing else that you shall think fit, and may even be set among the Out-works of Intermesses.

A piece of refined Cheese may also be taken, with a Lump of Butter, as much Flower as you can get up between your Fingers at twice, three Yolks of Eggs, a little Pepper and Lemmon-juice When the whole Mixture or Farce is well pounded together, let it be spread upon a Plate, and bak'd under the Lid of a Pie-pan, with Fire on the top; taking care that it do not burn.

R I S S O L E S.

Rissoles are proper for the Intermesses, and, to render them more delicious, ought to be made with Capons-breasts. As for the reſt, they may be ſeaſon'd and order'd almoſt after the ſame manner as the *Bouillans*, ſpecified under the Letter B; but they muſt be well fried and brought to a fine colour

They may alſo be made on Days of Abſtinence, of a delicious Fiſh-farce, and even of *Moußerons* and Spinage, for the Entertainments with Roots   As for the *Moußerons*, they muſt be dreſs'd before, with Butter, fine Herbs, Spice, the Juice of a Lemmon, and a little fried Flower: And the Spinage being boil'd, muſt be chopt ſmall, and ſeaſon'd with Salt, Sugar, Cinnamon and Lemmon-peel pounded or raſped   Theſe *Riſſoles* muſt be bak'd in an Oven, and ſerv'd up with Sugar and ſweet Water.

R O A C H E S.

A Side-diſh of marinated Roaches.

The Roaches, being firſt marinated in Oil, with Wine, Lemmon-juice, and the uſual ſeaſoning Ingredients, let them be well breaded, and gently bak'd in an Oven, till they come to a fine colour: Afterwards they muſt be neatly dreſs'd in a Diſh, and garniſh'd with fried Bread and Parſly.

Roaches dreſs'd in a Ragoo, and ſeveral other Ways.

Another Ragoo may be made of Roaches; broiling them upon the Grid-iron, after they have been ſoak'd in Butter; whilſt the Livers are fried with a little Butter; in order to be pounded, and ſtrain'd thro' the Hair-ſieve.   Let this Cullis be pour'd upon the Roaches, when ſeaſon'd with white Pepper, Salt, and Orange or Lemmon-juice, rubbing the Diſh or Plate, before it is dreſs'd, with a Shalot or Clove of Garlick

Roaches may alſo be farced, as well as many other ſorts of Fiſh; otherwiſe they may be dreſs d in *Caßerole*, or put into a Pie, for which laſt, ſee the fifteenth Article of Pies.

R O A S T - M E A T S.

Altho' there ſeems to be little or no difficulty, as to what relates to the Roaſt-meats; nevertheleſs it would be expedient to give ſome account of them; that is to ſay, not to ſhew the Degree of Heat, or the Time that is requiſite for the roaſting of every

parti-

particular Joint of Meat, or Fowl; becaufe thofe Circumftances may be fufficiently difcern'd by the Eye, and may be regulated according to the Thicknefs, or Nature of the Meats But only to explain the Manner of Dreffing, or Preparing them before they are fpitted, and the Sauces which are moft propei for them For example:

Large Quails and young Quails muft be drawn and eaten barded, with Pepper; or they may be larded, and ferv'd up with Orange

Pheafants and Pheafant-powts ought to be well pickt and drawn · They are ufually larded with thin Slips of Bacon, and eaten with Verjuice, Pepper and Salt, or with Orange

Large fat Partridges and young Partridges are ferv'd up in the fame manner, as well as Wood-hens

Wood-cocks and Snipes muft not be drawn, but only larded with very fmall Slips of Bacon: As they are roafting, a Sauce is to be prepar'd for them, with Orange, white Pepper, Salt, and a young Chibbol.

Plovers are drefs'd and eaten, after the fame manner.

Turkeys and Turkey-powts muft be bafted, as they are roafting, with a little Vinegar, Salt, Chibbols, and white Pepper

Ring-doves, or Wood-pigeons, and young Fowls of that fort, may be ferv'd up with Verjuice and the entire Grapes, or Orange, or elfe in Rofe-vinegar, with white Pepper and Salt

Turtle-doves are ufually order'd in the fame manner: They muft be drawn and larded with thin Slips of Bacon, as the foimer; as well as *Bifets*, which are a kind of Stock-doves, or Wood-pigeons.

Ducks, Teals, and other forts of Water-fowl, ought to be drawn and fpitted without larding When they are half-roafted, they may be bafted with Lard; and eaten all over bloody, with white Pepper, Salt and Orange-juice, or a natural Pepper and Vinegar-fauce. As for Barn-door Ducks, they may be larded with fome Rows of Bacon, and roafted fomewhat longer than the others.

Geefe, both wild and tame, muft be drawn, but not larded; if they are fat: They are to be bafted with Lard, and eaten with Pepper and Vinegar, or with Salt and Orange

Let green Geefe be drawn and barded, whilft a Farce is preparing for them, with the Livers, Bacon, chopt Herbs, young Chibbols, Pepper, Salt and Nutmeg; to which may be added,

Mut-

Mutton-gravy and Lemmon-juice, when ready to be ferv'd up to Table · Or elfe they may be eaten with Verjuice and the entire Grapes, or with Vinegar, Pepper and Salt

Thrufhes muft be bafted, and ftew'd with Bread and Salt, in order to be eaten, with Verjuice, Pepper, and a little Orange-juice; after having rubb'd the Difh, with a Shalot

Larks are ferv'd up in the fame manner, except that a little Sage may be put into the Sauce

Fat Capons ought to be drawn and barded; putting into the Body, an Onion ftuck with Cloves, with Salt and white Pepper · When they are ready, take off the *Bards*, or Slices of Bacon, bread them, and let them be eaten with Creffes fcalded in Vinegar, with Salt, or elfe with Orange and Salt, or with Oifters ftew'd in the Dripping As for the other Capons, they may be larded with fmall Slips of Bacon, and ferv'd up after the fame manner as the others, as well as large fat Pullets

Ortolans muft be drawn, and roafted on a fmall Spit, and bafted with a little Lard: Then they may be cover'd or ftrew'd with Bread and Salt, and eaten with Salt and Orange.

Mauviettes ought not to be drawn, but larded with thin Slips of Bacon; leaving the Feet. Then having made a Sauce of the Dripping, with Verjuice and Grapes, white Pepper and Salt, let them be eaten with Salt and Orange.

Beccafigo's require only to be well pickt, after having cut off their Heads and Feet · Then they are to be roafted on a little Spit, and ftrew'd with grated Bread and Salt, in order to be eaten with Orange, or with Verjuice with the Grapes entire and white Pepper

Hares and Leverets ought to be imbru'd with their own Blood, and larded with thin Slips of Bacon . They are ufually eaten with Pepper and Vinegar, or with fweet Sauce made of Sugar, Cinnamon, Pepper, Wine and Vinegar.

Large Rabbets and young ones are eaten with Water, white Pepper and Salt, or with Orange.

Lamb and Kid muft be parboil'd in Water, or broil'd a little upon the Coals, and larded with thin Slips of Bacon Then they may be eaten, with green Sauce, or with Orange, white Pepper and Salt, or with Rofe-vinegar.

A fucking Pig ought to be well fcalded in Water, taking out the Entrails, and putting into the Belly fome Pepper, Salt, Chibbols and a Lump of pounded Lard: When it is almoft roafted, let it be findg'd and bafted with Water and Salt. It may be eaten with white Pepper, Salt and Orange.

A

A young Wild Boar may be larded with thin Slips of Bacon, without cutting off the Head or Feet, and when well roasted, may be eaten with Pepper and Vinegar, or with Orange, Salt and Pepper.

An old Wild Boar must be dress'd after the same manner, and serv'd up with Pepper and Vinegar, or *Robert*-Sauce

A Roe-buck must likewise be larded with small Slips of Bacon, and as it is roasting, a Sauce must be prepar'd for it, with Onions fried in Lard, and afterwards strain'd thro' the Hair-sieve, with Vinegar, a little Broth, white Pepper and Salt; or it may be dress'd with sweet Sauce.

A Joint of a Stag or Hind ought to be larded with thin Slips of Bacon, and eaten with Pepper and Vinegar

Fallow Deer and Fawns must be larded in the same manner, as they are roasting, basted with a Liquor made of Vinegar, green Lemmon, a Bunch of Herbs, Pepper and Salt They are also eaten with Pepper and Vinegar.

Other Sauces proper for the Roast-meats.

Sauce made of Duck-gravy.
Wood-cock Sauce.
Sauce of Gravy of a Leg of Mutton, with a Shalot.
Sauce of Veal-gravy, with Orange.
Sauce of Veal-gravy, with a Shalot.
Sauce of chopt *Truffles* and fine Herbs.
Sauce of raw Gammon and Oisters.
Sauce of Onion and Veal-gravy
Sauce of a Partridge-cullis and Capers.
Sauce of Anchovies and Shalots.
Sauce of Oil and Mustard, after the Spanish Way.
Sauce of young Chibbols, fried brown.
Sauce of Verjuice with the entire Grapes and Veal-gravy.
Sauce of fresh *Mousserons* chopt
Poor Man's Sauce, with Garlick.
Poor Man's Sauce, with Oil.
Sauce of Gravy of a short Rib of Beef, with Garlick.
Sauce of Fennel and green Gooseberries.
Sauce of green Oisters and minc'd Gammon.
Ring-dove Sauce, with Pomegranate.
Sauce with Capons-livers.
Sauce of green Corn.
Sauce of new Verjuice, with a Shalot.

Ma-

Many other forts of Sauces may be found in their proper pla-ces, by the means of the General Table of the Meffes, at the end of this Volume.

ROE-BUCKS.

To dreſs a Roe-buck.

When it is larded with thin Slips of Bacon and roafted, it may be eaten with natural fweet Sauce ; or with Sweet-four Sauce ; or with a natural Pepper and Vinegar-fauce : Or elfe the Spleen of the Roe-buck may be fried in Lard, with an Onion ; after-wards pounded in a Mortar, and ſtrain'd thro' the Hair-fieve, with Mutton-gravy, the Juice of a Lemmon and Muſhrooms, and white Pepper.

Other Ways of dreſſing a Roe-buck.

Let the Fleſh of your Roe-buck be larded with thick Slips of Bacon, and fried for fome time in Lard. Then Stew it in a Sauce-pan, with Beef-broth or Water, feafon'd, with Pepper, Salt, Bay-leaves, Nutmeg, and a Faggot of Herbs ; adding alfo a Glafs of white Wine, and a piece of green Lemmon Let the Sauce be thicken'd with fried Flower, and ferv'd up with Lem-mon-juice and Capers

This fort of Meat, after it has been larded with thick Slips of Bacon, and drefs'd as before, may be left to cool in its own Broth, and brought to Table, upon a Napkin, with Slices of Lemmon, and Creffes boil'd in Vinegar and Salt.

ROULADES.

Take part of a Fillet of Veal with Beef-fewer, and mince them very fmall as it were a *Godivoe*, adding two Eggs with the Whites and fome Salt. Then having prepar'd a piece of a Leg of Mutton, or of Veal, or a Veal-caul, ſtrew it with Par-fly, and put feven or eight Slices of Lemmon in the Intervals : You muft alfo provide a Calve's Tongue, or a Sheep's Tongue boil'd, to be cut into fmall thin Slices, with little *Bards* of Bacon. Let your *Godivoe* be fpread over all, with Parfly, Pepper and Salt on the top ; and let all be roll'd up together and bound, in order to be ſtew'd as it were in a good *Court-bouillon*, with one piece, or feveral Slices of Bacon. Let the whole Mefs be ferv'd up among the Out-works or for a Side-difh, after having garnifh'd it, with whatfoever you fhall judge requifite.

See alfo the Article of *Beef-ftikes roll'd up*, under the Letter B. and that of *Poupiets*, under P.

S.

SALMON.

Several Ways of dreffing Salmon.

FRefh Salmon may be put into a Ragoo, made brown, as it were *Fricandoes*, with Veal-fweet-breads, *Truffles* and Mufhrooms ; adding good Broth or Beef-gravy, as it is ftewing, and fome Lemmon-juice, before it is ferv'd up to Table. The following Directions for the Trout may alfo be obferv'd, or elfe your Salmon, larded with middle-fiz'd Slips of Bacon and well feafon'd, may be roafted by a gentle Fire, bafting it with white Wine and Verjuice, and putting a Faggot of fine Herbs with a piece of green Lemmon into the Sauce You muft alfo temper with the Dripping, fome Oifters, boiled Mufhrooms, Capers, fried Flower and the Liver of the Salmon, adding fome white Pepper and Lemmon-juice, when the Difh is ready to be ferv'd up, among the Intermeffes.

A Tail-piece of Salmon in Cafferole.

See the Inftructions before given for the dreffing of a Codfifh-tail in the fecond Article of *Cod-fifh*, under the Letter C. and having farc'd your Tail-piece of Salmon in the fame manner, let it be breaded, and bak'd in an Oven, with white Wine, Salt, Chibbol, Thyme, a Bay-leaf or two, and Lemmon-peel When it is ready, pour a Ragoo upon it, and garnifh it with what you pleafe.

Salmon in a Ragoo.

Take a Joll or any other piece of Salmon, and having cut it into Slices, let it be bak'd in a cover'd Difh fet into the Oven, with a little Wine, Verjuice, Pepper, Salt, Cloves, a Bunch of fine Herbs, Nutmeg, Bay-leaves, green Lemmon and a little

Fifh-

Fish-broth. In the mean time, having prepar'd a good Ragoo of Oisters, Capers, fried Flower, Mushrooms, and the Liver of the Salmon, turn all upon it, and let it be serv'd up, with Lemmon-juice

Salmon dreß'd with sweet Sauce.

Having cut your Salmon into Slices and flower'd them, let them be fried in refined Butter: Then, soaking them a little while in a sweet Sauce made of red Wine, Sugar, Pepper, Salt, Cloves, Cinnamon, and green Lemmon, let them be serv'd up, with such Garniture as you shall think fit.

For the Salmon-sallet, see Pag 41 and for a Salmon-pie, the Letter P

SALPICON.

The *Salpicon* is a Ragoo usually made for large Joints of Beef, Veal, or Mutton, which are to be serv'd up roasted, for the principal Side-dishes To that purpose, having provided Cucumbers, boil'd Gammon, Capons-livers, the *Filets* of a fat Pullet, *Truffles*, Mushrooms, and Artichoke-bottoms, let all be cut into small square pieces: But the Cucumbers, being taken a-part, must be fried in Lard, and well clear'd from the Fat, throwing in a little Flower Afterwards, having fried them again a little while, they must be put to the rest of the above-mention'd Ingredients, with good Gravy, and all must be boil'd or stew'd together If you have any Gammon-essence, put in one Spoonful of it; and, to thicken the Sauce, prepare a good Cullis, to be sprinkled at last with a little Vinegar In the mean while, a Hole being made in a short Rib of Beef, or in the Leg of a Quarter of Veal, all that Meat must be taken away, which will serve for other Farces, and the Ragoo even now describ'd, must be substituted in its room.

A *Salpicon* may also be serv'd up separately for a Side dish

SANDLINGS, *see* DABS.

SAUSAGES

To make Sausages, let some Pork and Leaf-fat out of the Hog's Belly be chopt small, well season'd, and mixt with a little Parsly, other fine Herbs and a Shalot. If you would have

R them

them more delicious than ordinary; it will be requisite also to mince the Breasts of Capons, or fat Pullets, with a little raw Gammon and Anis, in the same manner as for white Hogspuddings. When the whole Mixture is well order'd and season'd, adding a little Gammon-essence, it may be bound with the Yolk of an Egg. Afterwards, having provided Sheeps-guts that are well cleans'd, according to the thickness that you would have your Sausages to be of, they may be made of a convenient length, and broil'd upon Paper, or fried; in order to be serv'd up to Table.

The same Compound or Farce may also be wrapt up in a Veal-caul and dress d as Capons-livers in a Caul; for which see the Article of *Livers* under the Letter L.

Veal-sausages are made in the same manner, after having minc'd part of a Fillet of Veal, with half as much Bacon, season'd with Pepper, Salt, Nutmeg and fine Herbs chopt very small. They may also be broil'd upon the Grid-iron, with thick Paper underneath, and serv'd up with Mustard, as the former, among the Side-dishes

Royal Sauciffons, *or thick Saufages.*

Having provided some Flesh of Partridges and of a fat Pullet or Capon, a little Gammon and other Bacon, and a piece of a Leg of Veal, all raw, with Parsly and Chibbols, let them be well chopt with Mushrooms and *Truffles*, and season'd with Pepper, Salt, beaten Spice, and a Clove of Garlick; adding also two whole Eggs, three or four Yolks and a little Milk-cream. Then roll up this Farce into thick pieces, according to the quantity that you have of it, and to the end that it may be dress'd, without breaking, let it be wrapt up in very thin Slices cut out of a Fillet of Veal, and beaten flat upon the Dresser, for that purpose; so as the Sausages may be made at least as thick as a Man's Arm, and of a convenient length. When they are thus order d, they must be put into an oval Stew-pan, with a great many *Bards* or thin Slices of Bacon at the bottom, and stopt up close; covering them with Beef-stakes, and other Bacon-*Bards* Afterwards, the Pan must be set between two Fires, taking care that they be not too quick, and the Sausages must be bak d or stew'd in this manner about eight or ten Hours As soon as they are ready, let them be remov'd from the Fire, and left to cool in the same Pan. Then they must be carefully taken out so as none be broken, and all the Meat round about muft be taken away, with the Fat˙ At laft you may cut the Saufages into Slices with a fharp Knife, and fet them in good order in a Difh or Plate, to be ferv'd up cold to Table If there be occafion to make a *Galantine* at the fame time, with the Royal Saufages, it may be drefs'd in the fame Stew-pan

SEA-DRAGONS, *fee* QUAVIVERS.

SHADS.

Broiled Shads.

When they are well fcal'd and cut, rub them with Butter and Salt, or elfe caufe them to take Salt in a Baking-pan, with Oil: Then they muft be broil'd upon the Grid-iron, over a gentle Fire, and brought to a fine colour They may be ferv'd up, with Sorrel and Cream; adding alfo fome Parfly, Chervil, Chibbol, Pepper, Salt, Nutmeg and fweet Butter. They may alfo be drefs'd in a Ragoo of Mufhrooms, or in a brown Sauce, with Capers.

Shads in a Court-bouillon.

After having fcal'd and cut your Shads, let them boil in white Wine, with Vinegar, Pepper, Salt, Cloves, Bay-leaves, Onions and green Lemmon, and let them be ferv'd up to Table upon a Napkin.

SIMNELS.

Iced Simnels.

Iced Simnels, may ferve either for Intermeffes, or to garnifh other Difhes, and are prepar'd after the following manner Having provided Simnels made of Water, according to the fize of your Difh, cut them into halves, as it were an Orange, leaving the Cruft on the top and underneath; and foak them in Milk, with Sugar, proportionably to the quantity of Simnels. Then let them be cover'd and laid under hot Embers, to be kept warm for the fpace of about four or five Hours, but they muft not be boil'd, left they turn to Pap Afterwards, having taken them out, let them be well drain'd and fried in frefh Lard As foon as they are colour'd, let them be ftrew'd with fine Sugar and iced over : At laft, after they have been turn'd and iced on the other Side, they may be brought hot to Table.

SMELTS.

We fhall not here infift on the manner of Dreffing Smelt-po-tages, with white and brown Broth, or of Filets of the fame Fifh, in regard that it is only requifite to obferve the Directi-ons already laid down for other forts of Fifh But it may not be improper to give fome account of the Side-difhes that are ufually made of Smelts

Several Ways of dreffing Smelts.

Smelts may be fried and ferv'd up in a Sauce made of dif-folv'd Anchovies, burnt Butter, Orange-juice and white Pepper.
At another time, They may be ftew'd in a Sauce-pan, with Butter, a little white Wine, Nutmeg, fried Flower and a piece of green Lemmon; adding fome Capers and Lemmon-juice, when ferv'd up to Table
Smelts may be alfo boil'd in a *Court-bouillon*, with white Wine, green Lemmon, Pepper, Salt and a Bay-leaf or two, and brought to Table, upon a Napkin, with Parfly and Slices of Lemmon, to be eaten with white Pepper and Vinegar, or elfe they may be drefs'd with the *Ramolade*-fauce defcribed Pag. 41.

SNIPES.

Snipes may be ferv'd up in a Ragoo, as well as roafted ; to which purpofe, they muft be flit into halves, without taking a-way any of their Entrails · Then let them be fried in Lard, and feafon'd with white Pepper, Salt, a Chibbol, and a little Juice of Mufhrooms and Lemmon The Difh may be garnifh'd, with Slices of Lemmon

SOLES.

Soles drefs'd after the Spanifh Way.

Let the Soles be fried, and afterwards cut into *Filets* ; whilft a Sauce is preparing for them, with good *Champagne*-wine, two
Cloves

Cloves of Garlick, Pepper, Salt, Thyme and a Bay-leaf Then foak them by degrees in this Sauce, and garnifh them, with what you fhall judge moft requifite.

A Side-difh of fried Soles.

Open the Back of your Soles, on both fides, and take away the Bone, till the white Flefh appears When they are fried, let them be garnifh'd with the Flefh of other Soles, and let a white Sauce be made with an Anchovie and Capers, or *Robert-*Sauce; or elfe a Ragoo of Mufhrooms with Pike-livers, Artichoke-bottoms chopp'd very fmall and Carp roes, fqueezing in fome Lemmon-juice, before the Difh is fet on the Table.

*Sole-*Filets *with Cucumbers.*

Having cut fried Soles into *Filets*, let them be mingled with Cucumbers drefs'd in the following manner: Let marinated Cucumbers cut into Slices, be fried and foak'd with Gravy or Broth ; in which they muft be afterwards ftew'd and well feafon'd, taking care that they do not ftick. The *Filets* being put to them, may be ferv'd up a little after, and garnifh'd with what you pleafe

Soles farced with fine Herbs, and dreß'd otherwife.

Let your Soles cool, after they have been fried, and let a Farce be made of fine Herbs, *viz* Parfly, Chibbol, Thyme, Savoury, and fweet Bafil, all chopt together, with Pepper, Salt, Cloves and Nutmeg Then drefs all thefe with a good Lump of Butter, and farce the Soles, taking out the Bones of every one, at the top of the Back Afterwards, foak them in melted Butter, and having breaded them, let them be broil'd upon the Grid-iron and brought to a fine colour. with the red-hot Fire-fhovel. They may be ferv'd up, with Lemmons cut into halves.

Other Soles are farced with Bread-crum, Anchovies, Parfly, Chibbols and fweet Butter, all well chopp'd, kneaded and feafon'd · When they are thus ftuff'd, let them be fteept in Oil, breaded and drefs'd as Pigs-pettitoes, *à la Sainte Menehout.* A little brown Sauce muft be prepar'd for them, and fome Lemmon-juice added, as they are ferving up to Table,

Other

Other Ways of farcing Soles for Potage may be feen in the 65th Article of *Potages*, under the Letter P and as many Side-dishes may be made of them; enriching them with Mushrooms, Oisters, Cray-fish and Capers, adding Lemmon-juice, when ferv'd up to Table.

In any feafon out of Lent, three or four Eggs may be mingled with the Farce, which is to be made of the Flesh of boned Soles, when they are half-fried, with fine Herbs and Bread-crum foak'd in Milk. Having stuff'd the Bones of your Soles with this Farce, bake them in an Oven, till they come to a fine colour, and fet out the Dish with Lemmon, or fome other proper Garniture.

Sole-Filets, *with a Lentil-cullis.*

After the Soles have been fried and cut into *Filets*, they muft be put into a good Ragoo of Lentils, fuch as is produc'd in the fifth Article of Potages, and gently boil'd a little while over the Fire. When the *Filets* are ready to be ferv'd up, let them be drefs'd in the Ragoo, or Cullis, and garnish'd with what you pleafe, for a Side-dish

Quavivers, Dabs and Perches may also be drefs'd in the fame manner, but the latter muft be handled more gently.

Other Ways of dreffing Soles.

Sole-*Filets* are likewife ferv'd up in a Cullis of Capers, others with *Truffles*, and others with *Robert*-Sauce, with fweet Bafil, or with Cray-fish: A *Pain*, or farced Loaf and *Gatoes*, may also be made of Soles, or they may be drefs'd in a *Court-bouil-lon*, or in a *Marinade*, as it has been obferv'd in the laft Article of *Marinades*. As for thofe that are fried, they may be eaten with Salt and Orange-juice.

SOUSCES.

To make an Intermefs of *Soufce*, let Hogs-ears and Feet be boil'd after the ufual manner, and left to cool in their own Li-quor: Then let them be cut into very fmall thin Slices, and let all the Bones be taken away; whilft fome of the beft fort of Vinegar is put into a Stew-pan, with Sugar, proportionably to the quantity of Meat: Let the Vinegar and Sugar be boil'd, with

a

a Stick of Cinnamon, three or four Cloves, a little Pepper and Salt, and two or three Slices of Lemmon. Let all be strain'd thro' the Hair-sieve, and when the Meat is cut into *Menus-droits*, let all boil together, till the Sauce becomes thick, as if it were for *Menus-droits* with Muftard. Afterwards, having remov'd the Stew-pan from the Fire, and having provided certain little fquare Boxes, of what fize you fhall think fit, all the Fat being alfo taken off with a Spoon, let the whole Mefs be turn'd into them, with fmall *Lardoons*, or Slices of Bacon, of the fame length as the Boxes. When they are fill'd, let them not be cover'd, till all be well coagulated. Afterwards, cover them with Paper, and the Lids of the fame Boxes. This Compound, or Jelly, may be kept during four or five Months, but the newer it is the better. It is ufually ferv'd up in thin Slices, and laid in good order, on a Difh or Plate, with a clean Napkin underneath.

STAG.

A Joint of Stag may be drefs'd feveral Ways; that is to fay, it may be larded with thick Slips of Bacon, and feafon'd with Pepper, Salt, Nutmeg, and beaten Cloves: Otherwife, having larded it with fmall Slips of Bacon, let it be fteept in white Wine and Verjuice, with Salt, a Faggot of Herbs, a piece of green Lemmon, and three or four Bay-leaves, and roafted at a gentle Fire; bafting it with its *Marinade*, or Pickle. When it is ready, let it be drefs'd in the Dripping, with fried Flower to thicken the Sauce, adding Capers, Vinegar, or Lemmon-juice, and white Pepper, when ferv'd up to Table.

Another Way of dreffing Stags-flefh.

Let the Loin or Shoulder of a Stag be larded with very thin Slips of Bacon, and cover'd with Paper. As it is roafting, let a Sauce be prepar'd for it, with Vinegar, Pepper, Salt, Nutmeg, fried Flower, Slices of Lemmon and Shalots.

Another Way.

After your Joint of Stag has been well roafted, it may be eaten with a fweet Sauce, made in this manner: Take a Glafs of Vinegar, with Sugar, a little Salt, three or four whole

R 4   Cloves,

Cloves, Cinnamon and a little Lemmon; and, when thefe Ingredients are boil'd together, put in a little fried Flower, white Pepper and Orange-juice.

Stag in a Ragoo.

Having larded a piece of Stags-flefh with thick Slips of Bacon, feafon'd with Pepper and Salt, let it be fried in Lard: Then let it boil for the fpace of three or four Hours in an earthen Pan, with Broth or Water, and two Glaffes of white Wine, feafon'd with Salt, Nutmeg, a Bunch of Herbs, three or four Bay-leaves, and a piece of green Lemmon When it is ready, let the Sauce be thicken'd with fried Flower, and add Capers and Lemmon-Juice as it is ferving up to Table.

Paft es are alfo made of Stags-flefh, which may be found in the Article of *Pafties,* under the Letter P.

Stock-fish, *fee* Cod-fish.

Sturgeon.

A Side-difh of Sturgeon for Flefh-days.

Sturgeon for Flefh-days may be drefs'd after different Manners; that is to fay, either in form of larded *Fricandoes* or Collops; or in thick Slices, *à la Sainte Menehout.* For the latter, let the Slices of Sturgeon be gently ftew'd in Milk and white Wine, well feafon'd, with a Bay-leaf and a little melted Lard · Then let them be breaded, and broil'd upon a Grid-iron; pouring a Sauce underneath, in the fame manner, as for Loins of Mutton, in order to be ferv'd up hot to Table

For Collops of the fame Sturgeon, after they have been cut and larded, they muft be flower'd a little, and brought to a colour with Lard · Then they are to be boil'd in a Sauce-pan, with good Gravy, fine Herbs, Slices of Lemmon, *Truffles,* Mufhrooms, Veal-fweet-breads, and a well-feafon'd Cullis Afterwards, the Fat being thoroughly drain'd from them, they may be fprinkled with a little Verjuice, and ferv'd up hot, as well as the other fort, among the Side-difhes and Out-works.

Ano-

Another Way of dreſſing Sturgeon.

Sturgeon may alſo be dreſs'd in *Haricot*, with Turneps; to which purpoſe, it muſt be boil'd in Water, with Pepper, Salt, Thyme, Onions and Cloves If you have any Broth at hand, ſome of it may be pour'd in, and then your Sturgeon muſt be fried brown in Lard · Afterwards, it muſt be clear'd from the Fat, and put into a prepared Cullis, with the Turneps, and a little Gammon cut into Slices, or chopt ſmall. It may be ſerv'd up, with Lemmon-juice, and ſet out with *Marinade*, or ſome other Garniture.

Sturgeon for Fiſh-days.

Let your Sturgeon be boil'd in a good *Court-bouillon*, and dreſs'd in a well-ſeaſon'd Ragoo of Muſhrooms, *&c*

A *Haricot* may alſo be made of Sturgeon, with Turneps, as on Fleſh-days, cutting it into pieces of the length of your Fin-'ger, in order to be boil'd in Water and Salt, and afterwards fried brown Then the Fat being drain'd off, it muſt be put into a Cullis of the ſame, and mingled with the Turneps, after they have been ſcalded and well ſeaſon'd

T.

T A R T S

Tarts made of Cherries and other ſorts of Fruit.

TAke preſerv'd Cherries, and let a piece of well-made Paſte, half puff'd be roll'd out very thin for an Under-cruſt, to be ſpread over the bottom of the Pie-pan · Then lay your Cherries in order, and roll out ſome Slips of Paſte, which can-not be made too ſmall With theſe, fine Ornaments may be made for your Tart, in form of a Star, a Basket, a Royal Banner, and ſeveral others, at pleaſure . Thus, having ſhap'd all with the Point of a Knife, the Tart muſt be bak'd, and afterwards ic'd with fine Sugar, paſſing the red-hot Fire-ſhovel over it It may be garniſh'd with *Feuillantins*, or ſmall *Fleurons* of all ſorts of Fruit. Tarts may alſo be made of other Fruits, and even of Cream, after the ſame manner : When Apricocks, Verjuice,

juice, &c are in feafon, they are natural; and at other times, Marmelade may be us'd. However, the Tarts may be always render'd more delicious, by making the Cruft, with Almond-pafte, or crackling Cruft, fuch as is defcrib'd in the firft Article of Paftes.

A Peach-tart.

Let ripe Peaches be fton'd, well pounded in a Mortar, and left in Heaps: In the mean while, having put fome Sugar, with candy'd Lemmon-peel cut fmall, into a Difh, let a fine Pafte be made fomewhat ftiff, with a little Butter, Flower, Salt, Water, and the Yolk of an Egg. Then roll out a round piece, very thin, for the Bottom-cruft, according to the fize of your Difh, and make a little Border of the fame Pafte, for the Side-cruft, about two Inches high: Afterwards, the Peaches being put into it in good order, the Pie may be fet into the Oven, and brought to a fine colour, with the red-hot Fire-fhovel, after having ftrew'd it with Sugar This is commonly call'd *a broiled Tart* by the French, and ought to be ferv'd up hot to Table.

Tarts of the like nature, may be prepar'd with Apples and other forts of Fruit; and, if you'll give your felf the trouble, they may be made of Pafte proper for crackling Cruft, neatly cut, dried in an Oven, and afterwards iced over with the Yolk of an Egg, fine Sugar and a little preferv'd Lemmon-peel, well temper'd together Having thus order'd your Pafte for the Lid, caufing it to be ic'd in the Oven, till it become very white, it muft be laid upon the Tart that is drefs'd in the Difh, a little before it is ferv'd up, and may be garnifh'd with *Meringues.*

A fweet-four Tart.

Take a Glafs of Verjuice, or Lemmon-juice, with a quarter of a Pound of Sugar, and when half is boil'd away, add fome Cream, with fix Yolks of Eggs, a little Butter, Orange-flowers, candy'd Lemmon-peel grated, and beaten Cinnamon: Let all be put into a Tart made of fine Pafte, and bak'd without a Lid.

Other forts of Tarts.

A kind of *Marmelade* or Cream, may be made of Apples, Beets, Melons, and other forts of Fruit; boiling them in white Wine,
and

and afterwards pounding them with Sugar, Cinnamon, Orange-flowers and Lemmon-peel · Then they muft be ftrain'd thro' the Hair-fieve, and put into a Tart made of very thin Cruft, with a little Butter, in order to be ferv'd up with musked Sugar and Orange flowers.

Tarts may alfo be made of all the different forts of artificial Creams fpecify'd under that Article.

TENCHES.

Tenches may be cut into pieces, and a white or brown Fricaffy may be made of them, with *Moufferons* or common Mufhrooms, *Truffles*, Artichoke-bottoms and fine Herbs, adding a thickening Liquor, as for Chickens, and an Anchovie chopt very fmall, as alfo fome Lemmon-juice, before it is ferv'd up to Table, fet out with *Marinade*

A Hafh may be alfo made of Tenches, garnifh'd with the Heads marinated and fried Or elfe they may be drefs'd in *Cafferole*, frying them, in burnt Butter, after they have been cut, and ftewing them in white Wine, with the fame Butter, Verjuice, a Faggot of Herbs, Pepper, Salt, Nutmeg, a Bay-leaf or two, and a little Flower When they are ready, let Oifters be put into the Sauce, with Capers, fome Juice of Mufhrooms and Lemmon, and let all be garnifh'd with fried Bread.

Moreover, Tenches may be farc'd, as Carps, or drefs'd in a Ragoo, cutting them into pieces, to be fried in refined Butter, in which an Anchovie is to be afterwards diffolv'd; adding Orange-juice, Pepper, Salt, Nutmeg and Capers · Then the Difh may be ferv'd up with fried Parfly and Slices of Lemmon.

As for thofe Tenches that are fet a-part for frying, they muft be flit on the Back, and ftrew'd with Salt and Flower When they are fufficiently fried, let them be ferv'd up to Table with Orange-juice.

TERRINE.

A *Terrine* is a very confiderable Side-difh, and may be thus prepar'd: Take fix Quails, four young Pigeons, two Chickens, and a Breaft of Mutton cut into pieces; and let all be bak'd or ftew'd in an earthen Pan, call'd *Terrine* in French, between two gentle Fires, with Bacon-*Bards* at the bottom to keep them from burning, or young ftreaked Bacon cut into pieces: Then

let

let the Fat be drain'd off, and some good Veal-gravy put in its place, with boil'd Lettice, a little green Peafe-foop, and green Peafe or Afparagus-tops · Let all be ftew'd again together for fome time, and thoroughly clear'd from the Fat, before they are ferv'd up to Table.

N. B Somewhat has been already deliver'd on this Subject, in the fecond Article of *Mirotons*, under the Letter M.

THRUSHES.

Amongft other Difhes, Thrufhes may be put into a Pie, to be ferv'd up hot, or into a Ragoo; frying them, for the latter, in Lard, with a little Flower, a Faggot of fine Herbs, Pepper, Salt, Nutmeg, a little white Wine and Capers; fqueezing in fome Lemmon-juice, as they are ferving up to Table

For Potage made of Thrufhes, let them likewife be fried in Lard, after they have been drawn, and then boil'd with brown Broth proper for that purpofe, as it has been already hinted, in the firft Article of *Broth*, under the Letter B The Livers being alfo fried in the fame Lard, muft be afterwards pounded, and ftrain'd thro' the Hair-fieve, with the fame Broth, in order to be put upon the Thrufhes, or into the Potage , which are to be drefs'd and garnifh'd with Mufhrooms.

TONGUES.

Having already explain'd divers Services of Neats-tongues, under the Letter N. let us now give fome Account of the other forts.

Calves-tongues.

To prepare farced Calves-tongues,

Let a Hole be made in the Tongues at the Root, with a little Knife; taking care that they be not cut in any part: Then thruft in your Finger quite thro', as if it were a Gut; fo as a Ragoo may be put into it, made of Veal-fweet-breads, Mufhrooms, *Truffles*, Parfly and Chibbol; all well feafon'd, and fried with a little Lard and Flower, that is not made brown. The Tongues, being farced with this Ragoo, muft be tied up very clofe at the Hole, and thrown into hot Water, to the end that

the

the firſt Skin may be peel'd off. Afterwards, they muſt be broil'd upon the Coals, or ſtew'd between two Fires, and when the Fat is thoroughly drain'd from them, they may be dreſs'd in a Diſh, with a good Ragoo, garniſh'd with *Fricandoes,* that are well larded but not farc'd

Another Way of dreſſing Calves-tongues.

Two other Side-diſhes may be made of Calves-tongues; that is to ſay, they may be dreſs'd in the ſame manner as the Neats-tongues, ſpecified in the third and fourth Articles, or elſe they may be roaſted after having been half done, and ſerv'd up with ſweet Sauce.

Hogs-tongues.

To dreß dried Hogs-tongues.

Take what quantity you pleaſe of Hog's-tongues, and ſcald them, only to get off the firſt Skin, but the Water muſt not be too hot: Then wipe them with a Cloath, and cut off a little of the thick End or Root To ſalt your Tongues, take green Juniper-berries, and dry them in an Oven, with two Bay-leaves, a little Coriander, Thyme, ſweet Baſil, and all ſorts of fine Herbs, except Roſemary, Sage, Parſly and Chib-bol: All theſe Herbs being well dried, muſt be pounded in a Mortar, and ſtrain'd thro' a Sieve Afterwards, having provided ſome pounded Salt and Salt-petre, mingle them together with the reſt, and let your Tongues be put into a Pail or Pot, laying them in order, one by one, as they are ſeparately ſalted; every Row of them being ſeaſon'd with all theſe Ingredients. They muſt be preſs'd cloſe together, and, when they are all ſalted, let a Slate be laid over them, and a great Stone on the top, leaving them thus cloſe ſtopt for ſix or ſeven Days Then take them out, drain them a little; and, having cut ſome Hogs-skirts, according to the length of the Tongues, let every one be put into its Caſe, made of thoſe Skirts, tying up both ends. When your Tongues are thus order'd, let them be faſten'd at the ſmall end or tip, to a Pole laid a-croſs the Chimny, at a convenient diſtance, ſo as they may not touch one another, and that they may be well ſmoak'd, for the ſpace of fifteen or twenty Days, till they become dry Thus they may be preſerv'd,

if

if well order'd, throughout the whole Year ; but in their beſt
condition, they muſt be eaten at the end of ſix Months . To
that purpoſe, they may be boil'd in Water, with a little red
Wine, a few Slices of Chibbol and Cloves When they are ready,
they may be cut into Slices or left entire, at pleaſure, and ſerv'd
up cold among the Intermeſſes

Sheeps-tongues.

Several Ways of dreſſing Sheeps-tongues.

Sheeps-tongues may be ſerv'd up with ſweet Sauce, in which,
after they have been flower'd and fried till they come to a fine
colour, they may be ſoak'd by degrees, with *Truffles* and *Mouſſerons.*

Sheeps-tongues may alſo be broil'd upon the Grid-iron, with
Salt and Bread-crum, in order to be ſtew'd in a Sauce, made of
Verjuice, Broth, Muſhrooms, Pepper, Salt, fried Flower, Nutmeg and green Lemmon ; or elſe a *Ramolade*-Sauce may be prepar'd for them, according to the Directions laid down, Pag 41.

Dried Sheeps-tongues may be order d after the ſame manner
as dried Calves-tongues above ſpecified.

TORTOISES.

Tortoiſes may be put into a Fricaſſy of Chickens ; and to that
purpoſe, having cut off their Heads, Feet and Tails, let them
boil in a Pot, with Pepper, Salt, Onion, Cloves, Thyme and
Bay-leaves Afterwards, having cut them into pieces, taking
care of the Gall, toſs them up in a Stew-pan, with fine Herbs,
Chibbols, Pepper, Salt, Artichoke-bottoms, *Morilles, Mouſſerons,*
common Muſhrooms and *Truffles* If you would have them
brown, let them be ſoak'd with Onion-juice, or elſe with good
Fiſh-broth and a little fried Flower. To dreſs Tortoiſes in a
white Fricaſſy, the Sauce muſt be thicken'd, with Yolks of
Eggs, adding ſome Verjuice and Lemmon-juice when ſerv'd
up to Table The Diſh may be garniſh'd with Roes, Lem-
mon-ſlices and Oiſters, either fried or raw, according to the
nature of the Fricaſſy

A *Poupeton* may alſo be made of Tortoiſes, or elſe they may
be ſteept for ſome time, in Vinegar, Pepper, Salt and Chibbols:
Afterwards they muſt be flower'd and fry'd, in order to be ſerv'd
up with fry d Parſly, Oranges and white Pepper.   TOSTS.

T o s t s.

Tosts may be serv'd up both on Flesh-days and those of Abstinence, and are very frequently us'd   For Flesh-days, boil'd Veal-kidneys chopt very small, with Chervil, Salt, Sugar, Cinnamon, and the Yolk of an Egg, may be laid upon the Tosts of Bread, and strew'd with other Bread, or else neatly ic'd over.

For Wood-cock Tosts, let the Flesh and Entrails of the Wood-cocks be likewise cut small, except the Ghizzard, and season'd with white Pepper, Salt and melted Lard. All being well mingled together, the Tosts may be made, and bak'd in a Pie-pan over a gentle Fire. They ought to be serv'd up without Sugar, only with Mutton-gravy and Orange-juice, or with a Shalot.

Tosts of the like nature may also be made, with Capons-livers fried in pounded Lard, three or four Mushrooms, fine Herbs and the usual seasoning Ingredients

For Fish-days, the Tosts are generally prepar'd with Butter, Oil of Olives or Hypocras; which manner of dressing is so easie and so well known, that it does not deserve to be any longer insisted upon.

T O U R T E S, *or* P A N - P I E S.

There are two sorts of *Tourtes* or Pies made in a *Tourtiere*, or Baking-pan, as well as of standing Pies both for Flesh-days and those of Abstinence , that is to say, one sort for Side dishes and the other for Intermesses. Some of the first Service have been already describ'd, particularly *Tourtes* or Pan-pies of Chickens and Pigeons in their respective Articles And as for the Intermesses, we have also produc'd Almond-pan-pies, Tarts of Cream, and of Fruit - Marmelades, and even some Fish-pan-pies; let us now proceed to explain the most considerable of those that remain.

A Quail-Tourte *or Pan-pie.*

After having well cleans'd and truss'd your Quails, let them be put into a Pan-pie made of beaten Paste, as the former, season'd with Pepper, Salt, Nutmeg and a Bunch of Herbs. This Pie must also be fill'd with Veal-sweet-breads, Mushrooms,
Truffles

Truffles cut into pieces, pounded or melted Lard underneath the Quails and Beef-fewet. Then it may be cover'd with a Lid, and bak'd during two Hours   Let fome Lemmon-juice be fqueez'd in, as it is ferving up hot to Table for a Side-difh.

A Tourte *or* Pan-pie, *after the Spanish Way for a Side-difh.*

Take Quails, Pigeons, *Mauviettes*, or *Ortolans*, that is to fay, any one of thefe forts, provided they be all fmall and tender Fowls : For example, if they are Pigeons, after they have been well trufs'd, a Farce muft be made of a little Marrow, Mufhrooms, *Truffles* a little piece of parboil'd Bacon, all well feafon'd with Spice and fine Herbs of all forts   Let your Pigeons be only flit on the Back to let in this Farce, and if they are fomewhat tough, they may be fcalded a little before they are ftuft 'd In the mean time, let fome Veal-fweet breads, Mufhrooms, Cockscombs and Artichoke-bottoms cut into Quarters be well feafon'd and ftew'd a-part ; whilft the Pafte is making, with Water, Flower, the Yolk of an Egg, a little Salt and Butter, but it muft not be too ftiff . Having fet it by a little, let it be beaten with the Rolling-pin, and divided into eight pieces, according to the bignefs of your Baking-pan   Of thefe eight pieces of Pafte, take four to ferve for the Bottom crufts , roll out every piece almoft as thin as Paper, rub the infide of the Pie-pan with Butter or Lard, and having put one piece of Pafte therein, wafh it over with melted Lard, to the end, that another may be laid upon it, and fo of the reft.   Then the Pigeons or other fmall Fowls, may be fet in order, with the Ragoo, and cover'd with *Bards* or thin Slices of Bacon.   Afterwards, taking the four pieces of Pafte that were left for the Lid, order them in the fame manner, as thofe for the Bottom-crufts, that is to fay, let them be wafh'd with Lard, before they are laid one upon another The Pie being thus cover'd muft be wafh'd over again on the top, and fet into the Oven, taking care that it be not of too brown a colour.   When it is bak'd , drefs it in a Difh or Plate, take off the Lid and *Bards*, pour in a good white Cullis, or one of Mufhrooms, according to the nature of the Fowls, and let all be ferv d up hot to Table.

A

A Tourte *or Pan-pie of a Capon's Breast for an Intermess.*

Take the Breast of a Capon or Pullet, and pound it in a Mortar with a little grated Lemmon-peel, a March pane, three or four Yolks of Eggs, Orange-flower-water, and a little beaten Cinnamon, all well thicken'd Let this Mixture be spread upon a piece of beaten Paste roll'd out for the Bottom-crust, and let the Pie be bak'd without the Lid. Then ice it over with fine Sugar, and having caus'd the Cover of a Pie-pan to be heated very hot, let it be laid upon the Pie, to give it a colour; adding a little sweet Water and Lemmon-juice, when ready to be brought to Table.

Another Pan-pie made of a Capon's Breast.

Let the Breast of a raw Capon, be minc'd, with as much Marrow or Beef-sewet Then let your Pie be made of beaten Paste, and the intervals stuff'd with Mushrooms, *Truffles,* Cocks-combs, Veal-sweet-breads, a little pounded Lard, Pepper, Salt and Nutmeg Let it be cover'd with a Lid of the same Paste, wash'd over, and bak'd for the space of an Hour and half Lastly, let some Pistachoes, with Mutton-gravy and Lemmon-juice be put into it at the instant of serving it up, and let it be set out with little Tarts, or some other sort of Garniture

A Pan-pie of Capons-livers.

Let the Livers be scalded in Water, and afterwards laid in Order in a Pie-pan upon fine Paste, with chopt Mushrooms, fine Herbs, Chibbol and pounded Lard, season'd with Pepper, Salt, Nutmeg, Cloves and a piece of green Lemmon · Then covering the Pie with a Lid of the same Paste, let it be wash'd over, and bak'd a full Hour. In the mean while, taking one of the Livers that were reserv'd, fry it with a little Lard and Flower; let it also be pounded and strain'd thro' the Hair-sieve, with Mutton-gravy and Lemmon-juice, after having rubb'd the bottom of the Dish with a Shalot Lastly, let all be put into the Pie, as it's serving up hot to Table

S

*Gammon-*Tourtes, *or Pan-pies.*

A piece of good Gammon may be cut into small Slices, and laid in order in the Pie-pan upon a piece of fine Paste, with Herbs chopt small, Pepper, Cinnamon, Nutmeg, fresh Butter and a Bay leaf. It must be cover'd, and wash'd over as the former, and only set into the Oven for half an Hour. When it is bak'd, let some Mutton-gravy be put into it, with Lemmon-juice and a Shalot.

The Gammon may be minc'd, if you shall think fit, to make a Pie of the like nature, adding Sugar, Cinnamon, white Pepper, candy'd Lemmon-peel and a little pounded Lard. When it is dress'd and bak'd as before, let Lemmon-juice and Sugar be put into it, in order to be set on the Table.

A Pan-pie of Sheeps-tongues.

Sheeps-tongues cut into Slices may be put into a Pie-pan, with candy'd Lemmon-peel, Currans, Dates, Pepper, Salt, Sugar, Cinnamon, two pounded Macaroons, some melted Lard, and a piece of green Lemmon. Then let your Pie be cover'd with a Lid, wash'd over, and bak'd for an Hour; putting into it some Lemmon-juice, Sugar and sweet Water, when serv'd up to Table.

A Pan-pie of a Neats-tongue.

Having cut a salted Neats-tongue into very thin Slices, as the former, let it be laid upon a piece of Paste in a Pie-pan, season'd with Cinnamon, Pepper, Sugar and melted Lard. Then cover it with a Lid of the same Paste, and when it is half bak'd, that is to say, about half an Hour after it was set into the Oven, pour in half a Glass of good Wine. Afterwards, let it be bak'd outright, and as it is serving up, put some Sugar into it, with Lemmon-juice and Pomegranate-kernels.

A Tourte, *or Pan-pie of Veal-sweet-breads.*

After having scalded the Sweet-breads in very hot Water, let them be put into a fine Paste, with small Mushrooms, *Truffles,* Pepper, Salt, Nutmeg, green Lemmon and pounded Lard. Then

cover-

covering the Pie with a Lid of the same Paste, wash it over, and set it into the Oven for an Hour When it is bak'd, pour in some Veal or Mutton gravy, adding Piftachoes and Lemmon-juice, a little before it is brought to Table.

A Pan-pie of Beatils.

The *Beatils* being well cleans'd in hot Water may be put into a Pie-pan, with Mushrooms, *Truffles*, Veal-fweet-breads, Arti-choke-bottoms and Beef-marrow, all well feafon'd, with Pepper, Salt, Nutmeg, a Faggot of Herbs, and pounded or melted Lard : Let it be cover'd with a Lid, and wash'd over as the others, and after it has been bak'd about two Hours in an Oven moderately heated, let some Mutton-gravy be pour'd into it, with Lemmon-juice, in order to be ferv'd up to Table.

A Pan-pie of Veal-kidneys.

This *Tourte* or Pan-pie may be made two feveral Ways For the firft, let your Veal kidneys be chopt fmall, with a little Lard, feafoned with Pepper, Salt, Nutmeg, Cinnamon, Chibbols, fine Herbs, Mushrooms and Veal-fweet-breads The Pie being thus made of beaten Paste, must be cover'd, and bak'd as before, during a full Hour

For the other Way, let your Kidneys be boil'd, minc'd, and put in like manner between two pieces of fine Paste, with Sugar, Cinnamon, Lemmon-peel, Dates, a little Butter, two Ma-caroons, and the other neceffary feafoning Ingredients Three quarters of an Hour are fufficient for the baking of this fort of Pie, into which you must put some Lemmon-juice, Sugar and Orange-flower-water, when ready to be ferv'd up to Table.

Tourtes, *or Pan-pies made of Butter, Lard and Marrow.*

For the Butter Pan-pie, take very fresh Butter, to the quantity of eight Ounces, according to the bignefs of your Pie, let it be refin'd and well clear'd from the Scum ; adding a little chopt Marrow, if the Entertainment be prepar'd for a Flesh-day, otherwise, it must not be us'd. The Butter, being thus refin'd, must be taken off from the Fire, and set by for some time. Then, breaking three new laid Eggs, take the Whites, and make some Snow, into which you are to put fine Sugar, four Yolks of Eggs, candy'd Lemmon peel cut very fmall, green Lemmon peel grated, and a little Orange-flower-water, all proportionably beaten. Pour the Butter into the fame Farce, and let all be well whipt together. In the mean while, having provided a fine Pafte, let a piece of it be roll'd out very thin, to be laid on the Pie-pan that is butter'd a little, and let the fides of the Pie be fhap'd with the Point of a Knife. Afterwards, the Farce being put into it, it muft be bak'd with a little Fire on the top, only in the middle of the Pie-pan, left it fhould take too brown a colour. To know when thefe forts of Pies are fufficiently bak'd, 'tis requifite to obferve, whether they are ready to flip off from the Baking-pans, and before they are ferv'd up, they muft be ftrew'd with fine Sugar, and ic'd over with the red-hot Fire-fhovel. They may be garnifh'd with *Rif-foles.* Apple-fritters, or any thing elfe of the like nature.

The Lard Pan-pie is prepar'd after the fame manner, only making ufe of tried Lard inftead of Butter, but care muft be taken, that it have not the leaft ill tafte, and that the Eggs be always newly laid. If the Pies are large, a greater quantity of Eggs will be requifite.

As for the Marrow-pie, it may likewife be made as the former; that is to fay, when the Marrow is refined or well melted, the Eggs are to be beaten in the fame manner, and the Lemmon-peels, with the other Ingredients muft be added. Others pound tne Marrow, Sugar, and Lemmon-peel all together, with a little Flower and Orange-flower-water. Afterwards, they whip the Whites of the Eggs, with three or four Yolks, and mingle them with the reft in tne Mortar. However, a fine Pafte ought to be made as for the other Pies, and 'tis no great matter how different the Ways of making them may be, provided they tend to the producing of the fame good Effect.

A fugar'd Pan-pie for an Intermeß.

Take five or fix Biskets, March-panes or Macaroons, with Sugar, and four or five Yolks of Eggs; pound them in a Mortar, with a little Orange-flower-water, and let the whole Mafs be laid upon Puff pafte. Then let the Pie be bak'd with a gentle Fire, and Iced over, till it comes to a fine colour.

An

An *Artichoke*-Tourte, *or Pan-pie.*

When the Artichoke-bottoms are well boil'd, and become very white, they may be put into a Pie, with fine Herbs, Chibbols chopt small, Pepper, Salt, Nutmeg and Butter Cover your Pie with a Lid, and put into it a white Sauce, with a little Vinegar, when ready to be serv'd up to Table

Otherwise, the Artichoke-bottoms may be pounded and strain'd thro' the Hair-fieve, with melted Butter or Lard, to make as it were a kind of Cream , adding two raw Yolks of Eggs, with Salt and Nutmeg Let all be put into a very fine thin Paste, and when bak'd, serv'd up with Mutton-gravy and Lemmon-juice.

A pounded Macaroon may also be put into the Artichoke-cream, with Sugar, Cinnamon, candy'd Lemmon-peel, a little Milk-cream and Salt. This Pie may be made without a Lid, but before it is brought to Table, it must be ic'd over with Sugar, and Orange-flower-water.

An *Asparagus-pan-pie.*

Let the tender part of the Afparagus be cut, and the Tops referv'd for garnifhing Afterwards, they muft be fcalded in Water, and drefs'd in a Pie, with melted Lard, Marrow, or Butter, fine Herbs, Chibbols, Pepper, Salt and Nutmeg This Pie ought to be cover'd with a Lid, and when bak'd, fome Cream may be put into it, or Mutton-gravy, and the Yolk of an Egg.

A *Spinage-pan-pie.*

Take Spinage-leaves, and fcald them in Water, or elfe ftew them in an earthen Pot, with half a Glafs of white Wine, to take away their Crudity As foon as the Wine is confum'd, let the Spinage be drain'd, and chopt very fmall, feafon'd with a little Salt, Cinnamon, Sugar, Lemmon-peel, two Macaroons and fweet Butter. Then let them be put into fine Paste, and, cover'd with Slips of cut Pastry-work ; adding fome Sugar and Orange-flower, as it is ferving up to Table.

A Truffle-*pan-pie.*

Having cut the *Truffles* into Slices, and caus'd the Skin to be well peel'd off, they may be laid in order on a piece of fine Paste roll'd out for the Bottom-crust . Then let a little Flower be fried in Butter, with fine Herbs chopt small, and a whole Chibbol, and let all be put into the Pie ; seasoned with Pepper, Salt and Nutmeg   This sort of Pies is not usually cover'd, but must be serv'd up with Lemmon-juice.

A Tourte *or Pan-pie made of* Mousserons, Morilles *and common Mushrooms.*

Let your Mushrooms be cut into Slices and laid upon a piece of fine Paste in the bottom of a Pie-pan, with fine Herbs, Chibbols, Salt, Nutmeg, fried Flower and Butter   Then cover your Pie with a Lid, wash it over, and when bak'd, serve it up, with Mutton-gravy and Lemmon-juice, after having taken away the Chibbols . A thickening Liquor may also be added with burnt Butter

The Pan-pies of *Morilles* and *Mousserons* are usually made after the same manner.

An Egg-par-pie.

Take the Yolks of Eggs, a Lump of Sugar, a little Butter and Orange-flower-water, make as it were a kind of Cream ; and put it into a piece of very thin fine Paste rais'd with a little Border for the Side-crust : Then having grated some Lemmon-peel upon it. let it be bak'd and ic'd over, when ready to be brought to Table

A Pan-pie, *with Sorrel-juice.*

After having pounded the Sorrel, to get the Juice, let it be put into a Dish, with Sugar, Cinnamon, Macaroons, a Lump of Butter, three Yolks of Eggs, candy'd Lemmon-peel grated and Orange-flowers: Then let all be boil'd together, as it were Cream, and afterwards laid upon a piece of very fine Paste in the bottom of a Baking-pan.   When the Pie is bak'd, it may be serv'd up, with Sugar.

Pan-pies of divers Colours.

Another Pan-pie may be made of a kind of green Cream; mingling some Beet-juice with Pistachoes and Almonds, as they are straining thro' the Hair-sieve: For all the other sorts of Colours, see what has been deliver'd on that Subject, for Jellies and *Blanc-mangers*, in the second Article of *Jellies* under the Letter I.

Other sorts of Tourtes, *or Pan-pies.*

Many other sorts of Pan-pies may also be prepar'd, to be serv'd up, as the former, among the Intermesses, as well for Flesh-days, as those of Abstinence, particularly, Pies made of the Pulp of Oranges cut into Slices and laid upon fine Paste, with Sugar, a pounded Macaroon, Cinnamon and Pistachoes. The same thing may be done with green Lemmons, only some candy'd Lemmon-peel grated must be us'd instead of Pistachoes. Both these sorts of Pies are to be serv'd up, with Musked Sugar Others may likewise be made of Pomegranate-kernels, candy'd Lemmon-peels, preserv'd Plums, cut Pistachoes, &c. For Almond-pies, it would be only requisite to follow the Directions, as well for the most proper Pastes to be used for that purpose, as the rest of the Managery, which have been laid down in the first and fourth Articles of *Almonds*, under the Letter A.

It may not be improper here to subjoin some other Pan-pies made of Fish, that are generally provided for Side-dishes, on Fish-days, *viz.*

*A Cray-fish-*Tourte, *or Pan-pie.*

Let the Cray-fish be stew'd in a Glass of white Wine, after they have been well wash'd; reserving the Claws and Tails: Let all the rest be pounded in a Mortar, to be strain'd thro' the Hair-sieve, with a little Broth, and melted Butter: Then the whole Mixture may be put into a Pan-pie, with Pepper, Salt, Nutmeg, young Chibbols and Mushrooms cut into pieces, and when the Pie is cover'd with a Lid, it must be wash'd over, in order to be bak'd, and serv'd up with Lemmon-juice.

Otherwise, the Flesh of the Cray-fish may be minc'd and put

into

into a Pie, with Carps-roes, Pikes-livers, *Morilles*, common Mushrooms, *Truffles*, Butter and the other feasoning Ingredients, in order to be ferv'd up with Lemmon or Orange-juice.

A Pan-pie made of Carps-roes and Tongues.

The Tongues and Roes of the Carps must be laid in order upon a piece of fine Paste, in the bottom of the Pan, feafon'd with Pepper, Salt, Nutmeg, fine Herbs, Chibbols, *Morilles*, common Mushrooms, *Truffles* and fweet Butter. Then, all being cover'd with a Lid of the fame Paste, let the Pie be bak'd with a gentle Fire, and ferv'd up with Lemmon-juice.

Pan-pies made of Pikes-livers.

These are to be feafon'd as the former, except that burnt Butter must be us'd, and a diffolved Anchovie put into them, with Capers and Lemmon juice, before they are brought to Table.

A Salmon-pan-pie.

After having ftew'd the Salmon for a while in Claret, it must be cut into Slices or *Filets*, and drefs'd in the Pie, with candy'd Lemmon peel, Dates, Sugar, Cinnamon, a little Pepper, Salt and Butter. When the Pie is half bak'd, pour in the Wine in which the Salmon was ftew'd; let it also be ic'd over, and ferv'd up, with Lemmon-juice.

Otherwife, the Salmon may be chopt fmall, with Mushrooms, fine Herbs, Chibbols, Artichoke-bottoms, Pepper, Salt and Nutmeg, and ferv'd up in the fame manner.

A Tourte, or Pan-pie made of Smelts, Pike, Soles, and other forts of Fish.

Let your Fish be cut into *Filets*, with chopt *Morilles*, common Mushrooms and *Truffles*, to be laid on the bottom of the Pie, feafon'd with Pepper, Salt, Nutmeg, fine Herbs, Chibbols and pieces of Mushrooms. Or elfe the Bones and Heads of the Fish may be taken away and fried, to ferve for Garniture. But the Pies must always be fet on the Table, with Orange or Lemmon-juice.

An

An Oiſter-pan-pie.

This Pie is uſually made after the ſame manner, only it will be requiſite to add a little Bread-chippings, with Capers and a Slice of green Lemmon, as alſo the Liquor of the Oiſters, before it is ſerv'd up to Table.

A Muſcle-pan-pie.

The Muſcles, being well cleans'd and waſh'd, muſt be fried in a Pan, and clear'd from their Shells, in order to be dreſs'd in a Pie, with Muſhrooms cut into pieces, *Morilles*, Pepper, Salt, Nutmeg, Thyme and Butter. When the Pie is half bak'd, the Muſcle-liquor muſt be put into it, with Bread-chippings, as alſo Lemmon-juice, at the inſtant of ſerving it up to Table.

A Pan-pie of farced Tench.

When your Tenches are well cleans'd from their Slime, ſlit them on the Back, and take away the Fleſh, ſo as the Head and Tail may ſtick to the Skin. Then mince this Fleſh with Muſhrooms, Carps-roes, fine Herbs, Pepper, Salt, Nutmeg and beaten Cloves; and, having ſtuff'd the Bones of the Fiſh with the ſame Farce, dreſs them in a Pie, with Oiſters, Muſhrooms, Carps-roes, Pikes-livers and Butter, adding half a Glaſs of white Wine, when the Pie is half-bak'd, and ſome Lemmon-juice, as it is ſerving up to Table.

Other Tourtes, *or Pan-pies made of Fiſh,* &c.

Tourtes, or Pan-pies, are likewiſe made of Perches, Tortoiſes, and many other Fiſhes, for which due Meaſures may be eaſily taken from the former, or from the particular Inſtructions given in their proper places, for the dreſſing of thoſe ſorts of Fiſh. To theſe may be added Pan-pies of *Beatils*, and others of Pigeons dreſs'd with a good Fiſh-farce, prepar'd with the Fleſh of Eels, Pikes and Carps, with pounded Roes. To that purpoſe, the Rumps of thoſe Pigeons muſt be made hollow, and a piece of a Pike's Liver, or ſome other ſtuff'd into it. Then they are to be ſtew'd a little in melted Butter, and put into a Pie, with artificial Cocks combs and Veal-ſweet-breads, made of of the fame Compound or Farce, and fcalded feparately in a Ladle. This Pie muft be feafon'd with Pepper, Salt, Nutmeg, Mufhrooms, Fifh-roes, *Morilles* and fweet Butter; adding a little white Wine at laft, and Lemmon-juice when ferv'd up to Table.

TROTTERS.

A Side-difh of Sheeps-trotters farced.

Let the Trotters be well fcalded, and afterwards ftew'd in good Broth, with a little Parfly and Chibbol; taking care that they be not over-done. As foon as they are taken out, let the Feet be cut off, leaving the Legs; the Bones of which muft be taken away, and the Skins fpread upon the Table or Dreffer, in order to be ftuff'd with a little of the *Farce of Croquets,* or fome other, and roll'd up one by one: Then, after having laid them in a Difh, and fprinkled them with a little melted Fat, they muft be neatly breaded on the top, and brought to a Colour in the Oven. When they are colour'd, let the Fat be drain'd from them, and let the fide of the Difh be rubb'd with a Shalot; pouring a little Ragoo upon them, or a Mufhroom-cullis, before they are ferv'd up hot to Table.

Another Way of dreffing Sheeps-trotters.

Sheeps-trotters may alfo be drefs'd with white Sauce, frying them in Lard, with fine Herbs, young Chibbols, Pepper, Salt and Nutmeg. The Sauce muft be thicken'd with Yolks of Eggs and Rofe-vinegar; garnifhing the Difh with the Trotter-bones fried in Pafte and Parfly.

TROUTS.

A Side-difh of broil'd Trouts.

The Trouts may be either breaded, or left in their natural condition; for the latter, a Ragoo may be prepar'd, with *Mouf-ferons, Truffles,* Fifh-roes, and Pikes-livers fried brown, alfo an Anchovie, fine Herbs, and a few Capers. Let the Trouts be laid a foaking for fome time in this Sauce, and afterwards ferv'd up, with Lemmon-juice.

For

For the others, that you would have breaded, they ought to
be steept in a good *Marinade*, for the space of a full Hour, after having cut them into pieces, to the end that they may take
the whole relish Then they may be broil'd over a gentle Fire,
and sprinkled with Lemmon-juice, whilst the Dish is garnish'd
with *Petits-patez*, *i. e.* little Pies made of Fish, or with *Marinade*.

An Intermeß of Trouts on Flesh-days.

Having provided two or three good Trouts, let them be neatly gutted at the Gills, scrap'd and well wipt Then, laying
them on the Dresser, let the red-hot Fire-shovel be gently pass'd
over them, yet so as not to touch them, and let it be re-iterated
from time to time . When they are sufficiently harden'd by this
means, they may be larded with small Slips of Bacon in rows.
Afterwards, some good *Bards*, or thin Slices of Bacon being laid
on the bottom of an oval Stew-pan, the larded Trouts must be
set in order upon them , kindling a little Fire underneath, and
putting some live Coals on the top of the Cover, to give the
Fish a fine colour · They must also be stirr'd at several times,
lest they should stick to the bottom.   When they are well colour'd, take away all the Bacon, soak your Trouts in good
Gravy, with a little *Champagne*-wine, and an Onion stuck with
Cloves, and let all be gently stew'd together, and well season'd
in the same Pan As soon as they are almost done enough, and
little Sauce is left, let some *Truffles*, Mushrooms and all sorts of
Garniture, according to the Season, be put into a little Gammon-essence, in order to make a well-season'd and somewhat
thick Ragoo   Then dress your Trouts in a large Dish, either
of an Oval or round Figure, and pour the Ragoo round about,
after the Fat has been thoroughly drain'd off The Dish may
be garnish'd, if you please, with Artichoke-bottoms, *Andouillets*,
or small Trout-collops well larded and order'd as those of Soles.

As for the large Sea-fish, they must be larded with thick Slips
of Bacon, and when well tied up, they may be boil'd in a good
Court-bouillon, proper for Flesh-days, that is well season'd, and
enrich d with all sorts of exquisite Ingredients , adding a little
Champagne-wine When the Fish are ready, let them be dress'd
in Oval Dishes, and let a Ragoo be turn'd upon them, made of
all sorts of Garnitures. Some fresh Oisters may also be added, with
their Liquor, or else a Carp-sauce, or one of Gammon-essence,

may

may be prepar'd for that purpofe, taking care that all be well clear'd from the Fat, and ferv d up hot to Table

TRUFFLES.

The Way of dreffing *Truffles* moft in vogue, is that of a *Court-bouillon*, fo as they may be ftew'd in white Wine or Claret, and feafon'd with Pepper, Salt and Bay-leaves.

They may alfo be broil'd upon the Coals, flitting them in half to put in fome white Pepper and Salt, and clofing them up again, in order to be wrapt up in wet Paper and laid over a Fire that is not too quick : Then they may be ferv'd up to Table, on a folded Napkin

Or elfe, after having cleans'd your *Truffles*, cut them into Slices, and fry them in Lard or Butter, with Flower Then they muft be ftew'd in a little Broth, with fine Herbs, Pepper, Salt and Nutmeg, and laid a foaking in a Difh, till there be little Sauce left ; to be ferv d up, with Mutton-gravy and Lemmon-juice.

Otherwife, feveral Ragoo's may be made of *Truffles* and Capons-livers, as alfo *Tourtes* or Pan-pies ; as it has been before obferv'd : And in the Entertainments with Roots or Collations during the time of Lent, they may be eaten dry, with Oil, but they muft be always fet on the Table among the Intermeffes.

TUNNIES.

Tunnies may be drefs'd in Slices or *Filets*, with Poor Man's Sauce, and in a Sallet, with the *Ramolade* defcrib'd Pag 41. They may alfo be fried in round Slices, and ferv'd up in a kind of Fifh-*Marinade*, fuch as is fpecified in the laft Article of *Marinades* Or elfe, they may be broil'd upon a Grid-iron, after having rubb'd and ftrew'd them with Pepper, Salt and Butter, to be eaten with Orange and burnt Butter. Otherwife, a *Poupeton* may be made of them ; or they may be bak'd in a Pot-pie, putting the Flefh chopt fmall into a Pot, or earthen Pan, with burnt Butter and white Wine ; alfo a piece of green Lemmon, Pepper, Salt, Mufhrooms, or Chefnuts and Capers · The Difh may be garnifh d with Bread and Oifters fried, and Slices of Lemmon. For the other Tunny-pies, fee the eighteenth Article of *Pies*, under the Letter P

TUR·

T U R B O T.

A Side-difh of Turbot, in a Court-bouillon.

Let a well feafon'd *Court-bouillon* be prepar'd, with Vinegar, Verjuice, white Wine, Pepper, Salt, Cloves, Thyme, Onions, Lemmon and a Bay-leaf or two; let a little Water be alfo added, and at laft fome Milk, to render it very white : Then the Turbot muft be leafurely ftew'd in it, over a gentle Fire, and garnifh'd with Parfly, Lemmon-flices laid upon it, and Violets in their Seafon

A Turbot ferv'd up among the Intermeffes on Flefh-days.

Having fcal'd and wafh'd your Turbot, put it into a large Difh, with *Bards* or thin Slices of Bacon, feafoned with melted Lard, white Wine, Verjuice, a Faggot of Herbs, Bay-leaves, Pepper, Salt, Nutmeg, whole Cloves and green Lemmon: Then let it be cover'd with other *Bards*, and bak'd in a Pot between two Fires, or in an Oven In order to ferve it up to Table, take away the Bacon-*Bards*, drefs your Turbot in a Difh, pouring upon it a good Ragoo of Mufhrooms, made of the Sauce, and garnifh it with Slices of Lemmon.

T U R K E Y S

Among the feveral Ways of drefling Turkeys, either roafted or in a Ragoo, the two following are, without doubt, the moft modern, and confequently deferve to be firft taken notice of: One of thefe, is a Side-difh of Turkeys farced with fine Herbs, and the other a Side-difh of the fame, drefs d with Onion-effence. Turkeys are alfo ftew'd in a *Salmigund* or Hotch-potch, and with Gammon-fauce, as fome other Meffes fpecified in the General Table.

Turkeys farced with fine Herbs.

Let the Turkeys be trufs'd for roafting, but not parboil'd : The Skin on their Breaft muft alfo be loofen d, to the end that they may be conveniently ftuff'd with a Farce made of raw Bacon,

con, Parfly, Chibbol, and moft forts of fine Herbs, all chopt fmall, pounded a little in a Mortar and well feafon'd · The Turkeys being thus farced between the Skin and the Flefh, as alfo a little in the Body, muft be well fpitted and roafted. Afterwards, they are to be drefs'd in a Difh, pouring upon them a good Ragoo, of all forts of Garnitures, and ferv'd up hot to Table The fame thing may be done with Chickens, Pigeons and other forts of Fowl, and to diverfifie them on feveral Days, they may be bak d or ftew'd in a Pot between two Fires, after they have been ftuff'd, as before When they are ready, let them be well drain'd, and ferv'd up with a good Ragoo of *Truffles*, and Veal-fweet-breads; all well drefs'd, clear'd from the Fat, and garnifh'd with fmall *Croquets*.

A Side-difh of Turkeys, with Onion-effence.

The 'Onions muft be cut into Slices and fried in a Stew-pan, with Lard Then the Fat being drain'd a little from them, they muft be tofs'd up again, with as much Flower as can be got up between your Fingers; adding fome good Gravy, Cloves, and the other neceffary feafoning Ingredients. When all have been ftew'd together a little while, let them be ftrain d thro' the Hair-fieve, and afterwards put into the Stew-pan a third time, with a few drops of Verjuice and a little Bread-cullis. In the mean while, the Turkeys having their Wings, Breaft and Legs well tied up, ought to be roafted, and drefs'd in a Difh; pouring the Sauce upon them, before they are ferv'd up after the ufual manner.

Other Side-difhes of Turkeys.

Sometimes young Turkeys, one of them larded, and the other only barded, or cover'd with thin Slices of Bacon, without being breaded, are roafted and ferv'd up in Gravy

At another time, your Turkeys being barded and roafted, take away their Legs, Wings and Breafts, and cut them into *Filets*, to be put into a Ragoo of Cucumbers fried brown, with a brown thickening Liquor, and ˙ ˙˙˙ of Lemmon, as they are dreffing.

V.

V.

VEAL.

IN several places of this Book, we have taken occasion to shew, how Veal may be drefs'd in order to make a great number of Meffes and Dishes for every Service ; particularly, Veal-ftakes for Side-dishes, Veal-cutlets, Pies made of a Fillet of Veal, &c. not to mention, a very great number of other Dishes that are made of Veal, or at leaft, in which Veal is us'd : So that it remains only to produce fome other manners of dreffing this fort of Meat, for feparate Dishes.

A Side-dish of Veal, after the Italian Way.

Having provided fome Slices or Stakes of Veal that are very tender, and cut them as it were to make *Fricandoes* or Scotch-collops, let them be beaten a little with the Cleaving-knife. Then let fome good *Bards*, or thin Slices of Bacon be laid on the bottom of a Stew-pan ; let the Veal-ftakes be likewise laid in good order upon them ; and let all be well feafon'd The quantity of thefe Stakes muft be adjufted, according to the bignefs of your Dish or Plate , which being cover'd on the top, with other Bacon-*Bards*, the Pan muft be fet *à la Braife*, or between two Fires When all have been fufficiently bak'd in this manner, take out all the *Bards* and the Meat a-part, and drain off the Fat; only leaving as much as will ferve to make fome brown Sauce, with a little Flower, in the fame Stew-pan, but not too much Afterwards, foaking it with good Gravy, put your Veal-ftakes again into the Pan, and make an end of dreffing them ; with Veal-fweet-breads, *Truffles* cut into Slices, Mushrooms, boil'd Cockscombs, two Slices of Lemmon, a Faggot of fine Herbs, a few drops of Verjuice, a bit of Shalot, and a little Bread-cullis to thicken the Sauce But all muft be well clear'd from the Fat, and brought hot to Table.

To drefs Veal à la Bourgeoife.

Let fome Veal-ftakes be cut fomewhat thick, and larded with a fmall wooden Larding-pin , the *Lardoons* being feafon'd a little, with Parfly, Chibbols, beaten Spices, Pepper and Salt :
Then

Then let feveral fmall *Bards* of Bacon be put into a Stew-pan, and let the Veal-ftakes be laid in order upon them   The Fire ought to be very gentle at firft, to the end that the Meat may fweat, and may be brought to a Colour on both Sides, by putting in a little Flower   When it is fufficiently colour'd, let it lye a foaking, with good clear Broth and boil gently   Afterwards, the Sauce muft be thicken'd a little, and clear'd from the Fat, fprnkling it with a little Vinegar or Verjuice, fo as the whole Mefs may be conveniently drefs'd in a Difh and ferv'd up hot to Table.

A Loin of Veal in a Ragoo.

Lard your Loin with thick Slips of Bacon, feafon it with Pepper, Salt and Nutmeg, and when it is almoft roafted, put it into a Stew-pan clofe cover'd, with Broth, a Glafs of white Wine, fome of the Dripping, fried Flower, a Bunch of Herbs, Mufhrooms, and a piece of green Lemmon   Laftly, let all be ferv'd up with fhort Sauce, after having taken away fome of the Fat, and let the Difh be fet out with larded Veal-fweet-breads, Cutlets, or other forts of Garniture

Other Ways of drefsing a Quarter and Loin of Veal

A Quarter of Veal may be larded with fmall Slips of Bacon, except the thick end , which is to be well breaded and feafon'd   It muft be garnifh'd with *Riffoles* and Capons-breafts, and fome Veal-gravy muft be pour'd upon it, when ready to be fet on the Table

It may alfo be marinated in an oval Stew-pan, and well order'd with the ufual feafoning Ingredients. When it is roafted, take the Kidney to make farced Tofts to garnifh the whole Quarter, or elfe an *Omelet*, and let the Difh be fet out with *Marinades*, either of Cutlets or Chickens, or with farced Cutlets and fried Parfly

Another middling Side-difh may be made of half a Loin of Veal, boil'd in a *Court-bouillon* that is well feafon'd and enrich'd, wrapping it up in a Napkin, left it fhould break. It muft be garnifh'd with fried Bread, Parfly and Lemmon-flices.

A

A great Side-diſh of a Quarter, or Crupper of Veal farced upon the Leg.

For the Ragoo that is proper for the ſtuffing of this Joint of Meat, ſee the Article of *Salpicon,* where it is explain'd at large; or elſe make a well ſeaſon'd Haſh of the Fleſh that is taken out of the Leg, and cover it again neatly with the Skin. Then let that part, which is not larded, be breaded with Bread-crum; garniſhing the Diſh with Cutlets either faiced or unfarced, or with *Riſſoles* and Cruſts of fried Bread, all brought to a fine colour: A Quarter of Veal may alſo be larded with *Hatlets*

Several Ways of dreſſing a Breaſt of Veal.

A Side-diſh may be made of a farced Breaſt of Veal, garniſh'd with roaſted *Poupiets* in the form of Quails, and a good Ragoo pour'd on the top: This Joint muſt be firſt roaſted brown, and afterwards ſtew'd in a Pot A piece of a Beef-ſtake muſt alſo be added, as it is dreſſing, to enrich it, and a brown thickening Liquor with Gravy, when ready to be ſerv'd up to Table. As for the Farce, it muſt be made of other Veal, with Beef-ſewet or Marrow, Bacon, fine Herbs, Muſhrooms and Veal-ſweet-breads, and ſeaſon'd with Pepper, Salt and Nutmeg. A Breaſt of Veal may alſo be boil'd in an earthen Pan, or in a Stew-pan, with Broth and a Glaſs of white Wine. Then ſome Muſhrooms are to be fried in the ſame Lard, in which the Meat was dreſs'd, with a little Flower, and all muſt be mingled together

Another Side-diſh may be made of a Breaſt of Veal in a *Tourte* or Pan-pie, with a well ſeaſon'd *Godivoe,* and good Garnitures, as for other Pies, adding a proper thickening Liquor and ſome Lemmon-juice, before it is brought to Table Laſtly, another Diſh may be prepar'd of a farced or unfarced Breaſt of Veal, roaſted and put into a Ragoo, with Lemmon-juice, when ſerv'd up; garniſhing it with Veal-ſweet-breads, Cocks-combs and Muſhrooms fried. Or elſe the Breaſt of Veal being firſt par-boil'd, may be marinated in Vinegar, with Pepper, Salt and Bay-leaves: Afterwards it may be flower'd and well fried, in order to be ſerv'd up with fried Parſly and the reſt of the Sauce.

VEAL-SWEET-BREADS.

Befides the Place that Veal-fweet-breads have in all the beft forts of Ragoo's, as it plainly appears in very many Particulars; feveral feparate Difhes may be made of them, or Out-works, both for Side-difhes and Intermeffes, of which the following, is one of the moft confiderable.

Veal-fweet-breads farced à la Dauphine.

Let fome good Veal-fweet-breads be fcalded a little, and larded with boil'd Gammon. In the mean while, having prepar'd a delicious and fomewhat thick Farce, make a Hole with the point of a Knife on the Side of your Sweet-breads; but fo as it may not pafs quite thro' · Then they muft be neatly ftuff'd in that Hole and bak'd in a Pot, or Pan between two gentle Fires; whilft a good Ragoo is making for them, of *Moufferons*, common Mufhrooms, *Truffles* and Artichoke bottoms : All being well drefs d fome Cocks-combs ftuff'd with the fame Farce muft be added and a little Chicken-cullis, to the end that the Sauce may not turn black · Then having thoroughly clear'd the Sweet-breads from the Fat, let them be put into the Ragoo and ftew'd a little Afterwards the whole Mefs muft be drefs'd in a Difh, fqueezing in the Juice of an Orange, and fet hot on the Table

Other Ways of dreffing Veal-fweet-breads.

Otherwife the Veal-fweet-breads, being larded with thin Slips of Bacon and roafted, may be order'd with a good Ragoo, or Sauce pour'd upon them : Or elfe, after having been marinated, cut into Slices and flower'd, they may be fried, in order to be ferv'd up, with fried Parfly and Lemmon-juice · Or laftly, different Ragoo's may be made of them, *viz* fometimes with a white Sauce; fometimes with *Morilles*, and common Mufhrooms; and fometimes with *Truffles*; but they muft be always fet among the Intermeffes.

VENISON, *fee Deer, Hinds, Roe-bucks, Stags, wild Boars*, &c.

VENISON-PASTIES, *fee* PASTIES.

W.

W.

WHITINGS.

Whitings may be dress'd in *Casserole*, after the same manner as many other sorts of Fish : They may also be fried, and serv'd up with Orange-juice and white Pepper ; to which purpose, they must be slit on the Back, and strew'd with Pepper and Salt : They must also be steept in Vinegar, flower'd and dipt in a thin Paste or Batter, before they are put into the Frying-pan. Otherwise Whitings may be farced ; as it appears in the Article of a *Miroton* for Fish-days, and their *Filets* may not only be serv'd up in a Sallet, as it has been observ'd Pag. 41. but also in several sorts of Ragoo's and even in a Standing-pie, in a *Tourte*, or Pan-pie and in Potage ; for which see the respective Articles whereto they belong, as those of Pikes, Soles, &c.

WOOD-COCKS.

How to made a Side-dish of Wood-cocks, with Wine, &c.

Take Wood-cocks and cut them into Quarters, as it were Chickens for a white Fricassy, as also some *Truffles*, cut into Slices, with Veal-sweet-breads, *Moufferons* and common Mushrooms, all which are to be fried together, and soak'd with good Gravy : Afterwards, two Glasses of white or red Wine may be pour'd in, and when the whole Mess is well stew'd and season'd ; a Wood-cock-cullis, to thicken the Sauce, or some other good Cullis, accordingly as it may stand with your Convenience A Spoonful of Gammon essence may also be added, and all must be thoroughly clear'd from the Fat Then lay your Wood-cocks in order in a Dish, turn the Ragoo upon them, and squeez in the Juice of a Lemmon, before they are brought hot to Table

To make a Salmigund *or* Hotch-potch *of Wood-cocks, with Wine.*

When the Wood-cocks are half roasted, let them be cut into pieces, and put into a Stew-pan with Wine, proportionably to their quantity : Let some chopt Mushrooms and *Truffles* be also

T 2   thrown

thrown in, with a few Anchovies and Capers and let all be well stew'd together. Then the Sauce being thicken'd with a good Cullis, the Wood-cocks muft be drefs'd and kept hot, without boiling : Afterwards, having drain'd off all the Fat, and fqueez'd in the Juice of an Orange, they may be ferv'd up hot to Table.

A Side-difh may be alfo made of Wood-cocks in *Sur-tout* , for which fee the eighth Article of *Pigeons* drefs d in that manner, under the Letter P ; and for a hot Pie of Wood-cocks and Partridges, recourfe may be had to the firft Article of *Pies.*

The End of the Court and Country Cook.

N E W

NEW
INSTRUCTIONS
FOR
Confectioners;

DIRECTING

How to Preferve all forts of Fruits, as well dry, as liquid; alfo how to make divers Sugar-works, and other fine Pieces of Curiofity belonging to the Confectionary Art.

CHAP. I.

Of the different Ways of Boiling Sugar; of the Choice of it, and of the Manner of Clarifying it.

FOrafmuch as the Ground-work of the Confectioner's Art, depends upon the different Ways of Boiling Sugar, it is requifite in the firft place, to give a particular Account of them, to the end that the Reader may more readily apprehend the meaning of feveral Terms hereafter us'd to exprefs them, and that unprofitable Repetitions may be avoided; which would inevitably happen if they were explain'd in every diftinct Article, as the variety of Matter would require. Thefe Boilings then, are perform'd by degrees, and bear the following Denominations; that is to fay, Sugar

T 3   may

may be boil'd till it becomes *Smooth, Pearled, Blown, Feather'd, Crack'd* and *Caramel* These Degrees are also distinguish'd with respect to their proper Qualifications, as the lesser and the greater Smooth, the lesser and the greater Pearled, Feathered a little, and a great deal, and so of the rest.

The Boiling of Sugar call'd Smooth.

As soon as your Sugar is clarified, and set again on the Fire in order to be boil'd, you may know when it has attain'd to its smooth Quality, by dipping the Tip of your Fore-finger into it; afterwards applying it to your Thumb, and opening them a little, a small Thread or String sticks to both, which immediately breaks and remains in a Drop upon the Finger. When this String is almost imperceptible, the Sugar is only boil'd till it becomes a little smooth, and when it extends it self farther before it breaks, 'tis a sign that the Sugar is very smooth. To avoid scalding your self, in making this Experiment, as it may happen, if your Finger were directly dipt into the Sugar, you need only take out the Skimmer, which ought always to be kept in the Copper-pan to stir the Sugar from time to time, and to cause it to boil equally: Then holding it a little while on the top, after having shaken it, touching the Pan, with the Handle of the Skimmer, receive the Sugar that still runs from it, and only pass the tip of your Finger upon the edge of the said Skimmer, which is sufficient to know, whether the Sugar is become smooth, or not, by observing the former Directions.

The Pearled Boiling.

After having boil'd your Sugar, a little longer, re-iterate the same Experiment, and if in separating your Fingers, as before, the String continues sticking to both, the Sugar is Pearled The greater Pearled Boiling is when the String continues in like manner, altho' the Fingers were stretch'd out farther, by entirely spreading the Hand. This sort of Boiling may also be known by a kind of round Pearls that arise on the top of the Liquor.

The

The Blown Boiling

When your Sugar has boil'd a few more Walms, hold the Skimmer in your Hand, and having shaken it a little, as before, beating the side of the Pan, blow thro' the Holes of it, from one side to the other, and if certain Sparks as it were, or small Bubbles fly out, the Sugar is come to the degree of Boiling, call'd *Blown.*

The Feathered Boiling.

When after some other Seethings, you blow thro' the Skimmer, or shake the *Spatula* with a Back-stroke, till thicker and larger Bubbles rise up on high, then the Sugar is become Feathered And when after frequent Tryals, you perceive these Bubbles to be thicker, and in greater quantity, so that several of them stick together, and form as it were a flying Flake; then the Sugar is greatly Feathered.

The Crack'd Boiling.

To know when the Sugar has attain'd to this degree, a Pot or Pan, must be provided, with cold Water· Then dip the tip of your Finger into that Water, and having dextrously run it into the boiling Sugar, dip it again immediately into the Water, at least if you would avoid scalding your self: Thus keeping your Finger in the Water, rub off the Sugar, with the other two; and if it breaks afterwards, making a kind of crackling Noise, it is come to the point of Boiling, call'd *Crack'd.*

The Caramel Boiling.

If in the condition, to which the Sugar is reduc'd in the former Boiling, it be put between the Teeth, it would stick to them as it were Glue or Pitch; but when it is boil'd to *Caramel*, it breaks and cracks, without sticking in the least. Therefore care must be taken to observe every Moment, when it has attain'd to this last degree of Boiling, putting the preceding Directions into Practice, to know, when it is Crack'd, and afterwards biting the Sugar so order'd with your Teeth, to try whether it will stick to them. As soon as you perceive, that it does

T 4   not

not stick, but on the contrary, cracks and breaks clever, take it off immediately from the Fire, otherwise it would burn, and be no longer good for any manner of use, because it will always taste burnt: Whereas with respect to the other well-condition'd Boilings, if after having preserv'd any Sweet-meats, some Sugar be still left, that is Crack'd, for example, or greatly Feather-ed, and that is of no further use in that condition, it would be only requisite to put as much Water to it, as is needful to boil it over again, and then it may be brought to whatsoever degree you shall think fit, and even intermix'd with any other sort of Sugar, or Syrup

This last *Caramel*-boiling is proper for Barley-sugar, and for certain small Sugar-works call'd by that Name, which shall be hereafter explain'd: The Pearled Boiling is generally us'd for all sorts of Confits, that are to be kept for a considerable time: Some cause their Sugar to be boil'd to a higher degree, but it is soon undone and reduc'd to the Pearled Quality, by the Moisture and Coldness of the Fruits, that are thrown into it   The Use of the other Ways of Boiling shall be shewn in treating of the several sorts of Sweet-meats, for which they are requisite.

It is also necessary to understand, That sometimes Fruit may be preserv'd with thin Sugar, that is to say, when two Ladles full of clarified Sugar are put to one of Water, four to two, six to three, and so on proportionably to the quantity of the Fruit, that ought to be well soak'd in it · To that purpose, the Sugar and Water must be heated together somewhat more than luke-warm, to be poured upon them

The choice of Sugar.

For the best manner of Preserving Fruits, a Confectioner ought to make choice of the finest and whitest Loaf-sugar, that can be procur'd; such as is hard and ringing, nevertheless light and sweet, without the least sharpness   If there be occasion to use Powder-sugar, the whitest and cleanest must likewise be chosen: However both these sorts ought to be clarified, so that there will be much less Work to do than otherwise, if the Loaf-sugar or Powder-sugar were not well-conditioned.

How to clarifie Sugar.

The Confectioner's Work begins with the clarifying of Sugar; to which purpose; an earthen Pan must be provided with Water, into which an Egg is to be broken with the Shell, or more, according to the quantity of Sugar. Then let all be whipt together with Birchen Rods or a Whisk, and pour'd upon the Sugar that is to be melted: Afterwards, having set it over the Fire, stirr it continually and take off the Scum carefully when it boils· As often as the Sugar rises, a little cold Water must be pour'd in, to hinder it from running over and to raise the Scum; adding also the Froth of the White of an Egg, whipt a-part. When after having well scumm'd the Liquor, there is only left a small whitish Froth, and not black and foul, as before, and when you perceive the Sugar to be altogether clear upon the Skimmer, in laying it upon the Surface, it must be remov'd from the Fire, and being pass'd thro' the Straining-bag it will be perfectly clarified.

When a confiderable quantity of Sugar is clarified at once, and confequently a great deal of Scum rifes, which is always accompanied with a little Sugar; this Scum being temper'd with Water, may be boil'd in the fame Pan, into which it was put, and afterwards all strain'd thro' the Bag

Private Persons, who in preferving Fruits, ufe only four or five Pounds of Sugar at once, to avoid this trouble, and yet not lofe any Sugar, may clarifie it in the following manner. Let the Sugar be melted with Water, and fet over the Fire, with the White of a whipt Egg. As foon as it boils and fwells up ready to run over, a little cold Water must be pour'd in to give it a Check But when it rifes a fecond time, let it be remov'd from the Fire, and fet by about a quarter of an Hour, during which fpace, it will fink, and a black Scum will only fettle on the top, which is to be gently taken off with the Skimmer. Afterwards, strain it thro' the Bag and it will be fufficiently clarified. Indeed Sugar fo order'd is not fo clear nor fo white as the former, neverthelefs it will ferve to make all forts of good Comfits

The Water that is proper for the boiling of Sugar, ought to be taken out of a Spring or River, and very clear, altho' for many other Things Well-water may alfo be us'd: The leffer quantity of Water is put to the Sugar, which is to be melted and clarified, fo much the lefs time is requifite for the performing of
the

the necessary Boilings ; whereas the contrary happens, when there is a great deal of Water, because it must all evaporate As to this particular, no scruple ought to be made, concerning a Maxim deliver'd in some Books, *viz* That in causing Sugar to be boil'd a-part without the Fruit, its best Spirits exhale with the Water, and it becomes only capable of Preserving the upper Part of the Fruits, as being made greasie and thick by the Boiling ; whereas (in their Opinion) the Fruits are more easily penetrated, when both are boil'd together in the Beginning. For this Assertion is contrary, not only to the general Practice of Confectioners, but also to Experience and Truth ; since the Fruits always appear to have as much Sugar in the Inside, as on the Surface, provided they be well order'd, which may be done by working and boiling them, several Days, in the manner hereafter describ'd For altho' generally speaking, the Preserving of Fruit may be finish'd in one Day ; yet it is expedient that divers be taken up in carrying on the Work, if you would have them kept for any considerable time, and order'd as they ought to be.

The common People only judge the Sugar to be sufficiently boil'd, when the Drops that are put upon a Plate grow thick, as it were a Jelly and cease to run, any longer · Indeed this Way of boiling is proper for certain Jellies of Fruit, and for *Compotes* ; but no great Progress would be made in the Art of Preserving, if nothing else were known : So that it is absolutely necessary to understand all the different Degrees of boiling above-specified, and the distinction is only made by those Tryals, at least without a long Practice, and even the most skilful Confectioners know nothing otherwise, after the Feathered Boiling.

C H A P. II.

Of the Utensils and Instruments necessary for a Confectioner, and of their Use.

THe understanding of this Article ought also to be pre-suppos'd, without which what is hereafter laid down, cannot be well apprehended ; as neither is it possible to put those Directions jections into Practice, if the greater part of these Utensils be wanting Therefore it is requisite to provide Pans, with their Skimmers, and *Spatula's*, one or two Furnaces, Sieves, Grates, a Stove, a Campain-oven, a Cistern, several Mortars, a Marble-stone, and a Syringe, not to mention the Trunks, Boxes, Pots, Glasses, and some other little Knacks, that are very common

The Pans ought to be of several Sizes, some flat and others hollow, for different Uses. The flat Pans are for those Fruits that ought to be soak'd in their Syrup, without laying them in heaps one upon another, and the hollow ones, are us'd when any Thing is to be preserv'd dry, by boiling and working the Sugar, as for Oranges, Lemmons and Conserves All these Pans are usually made of red Copper, as also the Skimmers and *Spatula's*, and there are a few Houses of Persons of Quality, where they are wanting, otherwise such Pans may be us d as are at hand, and the ordinary hollow ones may serve well enough, for all sorts of Operations.

Upon this occasion, it may not be improper to undeceive those, who upon the Asseveration of some Writers, might be induc d to believe, That the Copper causes an ill Taste in preserved Fruits, when they are set by in a Pan, from the Fire; for as yet it could never be perceiv d, altho' it is very customary to leave them therein indifferently during several Days Indeed care ought to be taken to keep them clean, and not to follow the Example of some Slovenly Work-men who when they intermix some old Syrups, let in the green Rust that sticks on the sides of the Pan, with a great deal of other Filth, which does not hinder them from proceeding in their Work, and disposing of all Promiscuously with a great deal of Assurance

It is expedient, that all the Pans be stampt according to the Standard, or have the mark of their Weight engrav'd upon them, in order to know the quantity of Sugar that has been boil'd in them, when they are put into one Scale, and the Fruits, which are to be preserv'd into the other, with the Tare of what the Pan weighs, to regulate and proportion the Weight of both, conformably to the Directions hereafter given.

The management of a Furnace is sufficiently known, only those of Confectioners ought to be somewhat larger than the common ones, to the end that the Fire spreading itself in a greater extent round about the Pan, the Sugar and Fruits which are to be preserv'd may boil more equally on all sides

Upon

Upon any emergent Occaſion, almoſt all the Operations may be perform'd over the ordinary Kitchen-furnaces, if they may be freely us'd without any diſturbance

The Sieves are alſo a ſort of Inſtruments the uſe of which is not unknown: They ſerve to make an end of drying the Paſtes of Fruits, when they are turn'd ; to ſtrain Jellies and Syrups , to drain Fruits, that have been laid in Water, and for ſeveral other good purpoſes   A finer Sieve call'd a *Drum* muſt likewiſe be provided, to ſift powder'd Sugar, that is us'd in divers Works.

To theſe muſt be added a kind of Cullander to drain the Fruits, either after they have been ſcalded in Water, or when they are taken out of the Sugar.   This Inſtrument, for want of which an ordinary Cullander may be us'd, is a Piece of Copper or Tin ſomewhat hollow, bor'd thro' with many Holes, and flexible, ſo as the Fruits may be eaſily ſlipt into it at pleaſure.   When Fruits taken out of the Sugar are to be drain'd, it is requiſite to ſet this Cullander over a Pan to receive the Sugar that drops from it

The ſame thing may be done with the Grates, which are made of ſeveral Circles of Wires ſet very cloſe together in form of Croſs-bars , upon which thoſe Comfits are chiefly laid, that are to be preſerv'd dry, whilſt the Sugar is preparing to ice them over

The Stove is a little Cloſet, well ſtopt up on all ſides, where there are ſeveral Stories, or Rows of Shelves, one above another, made of the ſame ſort of Wires, to hold the Sweet-meats that are to be dried, and which are uſually laid upon Slates, pieces of Tin, ſmooth Boards, or Sieves , having firſt caus'd the Syrup out of which they were taken, to be drain'd off. Then a Pan, or large Chafing-diſh, with Fire, is to be ſet on the bottom, and ſometimes two, if there are many Things to be dried, or if the Buſineſs requires diſpatch   Thus the Stove muſt be ſhut up cloſe, and in the Evening, or the next Morning, the Sweet-meats contain'd in it, either Paſtes or Fruits, muſt be turn'd, to cauſe them to dry equally   The latter are to be ſtrew'd with Sugar, except ſome ſorts, as green Apricocks and green Almonds; but the Paſtes muſt not be turn'd again, till they become firm, ſome of which are alſo ſtrew'd with Sugar on one ſide: Then they may be gently remov'd from the Slates, with a Knife and laid upon others, or upon Sieves, as it has been already hinted: Afterwards they muſt be
put

put again into the Stove, changing the Stories, if it be judg'd expedient, and renewing the Fire · So that the Art of Preserving cannot be put into Practice, without one of these Stoves, or some other Machine of the like nature ; for in drying Sweetmeats at the Fire, they would not receive the heat equally on all sides, and the Fruits would be shrivell'd up It would also be too tedious to dry them in the Sun, because they would give, and grow soft during the *coolness of the Night*, and at other times, when depriv'd of the Raies of that great Luminary.

The Campain-oven is a portable Oven made of red Copper, three or four Inches high, of a convenient length, and raised a little upon Feet, so that a Fire may be kindled underneath, as occasion requires The Cover or Lid of it ought to have Ledges, to hold Fire likewise, when it is necessary to put some on the top, or on both sides : This Cover must be taken off from time to time, to see whether that which is contain'd in the Oven be sufficiently bak'd or brought to a good Colour For want of such an Instrument, the Kitchen-oven of Masons-work, or some other may be us'd, accordingly as a convenient opportunity may be found ; or else a Silver-dish and certain large Baking-pans that are order'd almost in the same manner

The Cistern is another kind of portable Instrument, in form of a Box, into which *Blanc-mangers*, Jellies, Creams, and more especially Liquors are put, in order to be iced The Construction and Use of it shall be hereafter explain'd, in treating of those respective Articles.

Besides the Stone-mortar, in which Sugar, Almonds and other necessary Ingredients are pounded, another little one of Brass or some other Metal must be also provided for the beating of Cinnamon, Cocheneal, Cloves, Amber and other Things that ought to be reduc'd to a finer Powder

The Marble-stone, which is much of the same nature as that us'd by Painters for the grinding of their Colours, serves only to prepare the Barley-sugar, that is rubb'd with Oil of Olives.

The little Trunks, Boxes, Pots and Glasses, are different Vessels proper to hold dry or wet Sweet-meats, and such may be us'd as are at hand.

A Confectioner ought also to be furnish'd with a Strainingbag, to clarifie his Sugar, and to strain other Liquors ; a Rolling-pin to roll out pieces of Paste for crackling Crusts and March-panes ; divers Tin-moulds to shape them, and to dress
the

the Paftes of Fruits; a Syringe made on purpofe for other forts of March-pane and Biskets; certain wooden Stamps, to make an Impreffion upon the *Paftils*, and feveral other little Knacks, by the means of which he may fet off his Work to the beft advantage.

C H A P. III.

Of the Confectioner's Employment throughout the whole Year, according to the Seafons of the Flowers and Fruits.

AFter the Inftructions contain'd in the fore-going Chapter, it is expedient, before we proceed to the main Body of the Work, to expofe to publick View every Thing that may be preferv'd, as well Fruits and Flowers as other forts of Works, to the end that the Confectioners and other Officers may have a general Idea of what they are to perform, and at the fame time, of what may be ferviceable in every particular Seafon.

January and *February.*

During thefe two Months *Sevil*-Oranges, thofe of the Port, and others, are ufually preferv'd Whole, in Quarters, or in Sticks Paftes, Conferves and Marmelades, are alfo made of them; and their Peels are candy'd either in *Zefts*, or in Faggots.

Lemmons, *Cedres*, and yellow Citrons, are preferv'd after the fame manner; and if the Provifions that were made of other forts of preferved Fruits are now confum'd, that Defect may be reciprocally fupply'd by thefe, the pleafant Variety of which will be very grateful, and give a great deal of fatisfaction

March and *April*

Thefe are the two firft Months of the Year that afford Matter for new Comfits, that is to fay, Violets, which are the firft Flowers of a fragrant fmell that the Earth brings forth, after

It has been deliver'd from the Tyranny of the sharp Winter
With these Flowers, Conserves and Pastes are made, as also
Syrup of Violets, the gross Substance of which may be kept in
Marmelade, to make dry Pastes, at other times For want of
these, when it is requisite to prepare any Thing, that has the
taste and smell of a Violet, Indigo and Powder of Orrice are
generally us'd, particularly for *Pastils* and Mosses, which are
Sugar-works that may be made in any Season.

May

In this Month green Goose-berries first appear, of which
Compotes and Jellies are made ⋅ They are also preserv'd liquid
for the rest of the Year, either for Tarts, or to be serv'd up
again in *Compote*, upon certain Occasions

Green Apricocks come about the same time; affording Matter likewise for *Compotes*, Pastes and Marmelades ⋅ But they
are chiefly preserv'd dry, and kept for a considerable time

Green Almonds, which belong to the same Season, may be
order'd after as many different manners, *viz* for *Compotes*,
Pastes and Marmelades, as well as preserv'd dry or liquid, in
order to be us'd upon any emergent Occasion

Straw berries begin likewise to appear, which may be serv'd
up, not only in their natural Condition, but also in *Compotes*,
to diversifie the former Banquets

June.

This Month affords good store of Rasberries, Cherries and
Currans⋅ *Compotes*, Conserves and Pastes are frequently made
of the first of these Fruits, and 'tis now a proper time to begin
to Preserve them dry and liquid.

Cherries, as soon as any ripe ones can be procur'd, are likewise put into *Compotes*, half Sugar and Conserves ⋅ They may
be iced over with Powder-sugar, and as this Fruit comes to a fuller
growth, or when better sorts of them may be gather'd, they
are preserv'd in Ears, in Bunches and after other manners:
Cakes or Pastes are then prepar'd with Cherries, as also Marmelade, and at last they are preserv'd liquid, in order to be
kept for a considerable time A Jelly may be also made of them,
and the Juice extracted from those that are boil'd for Pastes,
and of others out of which the Stones were taken, to be preserv'd,

ſerv'd, may be us'd to very good purpoſe, in that Jelly, and for the Liquor call'd *Ritafiaz*, as well as the Syrup of thoſe that are dried.

As for Currans; Paſtes, Conſerves and *Compotes*, are firſt made of them, beſides thoſe that are iced; others are preſerv'd in Bunches and liquid; and afterwards Marmelade is made of them, with Jellies of ſeveral ſorts. Moreover, Syrups and Liquors are prepar d with all theſe ſorts of Fruit

This is alſo a proper time for the Preſerving of Orange-flowers dry, and for the making of Conſerves, Paſtes and Marmelade of them, which may be ſerviceable during the reſt of the Year, becauſe now there is the greateſt plenty of theſe Flowers

Conſerves and Syrup of Roſes are likewiſe made, ſo that this is one of the Months, in which the moſt Pains is to be taken, and that affords the greateſt Variety of Fruits and Flowers at once.

July.

The Fruits of the former Month ſtill take up the greater part of this, and the Preſerving of them is continu'd, after the above-mentioned Ways. This is the chief time for wet and dry Cherries, as alſo for the Jellies and Marmelades of Currans and Rasberries

In the beginning of the Month, white Walnuts are preſerv'd, either liquid or dry, to be kept during the whole Year, and a little afterwards ripe Apricocks, of which *Compotes* and Paſtes are firſt made: Others are par'd in order to be preſerv'd with half Sugar, or in Ears, and Marmelade is made of them, which is us'd in many Things, out of the Seaſon, particularly, for drying the Paſte; for Apricock-paſtils, or the Royal March-pane. At the ſame time, the Syrup and *Ratafiaz* of Apricocks are uſually prepar d

Pears now begin to provide Employment for the Confectioner, and to afford an agreeable Variety So that *Compotes* may be made of them, and Muſcadine-pears may be iced, to the number of ſix or ſeven in Cluſters, as they are; whilſt the *Blanquets* are preſerv'd, and ſome few other ſorts dried

There are alſo Plums and Grapes in the end of the Month, and altho' the latter are fine enough then to appear in their natural Colour, yet they are ſometimes iced with powder'd Sugar. The ſame thing is done with Plums; beſides that Paſtes

are

are already made of them, and they may be put into *Compotes*, or into half-Sugar, to be dried

August.

Much more Pains may be taken in this Month, in ordering these latter Fruits, because they are successively renew'd, by other kinds that are more proper for Preserving   Thus Orange-plums and Amber-plums, those of *Isle-verd* and others are preserv'd dry to be kept   Pastes and Marmelades are made of them, and they are still iced, and put into *Compotes*

The same thing is done with the Pears in their Season, more especially the *Rousselet*, or Russetin, and some others, that are of an exquisite taste

There are also certain Plums, proper for drying, in order to make Prunes, as occasion serves

Figs are preserv'd and dried in the same Month, and they may be iced with Powder-sugar, as well as Grapes   Syrup of Mulberries is likewise prepai d, and some th nk fit to preserve them   Apples are put into *Compotes*, and preserv d after some other manners

About the end of the Month, Girkins or small Cucumbers, Samphire, Purslain and other Herbs are pickled with Vinegar and Salt, for the Winter-sallets.

September.

Plums continue still, for a considerable time, ard Apples and Pears much longer : So that new *Compotes*, Pastes and Marmelades may be made of them, and the best ough to be chosen for that purpose ; such as the *Bon-chretien*, the *Bergamot*, and the Summer-*Certoe*, among the Pears   This last is also preserv'd dry

Peaches, which continue for a long while, likewise furnish Matter for Pastes, *Compotes* and Marmelade, and they may be order'd so as to make dry Sweet meats

Moreover, Bell-grapes are then preserv'd liquid, and Pastes, Jellies and *Compotes* are made of them   Muscadine-grapes are order'd in the same manner, and serve to make a very delicious sort of *Ratafiaz*

Barberries, which are generally ripe at the same time, are proper for Conserves.

V   *Octo-*

October.

In this Month and the following, you have other sorts of Apples and Pears, for all the above-mentioned Uses, and also for Jellies, if you shall think fit to prepare them

But this is the chief time, for making the Pastes, Jellies and Marmelade of Quinces, as also Comfits with *Must* or sweet Wine and others, which neverthelefs only fall under the management of the Country People

The Officers and Butlers are otherwife employ'd in this Season, that is to say, in gathering the Fruits, that ought to be in their Cuftody, which requires a more than ordinary Skill and Precaution

November and *December.*

Forafmuch as the Fruits of the Earth now ceafe, recourfe muft be had to the Provifions that have been made during the preceding Months; as well with refpect to dry and wet Sweet-meats, as to Jellies and Marmelades, which may be dried, in order to make Paftes that are wanting: A greater quantity of roafted Apples and Pears are likewife prepar'd, from time to time, with fome *Compotes* of Chefnuts, which may alfo be iced and dried

Laftly, The affiftance of Oranges and Lemmons, which are brought over at this time, is confiderable, more efpecially *China-*Oranges; but the others are not preferv'd till the following Months.

During the whole Year.

Befides all thefe forts of Sweet-meats, that depend on the Seafon of every particular kind of Fruit, there are divers Sugar-works and others, that may be prepar'd throughout all the Year: Such are feveral forts of Almonds, Biskets, March-panes, *Meringues,* and Paftils; as alfo, the *Caramel, Sultans,* Moffes, candy'd Comfits, and fome others, which with the raw Fruits, ferve at all times, for the better filling up of a Defert, more efpecially in Winter, and upon other Occafions, when preferved Fruits are wanting.

Befides

Besides these Employments, the Confectioners and other Officers, ought to be diligent in keeping their Sweet-meats in good order; and to that purpose, it is requisite from time to time, to infpect thofe that are liquid, to fee whether they are not grown four or mufty, and to remedy fuch Accidents, as alfo to change the Papers of thofe that are in the Boxes; and to take care that they be not laid up in any Place that is too moift, obferving many other Precautions which their own Difcretion, may fufficiently fuggeft to them.

Thofe Officers that are entrufted with the management of the raw Fruits, ought in like manner to apply themfelves to that purpose, and thus there is no time, but what may be taken up, in fome of thefe Employments, if to them be added, what is requifite for the preparing of the Sallets, dreffing of Deferts, and performing the other Duties incumbent on fuch Officers, efpecially in Noble mens Houfes.

In the Confectioners Apartment, inftead of fome part of the latter Functions, they may be employ'd to very good purpofe, in the making of Sugar-plums, but it would be needlefs to fhew the manner of carrying on that Work, becaufe it depends upon an habitual Practice, that is not exercifed in an Office, nor in the Houfes of private Perfons, where this Book may give fufficient Drections for managing all the other Concerns: Therefore, the Utenfils proper for that Bufinefs, are not explain'd among the others in the fore going Chapter. So that all this Tackle is left to thofe who are Confectioners by Trade; and if any Perfons are defirous to be of that Number, the Apprenticefhip that ought to be ferv'd, well fupply the defect of our Silence as to thefe Matters.

Let us now proceed to fhew the beft Method of managing all the reft, and begin with the Fruits, that are to be preferv'd dry or liquid, almoft according to the natural Order of their Seafons. Afterwards, the fame Order fhall be obferv'd in treating of the *Compotes,* Marmelades and Paftes, which we have thought fit to defcribe all together under their refpective Articles. Laftly, a particular Account fhall be given of the Sugar-works and others, that may be made in any Seafon of the Year; comprehending in general, every Thing that relates to the Art of preferving of Sweet-meats with Sugar, and even difcovering the choiceft Secrets of the Confectioner's Trade. As it appears from the Contents of the Chapters, and the general Table of the principal Matters.

C H A P. IV.

Of green Apricocks.

THe first Fruits that present themselves to be preserv'd, after green Goose berries, which do not properly belong to this Place, are green Apricocks: To that purpose, they are usually taken, before their Stones begin to grow hard, and they are preserv'd with their Skin, as also others pared, which appear much more fine and clear. Both these Ways may be perform'd according to the following Method

How to prepare and boil green Apricocks.

Those Apricocks that are design'd to be preserv'd with their Skin, ought first to be well clear'd from the soft Hair, or Down with which they are cover'd, and this may be done by the means of a good Lye, in which they are to to be scalded after the same manner as green Almonds   To that purpose, let some Water with new Ashes be pour'd into a large Pan, and set over the Fire, scumming off all the Coals that rise on the top   When this Lye has boil'd for some time, and you perceive by the Taste, that it is become sweet and oily, remove it from the Fire, and having set it by for a while, take all the clear Liquor   Then set it over the Fire again, and as soon as it begins to boil, put three or four Apricocks into it, observing whether they be well cleans'd, by that means   If the Experiment succeeds, the rest may be thrown in, but care must be taken to keep them from boiling, by stirring them about continually with the Handle of the Skimmer. The Apricocks being thus sufficiently scalded, must be taken out, tofs'd a little in a Cloth, and wash'd in fair Water: Afterwards, you must run them thro' the middle with a Knitting-needle, and throw them as they are so order'd, into other fresh Water   To cause them to recover their green Colour, the Water is to be chang'd again, and they must be boil'd over a quick Fire; taking out some of them from time to time, and pricking them with a Pin: If they stick to the Pin, 'tis a sign that they are not done enough; but as soon as they slip off from it, they must be taken away and carefully cool'd, by steeping them in cold Water.

Ano-

Another Way of preparing green Apricocks.

Having provided green Apricocks, before their Stones are grown hard, let two Handfuls of Salt, more or lefs, according to the quantity of your Apricocks, be pounded in a Mortar to a very fine Powder · Then let the Apricocks be put into a Napkin, with the Salt, and let all be well ftirr'd about, from one end to the other, fprinkling them with a little Vinegar As foon as you perceive, that they are clear'd from the Mofs or Down, rub them a little with your Hands to get off the Salt; wafh them in fair Water, and fcald them immediately As foon as they are fcalded (which may be known, by pricking them with a Pin, or when they eafily receive an impreffion from the Finger) let them be thrown into frefh Water In the mean while, take as much clarified Sugar, as will be requifite, and fet it in a Pan over the Fire. When the Sugar begins to boil, put in your Apricocks, after having drain'd them from the Water, and ftew them over a gentle Fire, till they begin to grow green: When they are well impregnated with the Sugar, let them be laid on a Grate, to be dryed, and afterwards fet in order upon Slates, ftrewing them lightly with powder'd Sugar, put into a Napkin Then being dried for fome time in the Stove, they muft be taken off from the Slates, and put into Sieves to be more thoroughly dried · At laft, they are to be laid up dry in Boxes, and kept for Ufe. This fort of Fruit is very good, when Preferv'd

To preferve green Apricocks.

Thefe Apricocks muft be firft order'd with thin Sugar, that is to fay, for every two Ladlesful of clarified Sugar, one of Water is to be allow'd, and all made luke warm together Having put your Apricocks well drain'd, into an earthen Pan, pour this Syrup upon them, and let them be foak'd in it till the next Day · Then fetting all over the Fire, in a Copper-pan, caufe them to Simper, ftirring them about gently from time to time. Afterwards, they muft be turn'd again into the earthen, Pan, or even left in the Copper pan, and may be fo order'd at any other time The next day, let the Apricocks be drain'd on a Cullander, and give the Syrup feven or eight Boilings; adding a little more Sugar; then throw in your Fruit, and let all

V 3

fimper

ſimper together   The ſame thing is to be re-iterated for four or five Days; giving your Syrup fifteen, ſixteen, or twenty ſeveral Boilings; and always augmenting it with a little Sugar, by reaſon of its diminution, and to the end that the Fruit may be equally ſoak'd therein   Afterwards, the Apricocks muſt be put into the Syrup, and made to ſimper at every time   To bring them to perfection, boil your Syrup till it becomes pearled, adding alſo ſome other Sugar likewiſe Pearled, and having turn'd in the Fruit, let all have a cover'd Boiling   Then remove the Pan from the Fire, and take off the Scum   As ſoon as the Apricocks are cool'd, let them be drain'd in a Cullander and laid upon Slates or Boards, in order to be dried in the Stove.   The next Morning, they may be turn'd, if it be requiſite, and in the Evening, ſhut up in Boxes, or little Trunks, with Paper between every Row

If you would have green Apricocks preſerv'd liquid, put them into a Pot, with their Syrup, when the whole Work is finiſh'd, and they may be dried at any time, as occaſion requires To that purpoſe, you need only heat Water over the Fire, and ſet your Pot of Apricocks into it, as it were in *Balneo Mariæ*, to the end that, by the heat of the Water, which is to boil, the Syrup may become liquid again, as if it were newly made, and by that means, the Apricocks may be taken out to be dried in the Stove, as before, after they have been drain'd.   But this is uſually done at once, becauſe they are apt to grow greaſy, and on the contrary, they keep very well dry.

Green Apricocks peeled.

Theſe Apricocks after they have been neatly peel'd, muſt be likewiſe pierc'd thro' the middle and thrown into fair Water : They ought alſo to boil in other Water, but when they riſe on the top, they muſt be thruſt down, and left to cool in their own Liquor.   Afterwards, being ſet on the Fire again, to recover their green Colour, they muſt be boil'd till they ſlip off from the Pin, and put into Sugar in the ſame manner as the former, as well to be kept dry as liquid.

For the *Compotes*, Paſtes and Marmelades of green Apricocks, See thoſe Articles, which are hereafter deſcrib'd together, for every kind of Fruit.

C H A P.

CHAP. V.
Of ripe Apricocks.

ALtho' there is a confiderable fpace of Time, between the Seafons in which green and ripe Apricocks are preferv'd ; neverthelefs, we fhall here continue the defcription of them to follow the Order of the Matter , having already accounted for what relates to the Lift of the Fruits according to their Seafons, in the third Chapter , to which the Reader is referr'd

Pared Apricocks

After having neatly par'd and fton'd the Apricocks, fhrting them on one Side, they are to be fcalded in Water, almoft boiling hot   As the Apricocks rife on the top, take them up with the Skimmer, and put them into fair Water to cool , if they are fomewhat foft · If they are otherwife, flip them into the Pan, again, continuing fo to do, till the end , except, when the Water being ready to boil, cafts them altogether on the top ; then let them all be taken out and cool'd   Afterwards, you are to pick out thofe that are fofteft, thofe that are indifferent foft, and thofe that are leaft fo · The firft fort muft be immediately put into Sugar, that has had three or four Boilings, the Second into Sugar, as it comes from the Straining-bag , and for the hardeft, the Sugar muft be boil'd again for a while, fetting it over the Fire, and adding a little Water.   When the Apricocks are all equally entire and foft, they muft be put into clarified Sugar, and boil'd, till no Scum or Froth arifes any longer, which muft be always carefully taken off.   The Apricocks being thus left in the Sugar, till the next Day, are to be drain'd ; whilft the Syrup is boil'd till it has attain'd to its fmooth Quality, augmenting it with Sugar · Then turn the Apricocks into the Pan, and having given them a Boiling, let them be fet by.   On the Day following, let them be drain'd, and let the Syrup be boil'd till it becomes Pearled : Afterwards, let them be flipt into the Pan again, adding fome Sugar likewife Pearled, and having given them a cover'd Boiling, let them be fet into the Stove, till the next Morning ; when they are to be taken out, and put into Pots, in order to be dried, or to be eaten in the fame condition, at pleafure.   V 4   To

To dry your Apricocks at all times, set a Copper-pan, with Water over the Fire, and the Pot or earthen Pan containing the Fruit, in the middle of the same Pan, which ought, upon that account, to be of a proportionable size: Let the Water boil about half an Hour, by which means, the Apricocks will be heated, and you'll have the liberty to take them out, to be drain'd Then they may be dress'd upon the Slates or Boards, in order to be set into the Stove, after they have been strew'd with Sugar

N B Forget not, in peeling or turning your Apricocks at first, to put them into fair Water.

Apricocks preserv'd in Half-Sugar.

Let four Pounds of Sugar be made Feathered, let four Pounds of Apricocks be put into it, and let all be boil'd a little, to cause them to cast their Juice. Then, having set them by to cool, bring them to the Fire again, and let them boil, till no Scum appear any longer: Having remov'd the Pan, let them be left in the Syrup, till the next Day; when they may be drain'd in a Cullander; whilst the Syrup is boil'd, till it become Pearled; at which instant it must be pour'd into an earthen Pan, and the Apricocks must be slipt into it: Afterwards, they must be scumm'd and set into the Stove, to be thoroughly soak'd: On the Day following, they are to be drain'd and dress'd upon the Slates, in order to be dried in the Stove, strew'd with Sugar. Otherwise, they may be kept liquid, till another time, and afterwards dried as the former

Apricocks in Ears.

Apricocks that have been order'd according to either of these Ways, may be dress'd in Ears; and to that purpose, it is only requisite, to turn one of the Halves, without loosening it altogether from the other; or to joyn the two Halves together, so as they may mutually touch one another at both ends, one on one side and the other on the other

'Tis observable, That ripe Apricocks are apt to grow greasie, as well as the green ones, so that they cannot be kept long liquid, because there is no way to prevent this Inconveniency: Then they require a great deal more pains in drying, and are less agreeable to the Palate. Therefore in regard that they keep

best

beft dry, it is moft expedient to order them fo at firft; or elfe the Confectioner or Officer will be oblig'd to alter their Property, making ufe of them for March-panes, or other forts of Works.

For the *Compotes*, Marmelades and Paftes of Apricocks, fee the particular Chapters, to which thefe Articles belong, as well as for thofe of all the other forts of Fruits, which fhall not be mention'd any longer for the future, in regard, that recourfe may be had to the Table or *Index* of the principal Matters, precifely fhewing the Page where thofe Matters are handled at large

C H A P. VI.

Of Green Almonds.

GReen Almonds follow the green Apricocks, as well with refpect to the Seafon, as to the manner of Preferving: However, we fhall here explain the feveral Ways of ordering them, at large; becaufe there are certain particular Circumftances to be obferved, that were not mention d in the preceding Articles.

How to cleanfe, and boil green Almonds.

Let Water, with new Afhes be fet over the Fire in a Pan, and let the Coals that rife on the top be fcumm'd off, when, after having boil'd for fome time, you perceive it to be fweet and flippery, as a good Lye ought to be, remove the Pan, and fet it by for a while, in order to get the clear Liquor Then bring it to the Fire again, and when the Lye begins to boil, throw in three or four Almonds; obferving, whether the Flocks or Husks that cover them, be well clear'd. If not, it is a fign, that the Lye is not good, and fome other muft be made, or that muft be recruited with new Afhes, otherwife the Almonds would only open and flit, and not be cleans'd. On the contrary, if the Husks flip off well, the reft of the Almonds may be turn'd into this Lye, but you muft hinder their boiling, by continually ftirring them about, with the Handle of the Skimmer.

As

As foon as it appears, that the Husks are eafily rubb'd off, take them out, and fhake them a little in a Cloth, holding it at both ends: Afterwards, one of the ends of the Cloth being open d, let your Almonds fall into a Pan full of fair Water. Thus having caus'd them to be well wafh'd, pierce them thro' the middle, with a Knitting-needle, or fome other Inftrument of the like nature; and as they are done, throw them into other frefh Water

This Way of preparing and cleanfing Almonds, is more certain, than to give them fome Boilings in the Lye, before they are taken out, or to put them into it with the Afhes, for it is to be feared, left that fhould caufe them to open, if care be not taken to prevent fuch Accidents. The fame Inconveniency of-
•ten happens, if according to any Method that is obferv'd, all the Fruit fhould be imprudently thrown into this Lye, without making the above-mentioned Tryal, at the hazard of two or three Almonds, to know, whether it be not too hot, or whether it be in its due Condition

To bring the Almonds again to their green Colour, it is requifite, that the fair Water be chang'd, and that they be boil'd in it, over a quick Fire: They may alfo be fcalded or ftew'd by degrees, without boiling to which purpofe, having put the Almonds into a Pan 'with Water, a Difh of almoft the fame breadth is to be thruft down into it, which may hinder them from rifing on the top, and confequently from turning black, and when the Liquor is ready to boil, fome cold Water muft be pour'd in by degrees. In following either of thefe Ways, it may be known, that the Almonds are fufficiently prepar'd, when they flip off from the Pin, at which inftant, they ought to be remov'd from the Fire, and fet by to cool.

To put *Almonds* into *Sugar.*

As to this particular, it is only requifite, to obferve the Directions already given for Apricocks Thus for every two Ladles ful of clarified Sugar, take one of Water, till you have a fufficient quantity for the foaking of your Almonds, or fomewhat more; becaufe it will afterwards ferve to augment the Syrup in other Boilings or for fome other Ufes. Let the Sugar and Water be heated as hot, as you can well endure to hold your Finger in it, and pour it upon the Almonds in an earthen Pan, leaving them thus till the next Day; when all muft be put into a Copper-pan fet over the Fire, and heated, till almoft ready to
boil·

boil Then they are to be turn'd again into the earthen Pans, or left in the Copper-pan, and the next Day, the Almonds muft be drain d in a Cullander, giving the Syrup feven or eight Boilings, and augmenting its quantity, with a little Sugar · Some time after, throw in your Fruit, and let all fimper together The fame thing is to be done for four or five Days fucceffively, caufing the Syrup to have fome other Boilings; which muft be ftill encreas'd with Sugar, every time, to the end, that the Fruit may always be equally foak'd. When you would have the Work finifh'd, let the Syrup be boil d, till it has attain'd to its Pearled Quality; adding, if it be requifite, fome other Sugar Pearled in like manner So as the Fruit may be conveniently flipt into the Pan, and have a cover'd Boiling. Afterwards, having remov'd it from the Fire, take off the Scum, on the top; and, as foon as the Almonds are cool'd, lay them a draining in a Cullander, in order to be drefs'd upon Slates or Boards, and dried in the Stove. Thefe Almonds are not ufually ftrew'd with Sugar, no more than green Apricocks, becaufe they appear finer in their natural Colour, and are very eafily dried. However, the Day following, they muft be turn'd on the other fide, if it be needful, and put into Boxes, when you perceive them to be very firm and dry.

Green Almonds may alfo be preferved liquid, as well as Apricocks, either to be eaten in that manner, or to be dried, as occafion requires, and to that purpofe recourfe may be had to the Directions before laid down, *Pag* 17 and 18 for green Apricocks.

C H A P. VII.

Several other Ways of Preferving Almonds.

BEfides new raw Almonds that are ferv'd up to Table, when ripe, there are feveral Ways of Drying them, which may be very ferviceable at thofe times, when there is no great variety of Fruits or Sweet-meats

Almonds order'd à la Siamoife.

Having dried and brought Almonds to a reddifh Colour in the Oven, let them be thrown into Sugar, boil'd till it becomes
Pearled;

Pearled , stirring them about well in the Pan, without setting it over the Fire : Then they must be laid in order upon a Grate, and put into the Stove, if you would have them serv'd up after that manner   Otherwise, being taken out of the Pan, they may be roll'd one by one, in powder'd Sugar or *Sedan-Nomparel* and continually stirr'd about, to the end that they may be cover'd, on all sides, with the Sugar or with the *Nomparel* Afterwards they must be taken out, and set into the Stove upon Papers.

Blown Almonds.

After having scalded and blanch'd your Almonds, let them be stirr'd about in the White of an Egg   Then let them be put into powder'd Sugar, and well roll'd in it   Having thus ic'd them over once, if you perceive that they are not done enough, dip them again into the White of an Egg, and afterwards into powder'd Sugar: At last, they may be laid upon a Sheet of Paper, and bak'd in an Oven, with a gentle Fire.

Iced Almonds.

Take blanched Almonds, and put them into an Ice that is ready prepared, with the White of an Egg, powder'd Sugar, Orange or Lemmon-flowers and *Sevil*-orange . Let them be well roll'd in this Compound, so as to be neatly iced, and afterwards dress'd on a Sheet of Paper, in order to be bak'd in the Campain-oven, with a gentle Fire, as well underneath, as on the top

Several sorts of crisp Almonds.

Crisp Almonds of a gray Colour.

Let a Pound of Loaf or Powder-sugar be melted, with a little Water, and let a Pound of Almonds be boil'd in it, till they crackle : Then remove the Pan from the Fire, and stir all about incessantly with the *Spatula*   If any Sugar be left, it must be heated again over the Fire, to the end that it may entirely stick to the Almonds ; continuing to stir them, without intermission, till the Work be finish'd.   Thus the Almonds will become crisp, and of a gray Colour.

Red

Red crisp Almonds.

To give your Almonds a red Colour; cause three quarters of a Pound of Sugar to be dissolv'd with a little Water, throw in the Almonds, and boil them as before, t'll they crackle, taking care to stir them from time to time, that they may not stick to the Pan Then remove them from the Fire, and keep stirring them continually, till they have taken up all the Sugar, without setting them any longer over the Fire Afterwards, having sifted them, the Sugar that runs thro' the Sieve, must be put again into the same Pan, with another quarter of a Pound of Sugar, and a little Water, to dissolve the whole Mass. The Sugar being boil'd till it become crack'd, add as much prepared Cocheneal, as will be requisite to give it a fine Colour, and let it boil again over the Fire, to cause it to return to its crack'd Quality; by reason that the Cocheneal brings it down from that degree of boiling. At that very instant toss in your Almonds, and at the same time take them off from the Fire; stirring them, without intermission, as at first, till they become dry

If you are minded to make a greater quantity of this sort of crisp Almonds at once; it will only be requisite to augment that of the Sugar proportionably, that is to say, allowing a Pound of one, for every Pound of the other.

As for the prepared Cocheneal; it is only the Liquor in which that Grain has been boil'd, with Allum and Cream of Tartar. It is generally us d for every thing that is to be brought to a fine red Colour, particularly *Blanc-mangers,* Creams, Jellies, Marmelades, Pastes, &c.

White crisp Almonds.

Crisp Almonds are also made white; to which purpose, after having scalded and blanch'd them, they must be thrown into Sugar boil'd till it become crack d Then let all have a Walm or two together, and for the rest, let the Almonds be order'd in the same manner as before, that is to say, stirr'd and turn'd continually, to the end that the Sugar may stick close to them, on all sides.

If you have at hand a Pearling-pot proper for Sugar-plums, or any other Vessel of the like nature, some boil'd sugar, that

1S

is Pearled, may also be pour'd into it, and dropt by degrees upon the Almonds, causing the Pot to be held by a Servant, till they are thoroughly soak'd and cover d over with it

Crisp Almonds of a Gold-colour.

There is another Way of Preparing crisp Almonds usually practis'd by Cooks, which may be perform d thus . When the Almonds are blanch'd, drain'd and roll'd in powder'd Sugar, let them be thrown into a Frying-pan, in which Oil has been heated : After having fried them in this manner, stirring them about, till they have acquir'd a fine Gold-colour, they must be speedily taken out with the Skimmer, in order to be dress'd in different Heaps   Some call these *Fried* Languedoc-*almonds,* and they are us'd for the Garnishing of Potages of Almond-milk, or other Messes of the like nature

Pistachoes *in* Sur-tout.

Take what quantity you please of Pistachoes, clear them from their Shells, and cause them to be made crisp, which may be done thus   When the Sugar is boil'd till it become Feather-ed, throw in your Pistachoes, and when they have continu'd a little while on the Fire, take them off, stirring them well with the *Spatula,* till they are all cover'd, but they must not be set again over the Fire.   Afterwards, having beat up the White of an Egg with a Spoon, add a little Orange-flower-water, and dip the Pistachoes into it : Then let them be taken out, and roll'd in Powder-sugar, that is very dry.   At last, being laid in order upon white Paper, they must be gently bak'd in a Cam pain-oven, with a little Fire underneath, and more on the top As soon as they are sufficiently bak'd, and brought to a good Co lour, they may be taken out of the Oven, and dried in the Stove.

C H A P.

C H A P. VIII.

Of Preserv'd Cherries, as well dry as liquid.

CHerries are the firft red Fruits that prefent themfelves to be preferv'd, at leaft thofe that appear early. Thefe forward ones are ufually put into Sugar with their Stones, becaufe they have as yet attain'd to little maturity, and ferve only as a Novelty : But it will be no difficult matter to take meafures in ordering all forts of Cherries, according to the following Directions.

Cherries in Ears.

Take fair Cherries, that are ftoned, put them into Blown Sugar, and give them fifteen cover'd Boilings. Then having fet them by, till the next Day, let them be drain'd in a Cullander, and let your Syrup boil till it be Pearled . Afterwards, throw in your Fruit, and let them have feven or eight cover'd Boilings; taking care that they be well fcumm'd, even after the Pan is remov'd from the Fire. When the Cherries are cool'd, take them out of their Syrup, to be dried in the Stove upon Slates, and ftrew'd with Sugar. They are call'd *Cherries in Ears*, by reafon of the manner of dreffing them ; which is to open and fpread them, joyning two together, fo as their Skins may remain on the out-fide and the Pulp on the infide. Then another Cherry of the fame nature is to be added on each fide, the Pulp of which is laid upon the Skin of the others.

Cherries preferv'd in half Loaf-fugar.

After having ftoned your Cherries, give them five or fix Boilings in Pearled Sugar, and then take off the Pan from the Fire. On the next Day, they are to be drain'd, whilft the Syrup is boil'd Smooth, and put into it : Then they ought to have twenty Boilings, as alfo to be well Scumm'd and to lye in the Stove, during the whole Night. Afterwards, they muft be drain'd in a Cullander, and drefs'd upon the Slates, to be dried in the fame Stove. One Pound and half of Sugar is fufficient at firft for fix Pounds of Fruit.

Cher-

Cherries in half Powder-sugar

Having provided four Pounds of stoned Cherries, with one Pound of Powder sugar, let all boil together over the Fire, taking care to stir the Fruit continually, till they have imbib'd the Sugar; which may be known, by touching them, when they are very soft and tender. Then being set by till the next Day, they may be drain'd, whilst the Syrup is boil'd smooth · Let the Cherries be thrown into it, and give them fifteen or twenty Boilings, always taking care, that they be well scumm'd: Afterwards, they must be remov'd from the Fire, and laid in earthen Pans, to continue in the Stove all Night On the next Day, they are to be drain'd, dress'd upon Sieves, and set into the Stove again, after they have been strew'd with fine Sugar

Cherries preserv'd liquid

Let Sugar be boil'd till it be Blown, and let the Cherries be slipt into it, having cut off part of the Stalks. They ought to have ten or twelve cover'd Boilings, before they are set by till the next Day Then they must be drain'd, and put into the Sugar again, when boil'd, till it become Pearled, augmenting it with some other Sugar likewise Pearled. At last, you may add some Syrup of Currans of the same Quality, to give them a finer Colour, and put them into Pots, to be kept for Use.

Another Way.

The Cherries may be order'd as the former, or as those that are preserv'd dry, except that a greater quantity of Sugar is to be added, and in finishing the Work, they must have some cover'd Boilings, after having brought the Sugar to the greater Pearled Quality. When they are cool'd, they may be put into Pots, and if you would have them tinctur'd with Straw-berries, some of that Fruit must be put amongst your Cherries, as they are preserving.

Cherries

Cherries preſerv'd dry, with Straw-berries.

You are to provide Cherries preſerv'd dry, out of which the Stones have been already taken, ſubſtituting in their room, as many Straw-berries likewiſe preſerv'd dry· Then let all be dried in the Stove, after they have been ſtrew'd with Sugar, as well in the dreſſing, as the turning of them.

Cherries in Bunches.

Take fair Cherries, that are of an equal bigneſs, and tye them up, with Thread, into little Bunches. Then put them into Blown Sugar of the ſame Weight, and give them about twenty Boilings. Afterwards, let them be taken off from the Fire, and ſcumm'd, and as ſoon as they are cool'd, put them into the Stove as they lye in their Pan, till the next Day; when they may be conveniently dried upon Slates.

Cherries booted, à la Royale.

Let *Kentiſh* Cherries, with ſhort Stalks, or others of the like nature, be thrown into Sugar, boil'd till it become Pearled. Some only cauſe it to ſimper, ſtirring the Fruit from time to time, and the next Day, having cauſ'd the Syrup to be Pearled, put the Cherries therein, adding other Sugar likewiſe Pearled. Before they are ſet into the Stove, other Cherries preſerv'd in Ears are alſo provided, which muſt be laid upon them croſs-wiſe, to the number, of three, four, or ſix, and afterwards ſet into the Stove. Theſe are commonly called *Booted Cherries.* The Cherries that are left with the Stalks, may alſo be order'd altogether after the ſame manner, as the others preſerved in Ears, and the ſame Method may be follow'd for the reſt.

Cherries preſerv'd liquid, after the manner of the City of Tours.

Having provided five Pounds of Cherries, with three Pounds of Feathered Sugar, throw your Fruit into it, give them fifteen Boilings, and afterwards add two other Pounds of Sugar likewiſe Feathered. The whole Work ought to be finiſh'd at once, without removing the Pan from the Fire, cauſing the Fruit to

X

be

be boil'd in the Syrup, till it has attain'd to its Pearled Quality
Cherries are preſerv'd after this manner, to very good purpoſe,
as alſo Straw-berries   If you would impregnate the latter, with
the Syrup of the Cherries, it muſt not boil with the Fruit, neither the one, nor the other ; but this Syrup muſt be pour'd upon
them, when they are quite done, and taken away from the Fire.
Currans may alſo be order'd after the ſame manner.

To make a Cake, or Paſte of Cherries

After having ſton d your Cherries, let them boil in a Pan, till
you perceive, that they have caſt their Juice : Then ſet them in
order in a Sieve, and let them be well drain'd : Afterwards, you
muſt pound them in a Mortar, and ſet them on the Fire again,
to be thoroughly dried In the mean time, having boil'd the Sugar, till it be Crack'd, pour it upon this dried Cherry-paſte, allowing a Pound of Sugar for every Pound of Paſte . Let all be
well temper'd together ſo as they may ſimper a little over the
Fire ; and let them be continually ſtirr d   A little while after,
they may be dreſs d upon the Slates, with a Spoon, and ſet into
the Stove. If you are of opinion, that the Paſte has not as yet
acquir'd a good Colour, a few Currans may be intermixt with
it, as it is drying ; having firſt caus'd thoſe Currans to caſt their
Juice, and then ſtrain'd them thro a Sieve

Other Ways of Preſerving and Ordering Cherries.

For *Compotes*, Conſerves and Marmelades of Cherries, recourſe may be had to thoſe Articles, relating to all ſorts of Fruits,
which are hereafter explain d
    As for Cherry-water, we ſhall only here obſerve , That
all the Juice of Cherries extracted, either in making Cakes,
Marmelades, Conſerves, or other Sweet-meats, may ſerve for
the preparing of *Ratifiaz*, ſo that nothing will be loſt, or thrown
away as uſeleſs.
    The Syrup of Cherries, that have been preſerv'd dry, may
alſo ſupply the place of Sugar , at leaſt, if you have no mind to
keep it, for the diverſifying of March-panes or other Comfits of
the like Nature; or to make uſe of it, in the preſerving of other
ſorts of Fruit. It may likewiſe be us'd to very good purpoſe,
in preparing the Jelly of Cherries , as to which Particular, it
will only be requiſite to obſerve the Directions hereafter laid
                                                    down,

down, for the different Jellies of Fruits, particularly for the quaking Jelly of Currans

As for Cherries that are serv'd up to Table in their natural Condition, there is a particular Way of embellishing them, hereafter explain'd in the 30th Chapter, under the Article of *Caramel*

C H A P. IX.

Of Strawberries and Rasberries.

STrawberries and Rasberries are very serviceable in Entertainments, and, when full ripe, afford Delight to three Senses, *viz* those of Seeing, Smelling and Tasting They have a vinous Taste, and serve to corroborate the Heart, Stomack and Brain, after the same manner as vinous Liquors. These good Qualities cause them to be so much esteem'd in their natural Condition, that they are seldom preserv'd, more especially Strawberries : They are usually eaten, soak'd in Water or Wine, and strew'd with Sugar · However they may be iced, as Cherries, Currans and Rasberries, and these last may be preserv'd as well dry as liquid

Rasberries preserv'd dry.

Having provided Rasberries that are not too ripe, let them be pick'd and put into Sugar that has attain'd to its Blown Quality, giving them a cover'd Boiling · Afterwards, being taken off from the Fire, they must be scumm'd, and slipt into an earthen Pan, to continue in the Stove during twenty four Hours. As great a quantity of Sugar is requisite as of Fruit, for example, about four Pounds of each When they are cool'd, drain them from their Syrup, and dress them as other Sweet-meats, in order to be strew'd with Sugar, and dried in the Stove after the usual manner.

Ras-

Rasberries preferv'd liquid.

Take four Pounds of good Rasberries, and put them, when pick'd, into three Pounds of Pearled Sugar Then give them a fmall Boiling lightly cover'd, and ftir them from time to time Afterwards, let them be cool'd, drain'd and dry'd as Cherries, but not to fo great a degree, becaufe they have not fo much Moifture: The quantity of Pearled Sugar ought alfo to be augmented, to the end that it may be fufficient for the foaking of the Fruit: But if the Rasberries are fomewhat greenifh or tart, they muft not be put at firft into Sugar fo boil'd, becaufe they would grow hard ; fo that it is expedient to make a due choice of them Rasberries with thick Grains are not fo fit for preferving, as being full of Juice, which foon turns to Marmelade Thofe that have fmall Grains, are moft proper for that purpofe, in regard that their Subftance is more firm and compact Rasberries that grow in moift Places, are not fo good as thofe brought forth in a dry Soil, neither is fo much Sugar requifite for the ordering of the latter fort ; by reafon that Fruits growing in marfhy Grounds always diffolve in Sugar.

Other Ways of ufing Strawberries and Rasberries.

For *Compotes* of thefe forts of Fruit, fee the Directions hereafter given under that Article Marmelades, Jellies and Paftes are likewife made of them, which fhall be explain'd among thofe of other Fruits

C H A P. X.
Of Goofeberries and Currans.

GOofeberries and Currans are ufually preferv'd at the fame time with Cherries and Strawberries, and green Goofeberries are the firft of all the Sweet-meats made in the Spring Among the different kinds of Currans, the common, which ripens foneft, is the moft proper for Preferving, as having more Subftance, and being moft agreeable, as well to healthy Perfons,

fons, as to thofe that are fick, by reafon of their grateful Tart-nefs The larger *Dutch* Currans are likewife preferrable on that account to the ordinary ones, which are very fweet, and better eaten raw, than when preferv'd, as being too full of Juice. Thefe Currans are generally ferv'd up to Table in iced Bunches, and if defign'd for Preferving, ought to be taken early, before they are grown ripe The fame thing is done in ordering the white *Dutch* Currans, which are likewife preferv'd in fingle Stalks, in Bunches, or in Jelly, as well as the common white Currans.

Green Goofeberries preferv'd liquid.

The Goofeberries muft be flit on one fide with a Pen-knife, and all the fmall Grains that are on the Infide muft be taken out . Then they are to be put into very clear Water, and fet over the Fire, which is to be kept moderate. As foon as they rife on the top of the Water, they are to be remov'd, and fet by in the fame Liquor: When they are cool'd, let them be put into other frefh Water, over a gentle Fire, till they recover their green Colour, and become very foft Afterwards, having cool'd them again in fair Water, let them be well drain'd, and put into Sugar, pafs'd thro' the Straining-bag · At the fame time, give them fourteen or fifteen Boilings, to the end that they may thoroughly imbibe the Sugar, and leave them till the next Day: Then, being drain'd, let them be flipt into the Syrup boil'd till it become Pearled, and let them have four or five cover'd Boilings At laft they may be put into Pots, and us'd as occafion fhall require

Jelly of green Goofeberries.

Your Goofeberries being prepar'd as before, boil an equal Quantity of Sugar, till it be Pearled · Throw in the Fruit, and let all boil together ; taking off the Scum, till they return to the Pearled Condition Then removing them from the Fire, ftrain them thro' a Sieve into a Copper-pan, and at the fame time, put the Jelly fo receiv'd into Pots in the fame manner, as other Jellies of that fort of Fruit.

Red

Red Currans preserv'd Liquid.

The Currans being pick'd, ought to be put into Pearled Sugar, and to have a light cover'd Boiling, Then they muſt be ſcumm'd, and brought to perfection the next Day ; to which purpoſe they are to be ſtrain'd thro a Sieve, whilſt the Syrup is boil'd to a Degree between Smooth and Pearled   Afterwards, let the Fruit be ſlipt in, and let as much other Pearled Sugar be added as is ſufficient for the well ſoaking of them They ought alſo to have ſeveral cover'd Boilings, between Smooth and P ailed, taking off the Scum, even after they have been remov'd from the Fire, and ſtirring them, from time to time, till they are cool d a little, left they ſhould turn to a Jelly   Laſtly, they muſt be put into Pots and cover d for ſome Days.

Currans preſerv'd in Bunches.

Take four Pounds of Currans tied up in Bunches, and boil your Sugar till it becomes Feathered   Then ſet them in Order in the Sugar, and let them have ſeveral cover'd Boilings · They muſt be ſpeedily ſcumm'd, and not ſuffer d to boil long, that is to ſay, only two or three ſeethings . Afterwards, let them be ſcummed again, and ſet into the Stove in the Copper-pan.   On the next Day, they may be cool'd and drain'd, dreſſing them in Bunches of a convenient thickneſs, in order to be well ſtrew'd and dried in the Stove

Jelly of Currens.

Take ſix Pounds of Currans and cauſe the like quantity of Sugar to be brought to its Crack'd Quality · Throw in your Currans, and let the Syrup boil to a Degree between Smooth and Pearled, and till the Scum ceaſes to riſe any longer   Then let them be laid in a fine Sieve, without preſſing them too much, and only left in it, to be thoroughly drain'd. Afterwards, having given the Jelly, a Boiling, let it be ſcumm'd, and put into ſeveral Pots   When it is pour'd into the Pots, another thin Scum will ariſe which muſt be taken off, to render the Liquor clear, and two or three Day after, it may be cover'd with Paper cut round, to be kept for Uſe.

A Jelly of the Like nature may be made of Pomegranates,

as alfo of Barberries, or elfe another fort of Curran-jelly, after the following manner.

Quaking Jelly of Currans.

Having provided fix Pounds and a half of Currans, let as much Juice be fqueez'd out of them, as is poffible, and let the Sugar be order'd, as before Then ftrain your Curran-juice thro' a fine Sieve, and pour it into the Sugar : Let all be lightly boil'd together to a Degree between Smooth and Pearled, and afterwards let the Jelly be conveniently difpofed of in Pots.

Jelly of Currans tinctur'd with Rafberries.

If you are defirous, that the Curran-jelly have a Tincture of Rasberries, a Handful or two of Rasberries may be added, according to the quantity of your Jelly And to make it chiefly of Rasberries, it will be requifite only to take four Pounds of Rasberries, two of Currans and five of Sugar, and to order all, after the fame manner, as for the former Jelly of Currans

Jelly of Currans, according to the Way of the City of Tours.

Having provided three Pounds of Currans, with two Pounds and a half of Sugar, boil'd till it be crack'd, throw in your Fruit, and give them feven or eight Boilings, till they return to the Pearled Quality, caufing the Scum to be carefully taken off: Then let them be ftrain'd thro' a Sieve, and pour'd into Pots, at the fame time

In ordering thefe forts of Jellies, whofoever defigns to play the good Husband, may take the Fruit or grofs Subftance, remaining on the Sieve, and boil it over again, with a little Water Afterwards, it muft be ftrongly fqueez d thro' the Hair-fieve, and by that means a great deal more good Jelly will be extracted But this is only requifite to be done, when a great quantity of the grofs Subftance is left, otherwife it would not quit coft, by reafon that the Profit will not countervail the Trouble

For the *Compotes,* Conferves, Marmelades and Paftes of Currans, recourfe may be had to thofe Articles hereafter defcribed in particular.

CHAP. XI.

Of Walnuts.

IN the Interval, or rather during the Season of red Fruits, and the first that succeed them, Walnuts are usually preserv'd, when they are come to their full Growth, nevertheless before the Wood is form'd ; which happens in the beginning of *July*, and a little after the Festival of St *John* Baptist.

White Walnuts

The Walnuts must be neatly par'd, till the White appears, and thrown into fair Water : Afterwards, they must be boil'd for some time in the same Water, whilst some other Water is set over another Furnace, into which the Walnuts are to be put, as soon as it begins to boil. It may be perceiv'd, whether they be done enough, by pricking them with a Pin, after the same manner, as green Almonds and green Apricocks, so that when they slip off from it, they ought to be remov'd from the Fire To render them White, it is requisite at first, to throw in a Handful of beaten Allum, and to give them one Boiling more Then they must be immediately cool'd, by turning them into fresh Water, in order to be put into thin Sugar, that is to say, allowing one Ladle-full of Water, for every two of Sugar

Some time after, having drain'd your Walnuts, slip them into earthen Pans, and having caus'd the Sugar and Water to be heated together, pour it upon them. On the next Day, let the Syrup be clear'd from the Pans, without removing the Walnuts, because they must not be set over the Fire, at all . Let this Syrup have five or six Boilings, augmenting it a little with Sugar, and let it be pour'd upon the Walnuts. On the next Day, it ought to have fifteen Boilings ; on the third Day, it must be boil'd, till it become somewhat Smooth ; as also on the following Days successively, till it be very Smooth, between Smooth and Pearled, and at last entirely Pearled ; encreasing the quantity of Sugar, at every time, to the end that the Walnuts may be always equally soak'd in the Syrup To bring the whole Work to perfection, let them continue in the Stove during the Night, and afterwards let them be put into Pots. By this means
the

the Walnuts will become very white, provided, that good fine Sugar be us'd in the Operation, and they may be dried in the Stove, at pleasure, as other sorts of Fruit For Walnuts preserv'd liquid, if some Syrup of Apricocks be added they'll keep much better

If you have a mind to stuff them with Lemmon-peel after the manner of *Roan*-walnuts, it may be done, before they are put into the Stove, to be dried · To that purpose, the necessary Opening may be made with the point of a Knife, either quite through, or on the top of the Walnut, and then the Lemmon-peel, issuing forth from thence, will appear, as if it were the real Stalk Some Amber may also be added, which will give it a Perfume very grateful both to the Taste and Smell.

C H A P. XII.

Of Plums.

AMong the different kinds of Plums, the most proper for Preserving, are the *Perdrigons*, or Orange-plums, Amber-plums, those of *Isle-verte* and some others, that have not only an exquisite and very sweet Taste, but also a Pulp that is of a more firm and durable Substance.

To Preserve white Orange-plums.

These forts of Plums must have three or four Pricks with a Pin, near the Stalk, and some others in several other Places, to the end that they may not afterwards be apt to tear, and that the Sugar may more easily penetrate their Body As they are done, they must be thrown into Water, whilst some other Water is boil'd, into which they are to be slipt When they begin to rise, they may be remov'd from the Fire, and set by to cool: Then let them be set again over a gentle Fire, to be brought to their former green Colour, and let them be cover'd ; taking care that they do not boil, lest they should turn to Marmelade. As soon as you perceive them to be very green, and somewhat soft, let them be cool'd in fresh Water and drain'd, in order to be put into thin Sugar, allowing, as it has been already hinted,

two

two Ladles full of Sugar, for one of Water, till the Fruit, being laid in earthen Pans, is well foak'd, without rifing on the top. On the next Day, they are to be flipt into a Copper pan, to fimper over the Fire, ftirring them gently from time to time, to hinder them from boiling; and, on the third Day, they may be drain'd on a Cullander or Sieve: Then flip them into the Syrup, that has had feven or eight Boilings, caufe them to fimper for a while, and fet all by, till the next Day, when the Syrup is to have fifteen or fixteen Boilings, augmented with Sugar, or Syrup of Apricocks, which is better for that purpofe, as preventing them from candying, fo that the Plums may be always equally foak'd. On the Day following, let the Syrup be boil'd Smooth, and on the next, between Smooth and Pearled, and having flipt in the Fruit; let it fimper every time, before it is taken off from the Fire. Laftly, Having boil'd your Syrup till it be Pearled, and flipt in the Plums, give them feven or eight cover'd Boilings, taking off the Scum, and drefs them, when you fhall think fit, in order to be dried in the Stove.

The Orange-plums muft be chofen, before they are altogether ripe, as well as the moft part of other forts of Fruits. The other kinds of Plums, that are of kin to thefe, are ufually preferv'd after the fame manner, and, among others, thofe of *Ifleverte* and the Mufcle-plums.

Amber-plums.

Let your Amber-plums be prickt with a Pin, in feveral Places, and boil'd in the fame Water into which they were thrown. As foon as they rife on the Surface of the Water, remove them from the Fire to be fpeedily cool'd in frefh Water: Then let them be drain'd, and foak'd in clarified Sugar, which is to be heated, and pour'd upon the Fruit lying in the earthen Pans. On the next Day, drain them again, and let the Syrup be boil'd a little Smooth. On the fecond Day, the Syrup muft be likewife boil'd till it become very Smooth, and on the third, till it be Pearled; when the Plums are to have feven or eight Boilings. As often as they are thus fet over the Fire, they muft be augmented with Sugar, which has attain'd to the fame Degree of Boiling, to the end that the Fruit may be always equally foak'd, in the earthen or Copper-pans, in which they are left, after they have fimper'd for fome time. When you have a mind to finifh the Work, let them lye in the Stove during the whole Night, so as they may be conveniently drain'd and dress'd the next Morning, in order to be dried in the same Stove, after the usual manner

Red Plums

Having provided these sorts of Plums, such as red Orange-plums, Bell-plums, Imperial, or Apricock-plums, or others of the like nature, let them be slit as it were Apricocks, and stoned. If you have four Pounds of Fruit, take the same quantity of Sugar, pass'd thro' the Straining-bag , put all together into a Copper-pan over the Fire, and keep continually stirring them, lest the Skins of the Plums should break, if they should happen to boil After having caus'd them to simper, for a while, set them by to cool · Then drain them on a Cullander or Sieve, whilst the Syrup is boil'd Smooth; slip your Fruit into the same Syrup; and give them seven or eight cover'd Boilings , carefully taking off the Scum, as well as when the Pan is remov'd from the Fire Afterwards the Plums, being put into earthen Pans, must continue in the Stove all Night , so that the next Morning they may be drain'd as soon as they are cold, and dress'd, to be dried in the Stove upon Slates, or Sieves

Plums preserv'd with half Sugar and otherwise.

Take four Pounds of Fruit, with the like quantity of Pearled Sugar ; give them one little Boiling, and set them by till they have cast their Juice Then let them be set again upon the Fire, and boil'd to the Pearled Quality Afterwards, they must lie in earthen Pans, till the next Day , when they may be drain'd, and dress'd as the others, for drying in the Stove All sorts of good Plums may be preserv'd after the same manner, and they may also be par'd, after having scalded them in Water: For the rest, the above-specified Directions may be observ'd in every Particular, only they must be strew'd with Sugar, before they are dried in the Stove

Moreover, there are *Compotes*, Pastes and Marmelades of Plums, which are explain'd among the others, under those Articles.

CHAP.

CHAP. XIII.

Of Pears preserv'd dry and liquid.

THere is a much greater variety of kinds of this Fruit; yet very few of them are commonly preserv'd, *viz.* the great Muscadine, the *Muscadil*, or lesser Muscadine, the *Blanquet*, the *Certoe*, the Orange-pear, and more especially the *Rousselet* or Russetin. The most part of the others, are either too soft, or too hard for that purpose; and if they are not eaten raw, Pastes, Marmelades and *Compotes* are only made of them, all which are hereafter describ'd under their respective Articles.

Rousselets, *or Russetins.*

Let these Pears be prickt round about the top, with a Bodkin, and set over the Fire, taking care that the Water do not boil, and pouring in fresh, from time to time, when it is ready to bubble up As soon as the Pears are become somewhat soft, let them be cool'd, par'd, and put into other fair Water Afterwards, being drain'd, they must be slipt into Sugar, newly pass'd through the Straining-bag, and ought to have between forty and fifty Boilings: On the next Day, they are to be drain'd again, whilst the Syrup is boil'd Smooth, in the which you are to slip the Fruit, and to give them one or two Boilings On the third Day, let the Syrup be boil'd to a Degree between Smooth and Pearled, and, on the fourth, till it be thoroughly Pearled, for the finishing of the whole Work; so as the Pears may have ten or twelve cover'd Boilings When they are cool'd, they may be put into Pots, and kept to be dried, as occasion shall require, which may be done in the same manner that has been before explain'd for Apricocks. To that purpose, some Water being boil'd in a Pan, the Pot must be set into it, and by the means of this kind of *Balneum Mariæ*, or vaporous Bath, the Syrup will be melted, so that the Fruits may be readily taken out and drain'd, in order to be dried in the Stove, upon Slates or Boards, after they have been strew'd with Sugar They are also dried at first, and keep very well when so order'd but care must be taken to turn and change them often, and at last to lock them up in Boxes, with Paper between every Row

Blan

Blanquets.

Forasmuch as this ſort of Fruit is ſooner ripe than the Ruſſetin, and very much eſteem'd; ſome of them are early preſerv'd for a Rarity, and immediately dried. To that purpoſe, they are uſually prepar'd in the ſame manner, that is to ſay, they are ſcalded after having been prick'd on the top; taking care that they do not boil· As ſoon as the Pears are made very ſoft, only by means of a gentle heat, they muſt be cool d and par'd, throwing them, as they are done, into freſh Water: Afterwards, they are to be put into Sugar newly clarified, and finiſh'd in the ſame manner as the Ruſſetins Both theſe ſorts muſt be ſtrew'd with fine Sugar, in an Handkerchief, when they are ſet into the Stove, or turn'd; in which Particular, 'twill only be expedient to follow the Inſtruct ons already given, for other ſorts of Fruits, as Apricocks, Plums, &c

Large Muſcadines, Orange-pears, Certoes, *and others.*

All theſe kinds of Pears and others, that are deſign'd to be preſerv'd entire, may be ſcalded and boil d in Water and Sugar, as the Ruſſetin; ſo that it would only be an unprofitable Repetition, to inſiſt any longer on them.

The muſked Bergamot

This ſort of Pear is likewiſe excellent, when preſerv'd, being a ſmall dry Pear, very much muſked 'Tis alſo call'd the Dovepear, the Sicilian Pear, or the little Autumn-muſcadine To order it to the beſt advantage, ſee what has been already laid down for the former, more eſpecially for the Ruſſetin, and take Meaſures, altogether according to that Method, which is as general as certain, for all theſe kinds of Summer-pears.

Pears preſerv'd in Quarters and otherwiſe.

Beſides the above-mentioned Pears, which may be preſerv'd whole and dry; there are others larger, that can only be ſo order'd in Quarters, as to be kept liquid: To that end, ſome Confectioners ſlit them into Halves, before they are ſcalded in Water, but it is more expedient to leave them entire, and not to pare them till afterwards, becauſe otherwiſe they would
be

be apt to grow black, being also more liable to be fill'd with Water, and to turn to Marmelade. For the rest, it is only requisite to follow the preceding Directions, relating to the other sorts of Pears

If you are desirous to preserve Pears of a somewhat large size, altogether entire, it would be expedient to scoop out their Core, with some of the Pulp in the middle, as it were that of an Orange · They are brought to perfection, by causing them to be boil'd in Sugar, at several times, and may also be dried

To these Ways of preserving Pears, may be added the Marmelades, Pastes and more especially the *Compotes* of them, that are kept even till the Season of new Fruit, and which shall be hereafter describ'd under those Articles.

C H A P. XIV.

Of Peaches and Figs.

THese two sorts of Fruit are so highly esteem'd in their natural Condition, that they are very seldom preserv'd As for the latter, this Care is left to the *Genoeses*, and to the Inhabitants of *Provence*, in *France*, in which Countries, they are more common, and even of a more exquisite and sweet Taste, by reason of the heat of those Climates, so that most People content themselves generally to make use of such as are brought from thence However, we shall not forbear here to subjoyn, what is most observable in the ordering of both, when they are design'd to be preserv'd.

Green Peaches.

When Peaches are yet green and small, they may be preserv'd as green Apricocks before specified in the fourth Chapter ; preparing them after the same manner, to get off the Flocks or Down, and to bring them again to a green Colour, before they are put into Sugar. But if they are larger, and the Stone is already form'd, they must be par'd and slit, to take it away Then they are to be scalded in Water, till they become very soft. As soon as they are cool'd and drain'd, let
them

them be made green again in other Water, set over a gentle Fire, and put into thin Sugar, allowing for every two Ladles full of clarified Sugar, one of Water, which being heated, the Peaches must be slipt in, and have some Boilings, carefully taking off the Scum On the Day following, the Syrup being boil'd somewhat Smooth, and the Fruit being turn'd into it, cause all to simper together for a while, and leave them till the third Day, when the Syrup is to be boil'd very Smooth, augmenting its quantity with Sugar, whilst you slip in the Peaches, and give them a Boiling Lastly, the whole Work may be finish'd, as soon as you perceive, that they have thoroughly imbib'd the Sugar, to which purpose, let the Syrup be boil'd, till it become Pearled, encreasing it with Sugar of the same Quality, and having slipt in the Fruit, let them have a cover'd Boiling Afterwards, removing the Pan from the Fire, clear all from the Scum, and in regard, that the Peaches have a somewhat cold and waterish Pulp, let them lye, during that Night in the Stove, to dry up all their moisture. On the next Day, you may dress them on Slates, glazed Tiles, or any thing else of the like nature, to be dried in the Stove, strew'd with Sugar Or else, they may be disposed of in Pots or Glasses, to be dried upon any emergent Occasion, according to the Instructions given, Pag. 17. Peaches that are preserv'd, before the Stone or Kernel is form'd, must be put into Sugar, no otherwise than green Apricocks, or green Almonds, and the same Precautions are to be us'd, for which see Pag 16. *Compotes,* Marmelades and Pastes may be also made of them, as well as of the following sorts, as it shall be observ'd in its proper Place

Ripe Peaches.

Altho' mention is made of ripe Peaches, yet when they are to be preserv'd, it is not expedient to stay, till they are absolutely so, but they must be taken, when they are half turn'd, by reason of their soft and clammy Pulp. They ought to be neatly par'd, as also slit, to get out the Stones, and scalded in Water: As they rise on the top of it, they must be taken out with the Skimmer, and turn'd into other Water to cool. Then, being drain'd, they are to be put into Sugar, as it runs from the Straining-bag, and boil'd till the Scum ceases to rise, which must be carefully taken off from time to time Having left them in this condition, till the next Day, let them be drain'd, whilst the Syrup is boil'd Smooth, augmenting it with Sugar   Afterwards ſlip in your Fruits, give them a Boiling, and take them off from the Fire   On the third Day, being drain'd again, as before, and the Syrup boil'd till Pearled ; let the Peaches be likewiſe ſl.pt into it, adding ſome Pearled Sugar   After they have had a co ver'd Boiling, let them continue in the Stove all Night, in or der to be dreſs'd upon the Slates, or Boards, and dried , ſtrew ing them with Sugar, on every ſide, as often as they are turn'd, unleſs you would have them kept liquid for ſome time.

Peaches may alſo be preſerv'd in half Sugar, as Apricocks, ſpecified Pag 20. and dreſs'd either way, in Ears, as that ſort of Fruit ; by turning one of the Halves, as they ſtick together , or by laying two, one upon another, ſo as they may be mutually conjoyn'd ; when they are ſmall.

Nectarins.

Nectarins may be preſerv'd, after the ſame manner as Peaches, following the Method already expreſs'd for the putting them into Sugar, and white Nectarins are more eſpecially proper, for this Sort of Sweet-meats.

Dried Figs.

Let the Figs be prick'd near the Stalk, with the point of a Knife, before they are ſcalded, which may be done by throw ing them into boiling Water, over the Fire, and a little while after, ſetting them by to cool   Some defer the pricking of them to that time, and bring them again to the Fire, without ſuffer ing the Water to boil; ſo as when they are become ſoft, and riſe on the top, they may be remov'd, and ſet a-part to cool. Afterwards, their green Colour muſt be recover'd, by ſcalding them once more in Water, over the Fire : Then being taken out, and drain'd, they may be preſerv'd with half Sugar, or at moſt, clar.fied, as it runs from the Straining-bag ; accordingly, as the Figs are either green, or ſomewhat ripe , which ought to ſimper in this Sugar, and to lye by during the whole Night On the next Morning, the Syrup muſt be boil'd Smooth, on the third Day, between Smooth and Pearled, and at laſt, quite Pearled, adding every time, as much Sugar as is needful   At thoſe ſeveral times, the Fruit muſt alſo be ſlipt into the Syrup that has attain'd to ſuch different Degrees of Boiling, and ought to fimper for a while Whenever you have a mind to difpatch the Work, let the Figs have fome cover'd Boilings, in order to be thoroughly fcumm'd, and laid up in Pots, or Glaffes; unlefs you would have them dried all at once To that purpofe, the Fruits muft be drefs'd upon Slates, after they have been well drain'd, and fet into the Stove, ftrewing them with fine Sugar, put into a Kandkerchief, for that purpofe

'Tis requifite to choofe fuch Figs, as are only half ripe, or even fomewhat green, provided they be of a fufficient thicknefs The *Genoa*-Fig, call'd *Aubicon* by the *French*, or the Feaver-fig, is the beft for this Ufe, and in regard that thefe Figs are of a dark Violet colour, if they were already turn'd, when defign'd to be preferv'd, they muft not be brought to a green Colour, nor any other forts of the like nature

CHAP. XV.

Of Apples.

THis Fruit is of no great Ufe in the Bufinefs of Preferving, and not very delicious, when fo order'd, at leaft with refpect to the drying of them *in Specie* For as for Paftes, Marmelades, and more efpecially *Compotes* of Apples, great quantities of them are ufually made, even till the new Fruits appear. However, fome may be preferv'd, after the two following Ways, when other forts of Fruit are wanting

Green Apples.

Any kind of Apples may be chofen that are fweet and very fmall; which are to be par'd, leaving the Stalks, and flit a little, to the end, that the Sugar may be more thoroughly imbib'd. Having thrown them into Water, to be cleans'd and fcalded, they muft be cool'd and afterwards brought again to a green Colour, in the fame, or other frefh Water · As foon as they are become very foft, let them be cool'd again, drain'd, and put into Sugar newly clarified, giving them fome Boilings: On the next Day, the Syrup muft be boil'd Smooth, at another time, between Smooth and Pearled, and at laft very much

Pearled;

Pearled , ſlipping in the Fruit, that all may ſimper together, and be ſet by, till the next Morning At this laſt time, the Apples ought to have a cover'd Boiling, before they are remov'd from the Fire, to be cool'd and drain'd , if it be requir'd to dry them : But they are moſt proper for liquid Sweet-meats, ſo that they may be immediately diſpoſed of in Pots, or Glaſſes, and kept to be us'd as occaſion may ſerve.

John-*apples and Pippins preſerv'd in Quarters.*

The former retain a very delightful red Colour, and the others may paſs for Apricocks, if ſome Syrup of Apricocks be pour'd upon them, as they are finiſhing.   Both theſe ſorts of Apples, after they have been par'd, are to be cut into two Parts, ſo as the Cores may be taken out of each Half , or elſe, the paring and cutting of them may be deferr'd, till they have been ſcalded in Water , to render them ſoft Afterwards, being cool'd and drain'd, they muſt be put into Sugar, newly paſs'd thro' the Straining-bag, in order, to have thirty Boilings On the next Day, they are to be ſtrain'd again, and the Syrup boil'd , till it has attain'd to its Smooth Quality Then ſlip in the Fruits, and let them have one or two Boilings. On the third Day, let the Syrup be boil'd to a Degree, between Smooth and Pearled ; and, on the fourth, till it be quite Pearled , cauſing the Apples to have ten, or twelve cover'd Boilings. As ſoon as they are cool'd, they may be dried, as all other ſorts of Fruit, ſetting them by to drain, for a while, dreſſing them upon the Slates, and ſtrewing them with fine Sugar, put into a Handkerchief : Otherwiſe, they may be kept liquid, and when, at another time, you are minded to dry them, boil ſome Sugar, till it be Pearled, and give them a few Boilings therein By this means they'll become more fair, in drying, as well as all other ſorts of Fruit, ſo order'd , becauſe it always happens, that their Moiſture, cauſes the Sugar to give, a little, in proceſs of time, which hinders them from being eaſily dried

C H A P. XVI.

Of Bell-grapes and Muscadine-grapes.

ALtho' these two kinds of Grapes are very different, yet they are no less esteem'd, amidst the great variety of Sweetmeats. The Bell-grape, well known at *Paris* by the Name of *Verjus*, is distinguish'd into three sorts, viz the White, the Red, and the Black For want of these, the *Pergoleise*, or *Italian* Grapes may be us'd, which are somewhat long and clear The best Muscadine-grapes for Preserving, are the long, or *Passemusque*, and the white Muscadine of *Frontignan*

Bell-grapes preserv'd liquid

Having caus'd some Water to simper over the Fire, throw in your Grapes, and set them by, as soon as it rises, in order to be cool'd, and afterwards brought again to a green Colour in the same, or other fresh Water Whilst the Fruit is draining, boil the Sugar, till it be Pearled, and slip in the Grapes, till all begin to simper At that instant, let them be remov'd and left in the Pan, till the next Day, when they are to be set over the Fire again, and gently stirr'd, till ready to boil On the third Day, having drain'd them, on a Cullander, and caus'd the Syrup to be somewhat Pearled, let the Grapes be slipt into it, and let all simper together a little while On the fourth Day, the Fruit must be drain'd again in the same manner, whilst the Syrup is brought to its Pearled Quality, then, the Grapes being turn'd into it, ought to have seven or eight Boilings At last, being taken off from the Fire, to cool, they may be put into Glasses, or Pots, and us'd as occasion requires

It would be expedient, to make choice of these Grapes, before they begin to grow ripe, and only to take the fairest, which are to be stoned, and slit on one side

Bell-grapes preserved dry.

They ought to be prepar'd, and put into Sugar, after the same manner, as the liquid Grapes, only the Sugar may be made somewhat more Pearled, for the last time of Boiling, be-

Y 2

fore

fore the Work is brought to perfection , to the end, that they may more easily be dried, after having caus'd them to be cool'd and drain'd, as the Cherries in Ears, described Pag 27.   They may also be dress'd in like manner, except that the Grapes must be clos'd again, and their Stalks left entire.   But you must not forget, either Way, to strew them lightly with Sugar, as they are set in the Stove and turn'd

Bell-grapes are most commonly preserv'd liquid, either entire, or after the Stones have been taken out   They are also preserv'd pared, and it is requisite only to observe, what has been before deliver'd, with respect to those that are otherwise order'd

The Pastes and *Compotes* of Bell grapes, are hereafter specified, under those Articles.

Jelly of Bell-grapes.

When the Grapes are prepar'd as before, let them be thrown into Pearled Sugar, and boil'd till it returns to the same Quality :   Then let all be pour'd into a Sieve, and let the Liquor that passes thro', without squeezing, or at least after a very little pressing, be conveniently dispofed of in Pots or Glasses. To this purpose, it is requisite, to produce as many Pounds of Sugar, as of Fruit.

Some make a Jelly of Bell-grapes, by squeezing them, after they have been scalded in Water, without opening them, and afterwards adding a Decoction of Apples   But the former Way is much better, and the Jelly so order'd will keep longer.

Muscadine-grapes preserv'd liquid.

You are to choose such Muscadine-grapes, as are only half ripe, or even somewhat greenish and tart, and to pare them, if you shall think fit; picking out the Stones, after they have been slit on one side ; or else they may be left entire   They may also be scalded in Water, over the Fire; but they may be very well preserv'd, without this particular Circumstance : To that end, let the Sugar be boil'd Smooth, and, having thrown in the Fruit, let all simper a little while, leaving them in the same condition, till the next Day   If you perceive, that they have sufficiently imbib'd the Sugar, compleat the Work, by causing the Syrup to be Pearled, and slip in the Grapes, in order to

. have

have ſome cover'd Boilings; taking off the Scum from time to time Then they muſt be neatly put into Glaſſes, or Pots, and cover'd as ſoon as they are cool'd.   Otherwiſe, the Muſcadines may have three Boilings, before they are brought to Perfection, the ſecond of which, is to be between Smooth and Pearled, but in the laſt, the Sugar muſt be always Pearled.   If it be melted at firſt with the Juice of other Muſcadine-grapes ſqueez'd for that purpoſe, the Perfume will be more fragrant and grateful to the Palate.

Muſcadine-grapes preſerv'd dry.

Let the Sugar be boil'd till it become Feathered, and let the Grapes be thrown into it, after having remov'd the Pan.   Then ſet it over the Fire again, and give the Fruit a cover'd Boiling ; taking off the Scum ; as in the preceding Article. Afterwards, the Syrup being only brought again to its Pearled Quality, it muſt be taken away, and ſet by to cool ; ſo as the Grapes may be conveniently drain'd and dreſs'd, in order to be dried in the Stove

Muſcadine-grapes ſo order'd, may be taken more ripe, than for liquid Sweet-meats, and thoſe that are thoroughly ripe, may be iced *Compotes* and Paſtes may be alſo made of them, which ſhall be hereafter explain'd under their reſpective Articles

C H A P. XVII.

Of Quinces and Marmelade made of them.

QUinces, when preſerv'd, are one of the domeſtick Sweet-meats moſt in vogue, as well upon account of their grateful Taſte, as by reaſon of their Uſefulneſs for certain Indiſpoſitions of the Body So that the Way of Preſerving them in Quarters, Marmelade or Jelly, is generally well known ; nevertheleſs, we ſhall here give a particular Deſcription of them, to the end, that it may be done after the beſt and ſureſt manner.

Quinces preserved liquid.

Having chosen the ripest, yelloweft and foundeft Quinces, let them be prick'd, and fcalded in Water, over the Fire. They muft also be par'd and cut into Quarters, taking out the Cores. Some order them thus, before they are fcalded, but it is more expedient, not to do it till afterwards, as well as with refpect to the other forts of Fruit; becaufe otherwife, being too much fill'd with Water, they would become foft and fpungy, and more apt to turn to Marmelade. However, care muft be taken to put the Quinces into fair Water, as they are par'd, whilft a Decoction is made of the Parings, Cores, and fome Parts of other Quinces. This Liquor being ftrain'd, will ferve for the ftewing of thofe that are defign'd to be preferv'd, till they become very foft, otherwife they may be fcalded after the ufual manner. Then they muft be remov'd from the Fire, in order to be cool'd and drain'd. In the mean while, fome clarified Sugar is to be heated fomewhat more than luke-warm, and pour'd upon the Quinces in an earthen or Copper-pan. On the fame Day, or the next, the Syrup being only made Smooth, the Fruit muft be flipt into it, and very gently boil'd, carefully taking off the Scum. It is fuppofed, that they may be brought to a redder Colour, by covering them, but this may be done by the means of prepared Cochineel, or even of Wine, which will make them red enough, if it be requifite. After the Quinces have had thirty or forty Boilings, fo as the Syrup may return at leaft to its Smooth Quality, they muft be taken off, and fet by till the next Day. Then, having boil'd the Syrup between Smooth and Pearled, flip in the Fruit, and give them fome Boilings, before they are remov'd from the Fire. To finifh the Work, the Syrup being Pearled, and the Quinces turn'd into it, let them have a cover'd Boiling, and let the Syrup be brought again to its Pearled Quality: At laft, when it begins to fink, all muft be taken out, and put into Pots or Glaffes, to be kept for Ufe.

The Quinces may alfo be drefs'd feparately in Boxes, and cool'd in that manner; whilft the Syrup is fet again over the Fire, till it become Pearled, in order to be pour'd upon the Fruit, fo as they may be cover'd with a fine Jelly: Then the prepar'd Cochineel may be added, or elfe, during the laft of the former Boilings, when they are potted, without any other Management.

Marme-

Marmelade of Quinces, according to the Mode of the City of Orleans.

Take the best sort of Quinces, and cut them into Pieces, which are to be par'd and clear'd from the Cores and Kernels: At the same time, having provided two Pounds of Sugar, boil'd till it is become Crack'd, throw in about six Pounds of Fruit and let all boil together, to a Pap. Afterwards, they must be turn'd into a new Cloth, to be well strain'd, and the Liquor which passes thro', will serve for the Marmelade. To that purpose, let this strained Liquor, be pour'd into other Pearled Sugar, to the quantity of four Pounds, and as soon as the whole Mess returns to the same Degree of Boiling, let it be carefully Scummed. Then you may remove it from the Fire, taking off the Scum again, if there be occasion, and pour it into Boxes, Pots or Glasses, which must be left in the Air, for some Days, before they are cover'd.

Other sorts of Marmelade of Quinces

Having cut the Quinces into Quarters, without Paring them, or taking away the Kernels, let them boil in Water, till they dissolve, and turn to Marmelade. Then let all be strain'd thro' a Linnen-cloath, or else thro' the Straining-bag, without squeezing, and let the Liquor be set by, whilst as much Sugar is boil'd, till it become Crack'd; into which it must be pour'd, with a little white Wine, or Claret, according to the Colour, that you would have given to the Marmelade. Some Sticks of Cinnamon beaten a little, may also be added, with Nutmeg, Cloves and Mace: Let all boil together gently, and take care to clear off the Scum, stirring them from time to time, with the *Spatula,* or with a Spoon. As soon as the Marmelade returns to its Pearled Quality, or is boil'd to the consistence of a fine Jelly, which falls in great Drops, when taken up with the Spoon, take it off from the Fire and pour it into a Sieve set over a Pan, or else strain it thro' a Linnen-cloath, in order to be put into Pots or Glasses, as before. The Marmelade may also be pour'd into leaden Moulds, and when it is cool'd, they may be put into hot Water, as it were in *Balneo Marie,* or a vaporous Bath, so as the Pieces of Marmelade may be easily loosen'd and let fall one upon another in the Boxes.

Y 4　　　　　　　　　　If

If you have a mind to give a finer Tincture to the red Marmelade, it may be done by the means of prepar'd Cocheneal, that is to say, such as has been boil'd in Water, with Allum and Cream of Tarter, and then all may be strain'd, to be us'd, as occasion requires.

Marmelade is also made, into which may be put a lesser quantity of Sugar than of Fruit, or of their Decoction, and this is all the difference, between these two Ways of preparing it

CHAP. XVIII.

Of Oranges and their Flowers.

WE are now come to the Winter fruits, and these are not of the least consequence, on the contrary, they hold one of the principal Ranks, among those that are proper for sweet-Meats. But it will be requisite at first, to give some Account of the Orange-flowers, which are chiefly preserved during the Summer, and then to procede in shewing the manner of preserving the Oranges themselves, according to their several kinds, *viz* those of *China*, *Sevil*, the Port and others ; which are either sweet or sour, or else both sweet and sour together

To preserve Orange-flowers.

The Orange-flowers must be thrown into Water and Salt, and left in that Pickle during five Days: Then they are to be scalded in two Waters, over the Fire, with a little Lemmon-juice, as the Orange-flower-buds hereafter described; in order to be put into Sugar, newly pass'd thro' the Straining-bag, and already heated : On the next Day, let the Sugar be boil'd, a little Smooth, and pour'd upon the Flowers, for they ought not to be set on the Fire, any longer   On the third Day, boil your Sugar quite Smooth, and pour it likewise upon the Flowers: Afterwards, having set all by to cool, let the Flowers be drain'd, and dried with Powder-sugar ; laying them in order, upon Sieves On the Day following, they must be turn'd on the other side, and strew'd likewise with Sugar put into a Handkerchief.

Orange-flower-Buds.

Let them be thrown into Water and Salt, as before. and continue therein, during eight Days I hen let them be drain'd, and prick'd in two places, with a Pin, that is to fay, on the Bottom, and thro' the Middle, to the end that they may more eafily imbibe the Sugar : In the mean while, fome Spring-water is to be fet over the Fire, and when it boils, the Flowers are to be put into it, with a little Lemmon-juice When they are half done, fome Water muft be fet over another Furnace, and the Buds laid a draining, which are to be thrown into it, as foon as it begins to boil: Afterwards, they muft be drain d again, and order'd with Sugar, as the former Orange-flowers, that is to fay, they muft be firft put into clarified Sugar, and then fcalded, three feveral times, without fetting them over the Fire, only pouring off the Sugar, from the earthen Pans, that contan the Buds, giving it the proper Boilings, above exprefs'd, and at laft turning it upon the fame Buds Then it being fet by to cool, they may be drain'd and dried with Powder-fugar

As for the Conferves, Marmelades, Paftes and Paftils made of Orange flowers, recourfe may be had to thofe different Articles hereafter fpecified, in their Order.

Sevil-*Oranges preferv'd in Quarters, or in Sticks*

The Oranges are firft to be Turn'd or elfe Zefted, after the fame manner, as Lemmons which fhall be explain'd Pag 57. except that the Surface of the Orange-peel, muft only be par d off very lightly The Oranges being thus prepar'd, may be cut either into Quarters, or into Sticks, accordingly, as you fhall think fit; but the Skin on the infide and the Juice muft be taken away. In the mean while, fome Water is to be fet over the Fire, and the Oranges are to be thrown in, as foon as it begins to boil: It may be perceiv d, that they are done enough, by their flipping off from the Pin, and then they may be cool'd, putting them into frefh Water; as alfo afterwards, into clarified Sugar. At the fame time, they ought to have feven, or eight cover'd Boilings, and to be fet by to cool However, they muft be boil'd over the Fire again, till the Syrup becomes almoft Smooth, and drain'd the next Day, to be put into Pots, whilft your Syrup is made Pearled; which being pour'd upon the Oranges, they

may

may be kept thus, till you shall judge it expedient to dry them, observing the Directions hereafter laid down for Lemmons, Pag 57 & 58

Sevil-*Oranges preserved entire*

As the Oranges are Turn'd or Zested they must be thrown into fair Water, and afterwards scalded over the Fire, till they become very soft, and slip off from the Pin Then they must be cool'd, and scoop'd with a little Spoon, made for that purpose, at a little Hole bor'd in the middle, where the Stalk grew They are usually put into Sugar, and dried after the same manner, as the Quinces and Sticks of Oranges, even now described

China-*Oranges preserved whole, or in Quarters.*

China-Oranges are preserv'd whole, as the former, except, that Part of them may be left without scooping, as being very delicious when done altogether entire, by reason of their sweetness: So that it is sufficient only to make a Hole on the top, as well to take away the inner Skin, as to the end that the Sugar may penetrate into the inside.

As for those that are preserv'd in Quarters, every Orange must be cut into three Parts, and the same Instructions must be follow'd, that were given a little before, for *Sevil*-Oranges

Oranges of the Port

This kind of Oranges, that are of a sweet-sour Taste, may likewise be preserv'd in Quarters, or in Sticks; in performing which Work, there is nothing else to be observ'd, but what has been already express'd for the other sorts of Oranges

Sour Oranges.

These are likewise preserv'd both in Quarters and in Sticks, but it is observable, That after having scalded them, they ought to be steept for one or two Days in certain Pails or other Vessels fill'd with Water, which is to be chang'd from time to time, to the end that their Bitterness may be taken away, as it may be perceiv'd by the green Tincture, which they give the Water.

Fo.

For the reft, it is expedient only to obferve, what has been already deliver'd, with refpect to the other forts of Oranges. Thefe laft are chofen either from among the *Bigarrades*, or the *Sevil*-Oranges, which are of that Nature

Faggots of Oranges.

The Orange-peels, that are turn'd or par'd very thin are often preferv'd, more efpecially thofe of fweet Oranges, drawing them out, to as great a length, as is poffible, and thefe are commonly call'd Faggots To that purpofe, they are to be fcalded in Water, over the Fire, till they become very foft, and put into Sugar newly clarified; giving them twenty Boilings Then they are to be remov'd, and fet by; but the next Day the Syrup muft be made Smooth and the Orange-parings flipt into it, that they may have two or three Boilings. On the third Day, let them be drain'd, whilft the Sugar is brought to its Pearled Quality, and let them have a cover'd Boiling, in order to be taken off, and diftributed into Pots, unlefs you are minded to dry them at the fame time This may be done, by caufing other Sugar to be made white, rubbing it on one fide of the Pan with the Skimmer, and boiling it till it be Feather'd. Then the Faggots are to be flipt into it and drefs d in Rocks. Otherwife, having caus'd the Sugar to be Blown, throw in your Orange-Parings, give them a cover'd Boiling, and fet them by, in order to be laid upon a Grate, or Hurdle, and dried in the Stove; which may be done in a fhort time, but the other Way is more preferrable.

Thus both yellow and white Faggots are made after the fame manner The former are thofe Parings which are made of the firft Peel of the Orange, and the others are taken off afterwards, by turning them a fecond time.

Zefts of *Sevil-Oranges.*

They are order'd altogether after the fame manner, as thofe of Lemmons, for which Directions fhall be given hereafter So that recourfe may be had to them, and it would be needlefs to anticipate the Matter in his Place.

Orange-

Orange-slips.

Small Slips may likewise be made of the same Oranges, and to that end, the same Method may be follow'd, which shall be anon explain'd for Lemmon-slips, of which a greater quantity is usually preserv'd.

Certain Slips of sour Oranges are generally put into a kind of Sugar-plums, call'd *Orangeaz*, which are very grateful to the Taste, when order'd with good Sugar. The same sort of Sugar-plums, are also made with Lemmon-slips.

C H A P. XIX.

Of Lemmons.

LEmmons may be preserv'd after different manners; and are of several sorts Certain green ones are sometimes brought over entire, which pass for *Indian* Lemmons: The ripe ones that come to our Hands, are frequently preserv'd whole, in Sticks, Slips, *Zests,* and otherwise; not to make mention of the Pasts, Marmelade and Conserves that are made of this Fruit. Let us begin with the first sort, altho' we have no longer an opportunity to preserve such in these Parts.

To preserve green Indian Lemmons.

These small Lemmons are to be lightly slit on one side, to the end, that the inside may be as much soak'd in the Sugar, as the other Parts: Then let them be thrown into Water over the Fire, but prevented from boiling, by pouring in fresh Water from time to time to cause it to sink. As soon as the Lemmons rise on the top, let them be taken off, and set by to cool: Afterwards their green Colour must be recover'd, by setting them over the Fire again in the same or other Water, which ought to boil by degrees, till the Lemmons become very soft, and slip off from the Pin. Then being taken out and cool'd again, nothing will remain to be done, only to put them into Sugar, after the same manner, as the following sorts of Lemmons.

Whi[

White Lemmons preferv'd in Sticks.

These Lemmons muft be Zefted or elfe Turn'd, according as your Intention is, either to preferve them in *Zefts* or Chips, or to make Faggots. To Turn, in this Senfe, is a Term of Art, fignifying to pare off the fuperficial Rind or Peel, on the out-fide, very thin and narrow, with a little Knife; turning it round about the Lemmon or Orange, fo as it may be extended to the length of feveral Fathoms To Zeft, is to cut the Peel, from top to bottom, into fmall Slips, as thin, as it can poffibly be done. The Lemmons thus order'd, are to be firft cut into Quarters, and then into Sticks, dividing thofe Quarters into two or three Parts, according to their Thicknefs. Afterwards, they muft be thrown into Water boiling over the Fire, and fcalded with their Juice and innermoft Skin, which keeps them whiter, and could not be got off from the Pulp, without difficulty, unlefs they were thus heated over the Fire : Care muft alfo be taken to throw them into fair Water, as they are Turn'd, or Zefted ; other-wife they would foon grow black

When you perceive, That the Lemmon pulp is become very foft, let it be cool'd, and afterwards put into Sugar, newly pafs'd thro' the Straining-bag : Then give it feven or eight Boilings, and pour all into earthen Pans. On the next Day, let the Sy-rup be pour'd off, without taking away the Fruit, and let it have twenty or thirty Boilings, having augmented it with a little Sugar Some time after, the Lemmons are to be put into it, and fo on the following Days fucceffively, as the Syrup is boil'd, firft a little Smooth, then altogether Smooth, at ano-ther time, between Smooth and Pearled, and at laft thoroughly Pearled ; always adding fome other Sugar, as often as the Pan is fet over the Fire.

As foon as the laft Boiling is perform'd, for bringing the Fruit to perfection, they may be drain'd and difpofed of in Pots or other Veffels, if they are defign'd for keeping. The Lemmons may alfo be dried at the fame time, or any other, at pleafure ; and for that purpofe, it is only requifite to cool them, which may be done more fpeedily, upon any urgent Oc-cafion, by fetting the bottom of the Pan into cold Water In the mean while, let fome Sugar be made Feathered ; and, ha-ving drain'd the Fruit, flip them into it, in order to have a cover'd Boiling. Then take all off from the Fire, and as foon

as

as the Boiling entirely ceafes, begin to work and make your
Sugar white, in a Corner, by rubbing it with the Back of a
Spoon, or Skimmer, againft the Side of the Pan   Afterwards
the Lemmons muft be boil'd in this clarified Sugar, and fet a
draining, upon Grates. Thus they'll become dry in a few Hour,
and at any other time, when you would have them dried, you
need only put the fame thing into practice

Lemmons *preferv'd in* Zefts, *or* Chips

As the Lemmons are Zefting, in the above-mention'd man
ner, let the *Zefts* be thrown into fair Water on one fide, and
the Quarters, on the other, to prevent them from turning Black
Afterwards, let the Water be heated, and the *Zefts* put into it,
to be fcalded, till they become very foft · Then, having turn'd
them into frefh Water, they muft be cool'd, and order'd with
thin Sugar, putting one Ladle full of Water into a Pan for
every two of clarified Sugar ; thus all muft be heated over the
Fire, as long as you can well endure to hold your Finger in
the Liquor. In the mean while, the Lemmon-chips being
drain'd, and flipt into an earthen Pan, the Sugar is to be pour'd
upon them, and they ought to be foak'd in it, fomewhat longer
than ordinary   They may be left in this condition, till the next
Day, when they are to be drain'd in a Cullander, whilft the
Syrup is boil'd, till it become a little Smooth   Some time after,
this Syrup muft be pour'd again upon the *Zefts* ; as alfo, on the
third Day, after having brought it to its Pearled Quality, and
augmented it with a little Sugar   On the fourth Day, the Lem
mon chips are to be drain'd again, and dried in the Sieve, upon
Hurdles, or upon the Grate, with a Pan underneath, to receive the Syrup that diftills from thence   They ought alfo to
be turn'd from time to time, till they become very dry, and at
laft fhut up in Boxes, to be kept for Ufe.

Lemmons *preferv'd in fmall Slips.*

Having Zefted your Lemmons, cut your Pulp into Slips,
which are to be flit again in their thicknefs, to render them very
thin, and by that means certain fmall Slips will be made, of the
length of *Lardoons,* or Slices of Bacon, that are proper for Larding   Thefe Lemmon flips, are to be fcalded, at firft, in Wa
ter over the Fire, till they become very foft. Then let fome
                                                            clari-

clarified Sugar, newly pafs'd thro' the Straining-bag, be likewife fet over the Fire, and, when it is ready to boil, throw in
your Slips, in order to have twenty Boilings They may alfo
be put into the Sugar all at once, without ftaying till it is hot.
On the next Day, having boil'd the Sugar Smooth, and flipt
them into it, let them have feven, or eight Boilings On the
third Day, or the Evening before, if they were made ready in
the Morning, you may bring your Sugar to its Pearled Quality,
and give the Lemmon-flips a cover'd Boiling. Afterwards, they
are to be put into Pots or other Veffels, according to the quantity, and dried, as occafion ferves; which is to be done after
the following manner:

Let your Lemmon-flips be well drain'd from their Syrup,
and put into Feather'd Sugar, giving them a cover'd Boiling,
and ftirring them from time to time. After this cover'd Boiling, remove the Pan from the Fire, and, as foon as you can
endure to touch the Handles, begin to work the Sugar, and
make it white, in a Corner, as before, by rubbing and beating
it by degrees, with the back of the Ladle or Skimmer, againft
the fide of the Pan Then, taking up the Slips, with two Forks,
let them be turn'd and foak'd in this Sugar, till they are well
ic'd over Laftly, they muft be laid a draining upon Hurdles, and
drefs'd in Rocks, by which means they will be fpeedily dried,
and brought to perfection. However, if the Bufinefs does not
require Difpatch, or if you have no mind to ice them in this
manner, fome Sugar may be boil'd till it has attain'd to its
Blown Quality, and the Lemmon flips may be put into it:
Then, having given them a cover'd Boiling, let them be taken
out, and drefs'd a little while after, upon a Grate, or Hurdle,
to be fet into the Stove But care muft be taken to turn them
on all fides, fo as they may be thoroughly dried, and at laft
laid up in Boxes, to be us'd as occafion fhall require

If the Lemmon flips fhould happen to puff, or turn four in
the Veffels, in which they are kept, they muft be fet over the
Fire, with a little Water to caufe them to give, and then boil'd,
till a thick and black Scum rifes on the top, which muft be taken off When they have recover'd their former Degree of Boiling, which is Pearled, their fournefs will be entirely taken
away, and they may be difpofed of at pleafure. To that purpofe, fome caufe the Syrup to be fift fet over the Fire, which
being fcumm'd, they turn in the Slips, to give them a Boiling;
but this Matter is altogether indifferent. The Management of
others

others is yet more inconsiderable, who, for fear of too much diminishing the quantity of their Sugar, defer the scumming of it till it settles when taken off from the Fire, and till the grossest Substance of the Scum is only left · For by that means, they run the hazard of being put to the trouble, to renew the same Work, within a very short time, and the same thing may be affirm'd, with respect to other sorts of Sweet-meats, that are to be clear'd from their sourness.

Faggots of Lemmon.

As to this Particular, it is only requisite to follow the Instructions given for the Ordering of Orange-faggots, Pag. 55. so that the Reader is referr'd to that Article, because few Lemmons are preserv'd after this manner, and a much greater quantity of Oranges, more especially the sweet ones

Lemmons preserv'd entire.

Having Zested, or else Turn'd your Lemmons, according to the Method explain'd in the second Article, throw them, as they are done, into fair Water, with some Juice of other Lemmons, to prevent them from turning Black. Let them also be scalded over the Fire, in Water, with Lemmon juice likewise, till they become soft and tender, and slip off from the Pin. Then, being cool'd in cold Water, they must be scoop'd with a little Spoon, made for that purpose, at a little Hole bor'd on the top. As soon as they are well scoop'd and cleans'd, they are to be put into Sugar, pass'd thro' the Straining-bag, and the whole Work is to be finish'd after the same manner, as Lemmons in Sticks. They may also be prepar'd for Drying thus. Let the Sugar be brought to its Feathered Quality, and made white in a Corner, according to the Directions elsewhere laid down. Then, having slipt in the Lemmons, let them be drain'd upon Hurdles, with the Hole underneath, after they have been taken out, with a Spoon and Fork

For Marmelade, and Pastes of Lemmon, see those Articles hereafter specified.

CHAP

C H A P. XX.
Of Cedres, *Limes, and yellow Citrons.*

THese three sorts of Fruit have so near a relation, one to another, that there is no difference in the preserving of them, and very little, with respect to the common Lemmons However, we shall here subjoin the particular Ways of ordering them to the best advantage.

Green Cedres *preserv'd in Sticks cr Quarters.*

In these Parts, only ripe *Cedres* are us'd, such as are brought over from beyond Sea , but in the Countries, where they grow, as in *Provence,* and on the Coasts of *Genoa* and *Nice,* great quantities of them are preserv'd Green, after having taken out the Juice, to make the Liquor call'd *Cedraz* To that purpose, they are usually cut into Quarters, to be reduc'd afterwards to Sticks, of any size that shall be thought fit They may also be cut according to their Thickness, and thro' the middle, by reason of the extreme largeness of this Fruit , by which means there will be two sorts, *viz* one entirely Green, and the other White They are generally preserv'd liquid, and transported in that condition , so that there is no more to be done, but to dry them, as Occasion serves, which may be perform'd in this manner : At first they must be drain'd from their former Syrup, and put into Feathered Sugar, in order to have a cover'd Boiling · As soon as they are somewhat cool'd, and you can endure to touch the Handles of the Pan, the Sugar may be work'd and made white, by beating and rubbing it by degrees against the side of the Pan Afterwards, your *Cedres* must be laid in the same Sugar and turn'd : Then they are to be taken out, and drain'd upon a Cullander, or Hurdle, so as their Pulp may lie downwards , by which means they will be finely ic'd over, and dried in a short time, without the help of a Stove

To preserve ripe Cedres *and* Limes *or* Pomecitrons.

They are usually cut, altogether as the green *Cedres,* or according to the following Method for Citrons, to which Article re-

Z

recourse may also be had, for the Way of ordering and putting them into Sugar, because it is absolutely the same, without any difference. The same thing may likewise be done, with respect to Limes, or great Lemmons, of which a kind of Syrup is also made, as well as Limonade.

Citrons.

Yellow Citrons are preserv'd either in Sticks, or in Slices, and sometimes without taking away the inner Skin and Juice As for those that are order'd after this last manner, it is only requisite to cut them into round Slices, of a convenient thickness, and afterwards to divide those Slices into two parts But the other Way is most usual, and to that purpose, after the Citrons have been Turn'd, or Zested, they are to be cut thro' the middle, and each half is to be divided into four Quarters: However, nothing but the Pulp ought to be taken, of which lesser Slices or Sticks are made, which may be cut again, according to their thickness, and preserv'd conformably to the following Directions.

To preserve the Pulp of yellow Citrons

Having cut the Citrons, as before, let them be thrown into boiling Water, and to facilitate the scalding of them, add an Handful of beaten Allum. As soon as you perceive the Fruit to be soft, let them be cool'd, and put into Sugar newly clarified: Afterwards let all have seven or eight Boilings, in order to be set by in earthen Pans till the next Day; when the Syrup being taken out, and boil'd somewhat smooth, must be augmented with other Sugar, and pour'd upon the Citrons. On the third Day, let the Syrup be made very Smooth, and likewise pour'd upon the Fruit To make them ready for the Repository, they are to be drain'd, and set in order in Pots, or other Vessels; whilst the Syrup is brought to its Pearled Quality, to be pour'd upon them When you would have your Citrons dried, you need only observe, what has been before laid down, for the ordering of *Cedres.*

Zests *of Citrons*, &c

The *Zests*, or Chips of yellow Citrons, *Cedres* and Limes, are preserv'd altogether after the same manner, as those of ordinary Lemmons, for which see Pag. 57

Chap. XXI.

Of Compotes *for the whole Year.*

WE have hitherto treated only of Fruits, as they are preserv'd in their natural Condition; either dry, or liquid; but now it is requisite to give some Account of the other sorts of Sweet-meats that may be made of them, observing likewise the Order and Season of every one of them, as before, of these, the most common are the *Compotes*. Neither is it difficult to prepare them duly, when the Method of Preserving all kinds of Fruit is well known; because, before they are entirely brought to perfection, they come to the Degree, which is sufficient for *Compotes* However, we shall not forbear here to express the best Manner of Ordering them, to the end, that the Reader may have greater Advantage in this Particular, and so much the rather, in regard, that, these sorts of Sweet-meats being design'd to be immediately eaten, or at least, in a short space of time, it is not necessary, to take so many Precautions, nor to observe so many nice Circumstances, as in the Managing of Fruits, that are to be thoroughly preserv'd

Compotes *of green Apricocks*

Having par'd your Apricocks, or put them into a Lie, such as is describ'd Pag 16. let them be cool'd and pierc'd thro' the middle; throwing them into other fresh Water. They must also be brought again to their green Colour, changing the Water once more, in which they are to be boil'd, till they slip off from the Pin. As soon as they are cool'd and drain'd, they must be put into thin Sugar, allowing one Ladle full of Water for every two of Sugar, and causing both to be made Luke-warm;

by which means they'll soon throw out all their Moisture, and imbibe the Sugar They may be left in this condition till Night, or the next Morning, according to the time, when they were put in, or as there may be occasion for the *Compote* Then bring all to the Fire, and give them thirty or forty Boilings, till the Apricocks are become soft, and have thoroughly imbib'd the Sugar. Afterwards, they must be set by to cool; but if you have only two or three *Compotes* of Fruit, and too much Syrup is still left, you may give it some Boilings a-part, and then pour it upon the Apricocks, dress'd in *China* dishes or Bowls provided for that purpose

But it is expedient to prepare a much greater quantity, at once, to serve from time to time, during the Season Besides, that what is left, may always be brought to perfection, by causing the other Boilings to attain to higher Degrees, which are necessary for the keeping of the Apricocks, as well liquid, as dry

Another Compote *of green Apricocks*

If you have a mind to make a *Compote* of green Apricocks, out of Season, it may be easily done, provided, there be some liquid ones at hand For you need only take such a quantity of Fruit as is requisite, with part of the Syrup, setting the latter over the Fire in a Copper-pan, with a little Water to cause it to give. Then let it have some Boilings, and pour it upon your Apricocks, in order to be serv'd up, either hot, or cold, accordingly as it shall be judg'd expedient.

Altho' dried Apricocks were only left in the Repository, nevertheless a very good *Compote* may be made of them; by putting them into a Pan, with some Syrup of other green Apricocks, or other Syrup of the like Nature, and causing them to give, as before Then after a few Boilings, you have no more to do, but to dress your *Compote* and serve it up to Table.

Compotes *of green Almonds.*

Having put Almonds into a Lie prepared according to the Directions in Pag 16 let them be brought again to their Colour, and boil'd Then they are to be put into Sugar, observing what has been even now deliver'd with respect to *Compotes* of green Apricocks, made ready at all times: So that the like may

bs

be prepared, with green Almonds, either in Seafon, or otherwife, when preferv'd wet, or dry.

Compotes *of green Gooseberries.*

Slit your Gooseberries on the fide, and pick out the fmall Grains that are enclos'd therein Then let them be fcalded in Water, over the Fire, and taken off, as foon as they rife on the top of the Water, fetting them by, to cool Afterwards, they muft be brought again to their Colour, and heated in other frefh Water, till they become very foft and tender At that inftant, they may be remov'd from the Fire, in order to be cool'd, drain'd, and put into Sugar newly clarified ; but they muft only be foak'd in it, and the fame thing is to be obferv'd, with refpect to other forts of Fruit Some time after, give them fourteen or fifteen Boilings, and if you percieve, that they have thoroughly imbib'd the Sugar, you may referve them, for the making of *Compotes*, at any time, till the Seafon is pafs'd So that the reft of the Work may be finifh'd, by giving them the Boiling, that is peculiar to this fort of Fruit, and fpecified in its proper Place, Pag 33

When thefe Boilings are perform'd, only for *Compotes*, if too much Syrup be left, it muft be boil'd feveral other times, after having taken out the Gooseberries, upon which it is to be pour'd, at laft At another time, if you are defirous to make a *Compote* of green Gooseberries, out of hand, take thofe that lie by liquid, and caufe them to give, with a little Water Then let them have a Boiling, with the Gooseberries, and drefs them, upon your *China*-difhes

Compotes *of Cherries.*

Having provided Cherries, and cut off part of their Stalks, take a quarter, or half a Pound of Sugar, which will be fufficient, if you defign only to make one or two *Compotes* Let it be melted, with a very little Water, becaufe the Cherries will yield a great deal of Juice, and let all boil together, carefully taking off the Scum, till the Cherries become foft, and have thoroughly imbib'd the Sugar If too much Syrup be left, give it fome other Boilings, and afterwards pour it upon your Fruit

Upon any emergent Occafion, even out of th Seafon, a *Compote* may be made of dried Cherries, or others, following

Z 3

the

the Instructions that have been given for the preceding Fruits

Compotes *of Rasberries.*

Having caus'd some Sugar to be brought to its Pearled Qua lity, let your Rasberries be thrown into it   Then give them a cover'd Boiling, and the Business will be effected.

Compotes *of Strawberries*

These *Compotes* are usually made after the same manner, but if the Strawberries are somewhat over-ripe, the Sugar must be boil d to a little higher Degree.

Compotes *of Currans.*

Take Sugar newly pass'd tho' the Straining-bag, and boil it till it is Blown: Then throw in your Currans, give them a Boiling, and remove them from the Fire   If you percieve, that they have thoroughly imbib'd the Sugar, they may be dress'd upon *China*-dishes, and serv'd up to Table   Otherwise, let them be brought to the Fire again, and have another Boiling

Compotes *of ripe Apricocks.*

When ripe Apricocks first begin to be in Season, they may be us'd without paring , but afterwards they must be Turn'd and Ston d, in order to be scalded over the Fire, as those that are design'd for Preserving   As soon as they rise on the top, and become soft, they must be taken off, and set by to cool . Then let them be put into Sugar, as it runs from the Straining-bag, and boil'd till the Scum ceases to rise any longer, which is a sign, that the Apricocks have cast all their Juice, and sufficiently imb.b'd the Sugar   But if they do not appear to be boil'd enough, you may give them a few more Boilings, as also the Syrup, in case, too great a quantity of it be left, so as it may be conveniently pour d upon the Fruit.

Another Way of making Compotes *of ripe Apricocks*

Compotes of Apricocks are likewise made without scalding so as to render them more delicious, and that they may retain a
greater

greater relish of the Fruit. Having par'd and ston'd them, you need
only put them all at once into clarified Sugar, or if that be wanting, into Sugar melted with Water, that is to say, a Quarter of
a Pound, or somewhat more, for every *Compote* Thus they are
to boil, till they become very soft; to which purpose, a sufficient quantity of Water must be put to them, altho' they also
yield some Juice. When the Scum ceases to rise, and the Apricocks have imbib'd the Sugar, take them off from the Fire, and
observe, whether it be not expedient to boil your Syrup, a little longer, that it may be sufficiently consum'd, and only so much
left, as is requisite for the soaking of your Fruit.

Compotes *of Plums.*

Let your Amber-plums, Orange-plums, or others, be prick'd
with a Pin, and thrown into Water. Then scald them over the
Fire, in the same, or other Water, and take them off, as soon
as they rise on the top, causing them to be speedily cool'd. Then
let them be brought again to their Colour, and made soft, according to their kind, and conformably to the Method explain'd
in the Article of *Plums.* Afterwards, they are to be put into
thin Sugar well heated, allowing one Ladle full of Water, to
two of Sugar. They are to be left in this condition till the next
Day, or only till the Evening, if Occasion require it, and then
they must be put again into a Copper-pan, in order to have as
many Boilings, as shall be judg'd expedient, till the Sugar be
thoroughly imbib'd. At that instant, it may be perceiv'd, that
the Scum does not rise any longer, and that the Plums are become soft and tender. A great quantity may be thus prepar'd
at once, and kept for a considerable time.

Another sort of Compote *of Plums.*

Compotes may also be made of Plums, without scalding, either leaving the Stones, or taking them away. Having put
them into thin Sugar, let all simper together, and after they
have been set by for some time, let them be brought to the Fire
again, to boil, till no Scum is left, and till they have thoroughly
imbib'd the Sugar. Or else, those Directions may be follow'd,
that are specified in the last Article of Apricock-*Compotes.*

Com-

Compotes *of Summer-pears.*

These sorts of Pears are to be scalded over the Fire, till they become somewhat soft, and prick'd on the top, with a Bodkin, even to the Core. Afterwards being cool'd, they must be par'd, and thrown into fresh Water, in order to be put into clarified Sugar; adding a little Water, to boil it   If the Pears are large, they may be cut into Halves or Quarters, so as they may simper in the Sugar, and cast their Juice.   Then let them boil, till the Scum ceases to rise, and your *Compote* will be made.   If too great a quantity of Syrup be left, let it be consum'd a little by boiling, and pour'd upon the Fruit   *Compotes* may be made after the same manner, of *Blanquets,* Russetins, Muscadines, and other sorts of Pears

The clarifying of the Sugar may also be dispens'd with, only throwing a Lump of Sugar of a convenient Thickness, into the Water, in which they are to be boil'd; and taking care that the whole be well Scumm'd: A good quarter of a Pound of Sugar may be sufficient for a *Compote* of the like Nature

Compotes *of other sorts of Pears.*

Winter-Pears may also be put into *Compotes,* in the same manner, particularly the *Bon-chretiens,* those of St. *Francis* and others   They must be first prick'd to the Core, with a Bodkin, and scalded in Water· Then they are to be cool'd, par'd and divided into Quarters, throwing them again into fresh Water Afterwards, they must be put into one half Sugar and the other Water, and boil'd, till they have thrown out all their Scum, which is to be carefully taken off, with the Skimmer.   Let the Pan be remov'd from time to time, and set aside, as soon as the Pears have thoroughly imbib'd the Sugar, and are become soft, otherwise they would turn to Marmelade: Then let the Pears be dress'd upon *China-*dishes, and having given the Syrup, some other Boilings, if it be requisite, pour it upon your Fruit, and squeez in the Juice of a Lemmon, or Orange: The same thing may also be done in the preceding *Compotes*

Com-

Compotes *of Pears made in a Bell.*

There are certain Pears, as the *Certoe*, the Pound-pear and some others, of which another sort of *Compote* may be made, by causing them to be stew'd in a Bell, thus. Having par'd and cut your Pears into Quarters, put them into an earthen Vessel, or one of Copper, made for that purpose, in form of a Bell, with Water, Sugar, Cinnamon and Cloves A quarter of a Pound of Sugar, or somewhat more, will be sufficient for a Pound of Fruit, and only so much Water, as may serve to soak them · Let them be stew'd over a gentle Fire, and when they are half done, let half a Glass of red Wine be added But the Pot must be kept close stopt, and the Fruit stir'd from time to time, lest they should stick to the Bottom Afterwards, the *Compote* is to be dress'd, and the Syrup pour'd upon it, if there be no more than is needful, otherwise it must be consum'd by degrees, because too great a quantity of it ought not to be left.

Compotes *of roasted Pears.*

Compotes may likewise be made of roasted Pears · When they are sufficiently done, and par'd as neatly as is possible, let them be slit and the Cores taken out : Then they are to be put into a Pan, with Sugar and a little Water, which is to be boil'd and and consum'd, till the Pears become very red, and till very little Syrup be left, but they ought to be often stirr'd, to hinder them from burning, and sticking to the Bottom. Afterwards, having dress'd them for your *Compote*, you may squeez in the Juice of an Orange, or Lemmon, which will wonderfully heighten their Relish

Pears may be also put into a Silver-dish or Plate, and bak'd in an Oven, or otherwise, with Powder-sugar, after they have been first scalded in Water, in order to be par'd; or else they may be par'd, without scalding Then let them be dress'd, strew'd again with Sugar, and brought to a Colour, with the red-hot Fire-shovel; adding the Juice of an Orange, when ready to be serv'd up to Table

See hereafter the *Compotes* of Peaches, among which mention is made, of another manner of diversifying these *Compotes*, accordingly as occasion may require.

Com-

Compotes *of Apples.*

Pare your Apples, cut them into Halves, or Quarters, take out the Cores, and, as they are done, throw them into fair Water: Then put a good Quarter of a Pound of Sugar, if it be only for one *Compote*, or a greater quantity, proportionably for several *Compotes*, into a Quart of Water, or more, and let all boil with the Apples As soon as they are become very soft, and have thoroughly imbib'd the Sugar, take them out, and lay them in order upon your *China*-dishes, whilst the rest of the Syrup is boil'd and consum'd, till it turn to a Jelly, which happens, when it falls from the Spoon, in thick drops, and does not run in Threads Then pour it upon your Fruit, and, if you please, squeez in the Juice of an Orange, or Lemmon

Other Ways of preparing Compotes *of Apples.*

Let a Decoction be made of the Parings and Cores, with some other Apples, which being strain'd will serve for the Boiling of your *Compote*, in the same manner as before. Or else, when the Apples are stew'd, and a great quantity of Syrup is still left, let the same Parings and Cores be boil'd in it, and let the Syrup be pass'd thro' a Sieve, before it be pour'd upon the Fruit

Compotes of roasted Apples may also be made, observing the Directions already laid down for Pears But you must remember, to cause your Fruit to be stew'd over a good Fire, and to turn them, from time to time, with the Ladle.

A Compote *of Apples* à la Dauphine.

Having cut your Apples into eight Quarters, every one of which is to be made round, in form of little Balls, as it were Plums; let them boil in a Decoction, of all the Parings, and some other Apples, with the necessary quantity of Sugar, as for other *Compotes*. At last, a little Cochineal is to be added, to give them a red Colour, and the Syrup must not be so much wasted; unless you would have the *Compotes* ic'd over, to diversifie them

Com-

Compotes *of farced Apples.*

Take about a quarter of a Pound of the dried Pulp of Oranges and Lemmons, and pound it in a Morter· Then let some Apples be chopt small, and mingled with Marmelade of Apricocks, or some other sort that is at Hand . Afterwards, having bor'd the Apples thro from top to bottom, without paring them, let the Hole, which ought to be wide enough to receive your Thumb, be fill'd with the said Marmelade, let all be gently bak'd, upon a Silver-plate, in the Oven, or else Fire may be put round about the said Plate, and when the Apples are done enough, they may be soak'd in a little Syrup, as the others.

Compotes *of Peaches.*

When the Peaches are full ripe, they can only be roasted ; because this sort of Fruit is too soft.   Therefore they must be neatly par'd ston'd and laid in Quarters, upon a Silver-dish, or Plate, with Sugar, and, if you think fit, with candy'd Lemmon-peel chopt small   Then, being bak'd in an Oven, let them be dress'd, if they are to be serv'd up with any Thing else, and let the red-hot Fire-shovel be pass'd over them, to give them a fine Colour, after they have been strew'd with Sugar.

This *Compote*, and others of the like nature, may be put into a *Tourte*, or Pan-pie, and to that end, a Border of Paste, and even the whole Furniture that is usually provided for other Pan-pies, must be laid in the Dish, in which the Peaches are to be roasted, and the Fruit must be set in order therein.   In the mean while, another Piece of Paste for Crackling Crust, being roll'd out, may be cut into slips, and separately bak'd in an Oven, in order to be ic'd over with the White of an Egg, and Powder-sugar, well temper'd together   This ic'd Crust must also be dried in the Oven, till it become very white, and laid upon the Pie, a little before it is serv'd up to Table

Other Compotes *of Peaches.*

Compotes may be made of Peaches that are less ripe, according to the Instructions before given for those of Apricocks, Pag 62. and others may likewise be prepar'd, upon occasion, of green Peaches, in their Season, or such as have been already preserv'd ;

in

in the ordering of which, it is only requisite to observe the Method laid down for *Compotes* of green Apricocks

Compotes *of Bell-grapes.*

The Bell-grapes must be first scalded in Water, and brought again to their Colour, as those that are design'd for preserving liquid, or otherwise To that purpose, let your Water simper over the Fire, throw the Fruit into it, and, as soon as they begin to rise, set all by to cool: Then cause them to become green again, in the same, or other Water, and when they are very soft, let them be laid a draining ; whilst some Sugar is boil'd Smooth, or only simpers a little Afterwards, having remov'd the Pan aside, till the Evening, or the next Day, accordingly as you have time, and, having set it again over the Fire, give the Fruit ten, or twelve Boilings, and your *Compote* will be brought to perfection.

Thus, if you think fit, a sufficient quantity for several Services, may be prepar'd, and kept for a considerable time If you have a mind to make a *Compote* of Bell-grapes, out of the Season, you need only take some of those that have been already preserv'd liquid, and cause the Syrup to give a little · Then let it have a Boiling, slip in the Grapes, and dress all upon your *China*-dishes.

Compotes *of Quinces.*

Let the Quinces be cut into Quarters, proportionably to their Thickness, without absolutely loosening them, one from another, so as they may stick together, as if the Fruit were still entire Or else, they may be only pierc'd to the Core, with a Bodkin, and scalded in Water, till they become soft At that instant, let them be remov'd from the Fire, to be cool'd and par'd, taking away the Kernels, and throwing them as they are done, into other fresh Water Then, putting them, as the Pears, into one half Sugar, and the other Water, let all simper together, and set them by for a while, accordingly as the time will permit. Afterwards, being set over the Fire again, they must be boil'd, and scumm'd, till they have thoroughly imbib'd the Sugar, in order to be dress'd for your *Compote*, with the Syrup, when only so much is left, as will be requisite for the soaking of them Lastly, let the Juice of an Orange, or Lemmon be squeez'd upon all, and let them be serv'd up hot to Table.   *O.*

Other Ways of making Compotes *of Quinces.*

The Quinces may be wrapp'd up in wet Paper, and roasted by degrees under hot Embers Then they are to be cut into Quarters, taking away the Cores, par'd, and put into a Copper-pan, with Sugar and a little Water; causing them thoroughly to imbibe it When the Syrup is sufficiently consum'd, they may be dress'd, and serv'd up hot, in the same manner, as the former

Or else, when your Quinces are roasted, pare them, and cut that part which is most done, into Slices. Then putting them into a Dish, or Plate, with Powder-sugar, and a little sweet Water, let them be cover'd, and laid upon the hot Embers, by which means they'll be well soak'd, by degrees, and a Syrup will be made of an exquisite Taste

Compotes *of Chesnuts.*

Having roasted and peel d your Chesnuts, let them be beaten flat, and put into a Dish, pouring upon them some Syrup of Fruits, or a Decoction of Apples, boil'd with Sugar, till it become Smooth Then cover the Chesnuts, and lay them a soaking, over a gentle Fire; adding other Syrup, from time to time; as the former is consum'd. They ought to be serv'd up hot, to Table; and to that end, the *China*-ware must be set in order upon a Dish, so as the Fruit may be turn'd upon them Then moisten all, with Syrup, if it be requisite, and squeez upon them the Juice of a Lemmon, or Orange

Compotes *of Lemmons, or Oranges.*

Let your Oranges, or Lemmons be Turn'd, or else Zested, and scalded in Water, over the Fire Then, having set them by, to cool, cut them into Slices, or Sticks, or into round Slices, cross-wise, and take out the Kernels, throwing the Fruits, as they are done, into fair Water Afterwards, having made a Decoction of Apples, with Sugar, let it be reduc'd almost to a Jelly, and let the Oranges, or Lemmons be slipt into it · Otherwise, let them be put into Sugar, newly pass'd thro' the Straining-bag, and have eight, or ten Boilings Then they may be set by, for some time, and finish'd at pleasure, by giving them
twen-

twenty other Boilings, in order to dress the *Compote*, and serve it up to Table.

C H A P. XXII.

Of the Conserves of Flowers and Fruits.

THis Article is as remarkable as the preceding, and of no less importance, in the Art of Preserving; more especially, for the preparing and dressing of a Desert, or Banquet of Sweet meats.

Conserves of Orange-flowers.

Take about three Pounds of Sugar, and boil it, till it becomes Feathered: Then, having pick'd a Handful of Orange-flowers, let them be chopt, and thrown into the Sugar, when the Boiling ceases. But care must be taken to temper and mingle them well with the Sugar, to the end, that they may be impregnated with it, on all sides. Afterwards, you are to work the Sugar, quite round about the Pan, till a small Ice be made on the top, and then speedily pour off your Conserve, into Paper-moulds, or others · When it is cold, that is to say, about two Hours after, it must be taken out of the said Moulds, and kept for Use To serve it up to Table, it may be cut after what manner you please, either into Lozenges, or otherwise, to which purpose, it is only requisite to mark it with the point of a Knife, and it will easily break. If you have a mind to dress it in an oval, or round Form, it may be done with a Spoon, when the Conserve is newly made, and so of the rest.

Conserve of Cherries

Let the Cherries be ston'd, scalded over the Fire, and well dried: Then boil the Sugar till it be Blown, and throw in the thick Substance of the Cherries; tempering it well with the Sugar, to the end that all may be thoroughly intermixed: Afterwards work the Sugar round about the Pan, till it makes a small Ice on the top, and then pour your Conserve into Moulds. This
Me-

Method is to be obſerv'd, when Cherries firſt appear, but when they are in their full Seaſon, you muſt cauſe them to caſt their Juice, and afterwards lay them upon a Sieve As ſoon as they are drain'd, they muſt be pounded in a Mortar, and ſet over the Fire again, to be well dried Some time after, then thick Subſtance muſt be put into Blown Sugar, as before, and order'd, after the ſame manner.

Conſerve of Currans.

Having pick'd your Currans, and put them into a Copper-pan, over the Fire, to cauſe them to caſt their Juice, let them be well drain'd on a Sieve. Then ſtrain them, and let that which runs thro' the Sieve be ſet again over the Fire, to be dried. In the mean while, let the Sugar boil, till it has attain'd to its Crack'd Quality, and throw in as much of the thick Subſtance of your Fruit, as will be ſufficient to give the Conſerve a good Colour and Taſte ; tempering all well with the Sugar After-wards, let the Sugar be work'd and made white, round about the Pan, as upon other Occaſions, and when you perceive a thin Ice, on the top, take off the Pan and dreſs your Conſerve in the Moulds.

Conſerve of Raſberies.

This ſort of Conſerve is uſually made as the former, only it muſt be mix'd with a few Rasberries to give it a Smell and Tincture, as if it were made altogether of that Fruit: To that purpoſe, a Handful of Rasberries may be added, with their Grains, but theſe Grains are ſomewhat troubleſome to the Teeth, and may ſpoil your Conſerve, when you are about to cut it.

Conſerve of Smallage.

Let the greeneſt Leaves of Smallage, or Celery be ſcalded over the Fire, and give them three or four Boilings Then let them be well drain'd, pounded in a Morter, and ſtrain'd thro' the Sieve; whilſt ſome Sugar is boil'd, till it be a little Feathered As ſoon as the Boiling ceaſes, throw in what was ſtrain'd, and temper it well with the Sugar, which muſt be work'd as before, and when an Ice appears on the top, the Conſerve may be pour'd into the Moulds

Winte

White Conserve.

For want of Orange-flowers, some Marmelade made of them may be us'd, if you have any at Hand; Otherwise, take a little Marmelade of Lemmons, with Orange-flower-water, or the Juice of a Lemmon, if you are minded to diversifie the Conserves. In the mean time, the Sugar being boil'd, till it become Feathered, temper your Marmelade with it, and for the rest, observe the Instructions given for the preceding Conserves.

Conserve of Violets.

Conserve of Violets is made in the same manner, as that of Orange-flowers; only the Violet-flowers must be pounded in a Mortar, after they have been pick'd, and you are to put into the Sugar, what is requisite to give your Conserve, the Colour and Taste of Violets. It may also be made, with Marmelade of Violets, if any of the gross Substance taken from your Syrup of Violets, be left; incorporating it with Pearled Sugar; For by that means, it will keep, as long as you shall think fit, and Pastes may likewise be made of the same Substance, mingling it with Marmelade of Lemmons, which easily imbibes its Tincture.

Other sorts of Conserves.

Many other Conserves may be made, in taking measures from the former; particularly of Barberries and Pomegranates, by observing the Directions before laid down for those of Currans; of Roses and Jessemin, imitating the Conserves of Violets, or Orange-flowers, and so of others, which may be prepar'd, according to Discretion.

C H A P. XXIII.

Of Marmelades.

AN Account might be given of what relates to this Article, in treating of every kind of Fruit in particular, but forasmuch as several sorts of Marmelade may be made at once it was judg'd more expedient, to comprise all in one Chapter, so as recourse may be more conveniently had thereto. These Marmelades are of great Use in an Office, for the making of Pan-pies, or Tarts, or else, by the Mixture and Distribution of their Colours, the Coats of Arms of several Families may be represented, as also, Flower-de-luces, Crosses and many other Devices. When you would have more than one sort of them made in one Day, and with the same Stock of Sugar, all these Fruits must be first pick'd, scalded in Water, or boil'd over the Fire, according to their Qualities, then strain'd thro' Sieves, and dried in different Copper-pans, or Silver-dishes: In the mean while, Sugar is to be boil'd, proportionably to the Quantity of Pastes, which are to be put in, when it has attain'd to the degrees of Boiling hereafter express'd. To that purpose, it is expedient to begin with those Pastes, or Marmelades that require a less strong Sugar, and whilst they are soaking and simpering over another Furnace, the Sugar may be brought to that degree of Boiling, which is necessary for the others, which afterwards are to be order'd in the same manner.

Marmelade of green Apricocks.

Let the Apricocks be put into a Lie, such as is describ'd Pag. 16 and cool'd in fresh Water, to take off the Skin. Then they must be well boil'd, till they become very soft, and being drained, pass'd thro' a Sieve, into a Pan. Afterwards, this Paste must be dried over the Fire, carefully stirring and turning it, on all sides, with the *Spatula*, so as no Moisture may be left, and till it begins to stick to the Pan. In the mean while, let some Sugar be boil'd, till it become Crack'd, which is to be temper'd with the Marmelade, after having weigh'd out as much as is needful, that is to say, a Pound of one, for every Pound of the other: When this is done, it remains only, to cause all to simper together, for a while, and to put your Marmelade into Pots, or Glasses, or else to procede to the drying of it.

Marmelade of Cherries.

The Cherries must be first ston'd, and set over the Fire in a Copper-pan to cause them to cast their Juice. Afterwards they are to be drain'd, bruis'd and pass'd thro' a Sieve, and the Marmelade muft be put again into the Pan, to be dried, over the Fire, as before   Then let fome Sugar be boil'd, till it be great ly Feathered ; allowing one Pound of it, for every Pound of Fruit, or Pafte · Let all be well intermix'd together, in order to fimper for fome time, and at laft let the Marmelade be put into Pots, or Glaffes ftrew'd with Sugar   They ought not to be left long upon the Fire, left they fhould become too black, and for that reafon, they muft be fet over one that is quick, in order to be thoroughly dried

Marmelade of Currans

Having provided Currans, and ftripp'd them off from the Bunches, foak them in boiling Water, till they break   Then removing them from the Fire, let them be drain d upon a Sieve, and as foon as they are cold, pafs'd thro' the fame Sieve, by reafon of the Grains , fome time after, they muft be dried over the Fire, according to the ufual Method , whilft the Sugar is brought to its Crack d Quality, allowing a Pound of it for every Pound of Fruit. Laftly, let it all be well temper'd together, and having caus'd them to fimper a little, let them be ftrew d with Sugar, in order to be conveniently difpos d of in Pots or Glaffes, as before Marmelade of Bell-grapes is made after the fame manner

Marmelade of Rafberries

The Body of this Marmelade is ufually made of very ripe Currans, to which is added a Handful of Rasberries, to make it appear as if it confifted altogether of the latter   For the reft, it is only requifite to obferve, what has been even now deli ver'd, with refpect to the preceding Marmelade

Marmelade of ripe Apricocks.

Take five Pounds of very ripe Apricocks, boil them in two Pounds of Pearled Sugar, till they have thrown out all their Scum, and then remove them from the Fire. When they are cold, fet them again over the Fire, to be broken and dried, till they do not run any longer. In the mean time, three Pounds and half of Sugar, being made Crack'd, let it be incorporated with the Pafte; let all fimper together for a while, and let the Marmelade, ftrew'd with fine Sugar, be difpos'd of in Pots, or Glaffes, as the others.   *Mar*

Marmelade of Plums.

If they are fuch Plums, as flip oft from their Stones, let thofe Stones be taken awa, Otherwife, let them be fcalded in Water, till they become very foft, let them alfo be drain'd and well fqueez'd thro' the Sieve Then dry your Marmelade over the Fire, and let it be incorporated, with the fame Weight of Crack'd Sugar Laftly, having caus'd it to fimper, for fome time, let it be put into Pots, or Glaffes, and ftrew'd with Sugar

Mirabolan Plums, as well red, as black, are very proper for this fort of Sweet-meats

Marmelade of Pears.

Let your Pears be fcalded in Water over the Fire, and when they are become very tendei, let them be taken out and drain'd: Then ftrain all thro' a Sieve, and let your Sugar boil, till it be very much Feathered, allowing three quarters of a Pound of it for every Pound of Fruit. Laftly, having temper'd it with the Pafte, which ought to be well dried, and having caus'd them to fimper for a while, pour the Marmelade into Pots or Glaffes ftrew'd with Sugar

Marmelade of Apples

Marmelade of Apples is made altogether according to the Method even now explain'd, as well for the manner of ordering the Fruit, as with refpect to the Quantity, and the Degree of boiling the Sugar, which is neceffary, for that purpofe.

Marmelade of Sevil-Oranges.

Having cut your Oranges into Quarters, without Turning or Zefting them, take away the Juice and the tops, where there is a tough Skin, which cannot eafily be foften'd: In the mean time, let fome Water be fet over the Fire, and when it is ready to boil, throw in your Orange-peels which muft boil, till they become very foft, and yield to the touch of your Finger: Then they are to be cool'd in frefh Water, drain'd, and ftrongly fqueez'd thro' a Linnen-cloath: This Pulp muft alfo be pound-

ed

ed in a Mortar, and paſs'd thro the Sieve; whilſt ſome Sugar is boil'd till it be Feathered, which is to be mingled with the Marmelade in the Copper-pan, into which it was put, to be heated again a little, to the End that the moiſtneſs may evaporate. The uſual quantity of Sugar is requiſite, as well that it may ſlip off, from the bottom of the Pan, as that, what is taken up with the *Spatula* may be entirely ſeparated from the reſt, without running. At laſt, ſet your Marmelade upon the Fire again, to ſimper, and let it be pour'd hot into Pots or other Veſſels.

Marmelade of Lemmons.

The Lemmons being Zeſted, cut into quarters, and clear'd from their Juice, muſt be thrown into Water, as they are done, to hinder them from turning black: Then having caus'd other Water to boil over the Fire, let them be put into it, and when they have had four or five Boilings, ſqueez in the Juice of a Lemmon, as alſo that of another, ſome time after. As ſoon as your Lemmon-pulp is become very ſoft, it muſt be cool'd, drain'd and ſqueez'd in a Linnen-cloath, before it is pounded in the Mortar, and paſs'd thro the Sieve. Laſtly, your Marmelade muſt be ſet over the Fire again, a little while, as the former, and the Sugar is to be order'd, after the ſame manner

Marmelade of Orange-flowers.

Take only the Leaves of your Orange-flowers, without the Yellow; or Stalks, and as they are pick'd, throw them into fair Water, into which the Juice of a Lemmon has been ſqueez'd Then ſcald them over the Fire, as it has been ſhewn, in the preceding Articles, till they become very ſoft, adding likewiſe, the Juice of another Lemmon Afterwards, being well preſs'd in a Linnen-cloath, or elſe with your Hands, they muſt be pounded in a Mortar, and ſtrain'd thro' a Sieve, if it be requiſite. As for the Sugar, it muſt be made greatly Feathered, and incorporated with the Marmelade, till it ſlips off from the bottom and ſides of the Pan. Laſtly, having caus'd all to ſimper, a little, the Marmelade may be pour'd into Pots, and kept for uſe; if you are not deſirous, to have it immediately dried.

This is the beſt Way of preparing the Marmelade of pure Orange-flowers; otherwiſe, to ſave ſome Charges, it may be

min

mingled, as Occafion requires, with a little Marmelade of Lemmons, which is equally white and of the fame Tafte · Infomuch, that fome Confectioners caufe it to pafs for the true Marmelade of Orange-flowers ; contenting themfeves only to throw in a Handful of Flowers, when it is made, to give it a little Smell, or Tincture of them

Obfervations upon the feveral forts of Marmelade.

The manner of drying all thefe different forts of Marmelades fhall be explain'd in the following Article of Paftes Thofe of green Apricocks, and green Almonds are apt to grow greafy, and will not keep very long , fo that it is requifite either to dry them immediately, or in lefs fpace of time, than three Months; otherwife they cannot be well dried The Marmelades of O-range flowers and Lemmons, generally candy within a little while, altho' they are duely prepar d, but that is no great dammage. Whenever you would have them dried, let all the Candy be put with a little Water into a Copper-pan, over the Fire, and let it be brought again, to the neceffary Degree of Boiling, with other Sugar, as much as is needful for the drying of your Pafte , fo as all may be mingled with the faid Pafte, according to the Method, hereafter fpecified

C H A P. XXIV.
Of the Paftes of Fruits.

IT is only requifite to have recourfe to the particular Marmelades, of every fort of Fruit, defcribed in the fore-going Chapter, to know how to make as many Paftes, in regard that it is almoft the fame thing, and the whole Work is brought to Perfection by drying thofe Marmelades. To that purpofe, when the Bufinefs requires difpatch, the Sugar muft boil, till it be crack'd, or at leaft, greatly Feathered; to be incorporated with the dried Fruit Afterwards, the Marmelade being made according to Art, may be taken up with a Spoon, and drefs'd upon Slates, or in Moulds, in order to be dried in the Stove, with a good Fire. In the Evening, or the next Day, they

A a 3   muft

muſt be turn d on the other ſide, and laid again upon the ſame Slates, or upon Sieves As ſoon as theſe Paſtes are become very firm and compact, they are to be lock d up in Boxes, and may be us'd, as Occaſion requires

At other times, when you would have any Paſte dryed, let as much Marmelade, as you ſhall think fit, be put into a Copper-pan, and having caus d ſome Sugar to be brought to its Feathered Quality, pour it in; tempering it well till it ſlips off from the bottom of the Pan, after the ſame manner, as in the making of Marmelade Then let all ſimper together, for a while, and let the Paſte be immediately dreſs'd upon Slates, or in Tin-moulds, made in form of a Heart, Square, Flower-de-luce, &c. which are uſually ſet into the Stove, to be dried as before Theſe are the general Directions that may be given, for the ordering of ſuch Fruit-paſtes as are made of Marmelades, allowing two Pounds of Sugar, for every Pound of Fruit But for other Paſtes, that are made on purpoſe, an equal quantity of each will be ſufficient, and the Sugar muſt be boil'd till it has attain'd to its Crack'd Quality.

Paſtes of green Apricocks.

Let your green Apricocks be prepar'd, and made into a Paſte according to the Method laid down for the Marmelade of the ſame Pag. 77. Then your Sugar being boil'd till it become Crack'd, muſt be incorporated with the Paſte, allowing a Pound of one, for the like quantity of the other Afterwards, let all ſimper together, and at the ſame time dreſs your Paſte, as before, in regard that it will not keep long, by reaſon of it aptneſs to grow greaſy

The Paſtes of green Almonds, if any are made, may be prepared after the ſame manner.

Cherry-paſtes.

The Cherry-cakes deſcribed under the Article of that Fruit Pag. 30 may be now us'd to very good purpoſe, but when they are out of Seaſon, ſome Marmelade of Cherries is to be taken, which, being cool'd and boil'd again in new Sugar, that is Feathered, as it has been already hinted, may be order'd with a Spoon, and ſet into the Stove to be dried. When this Paſte is turn'd on the other ſide, it muſt be lightly ſtrew'd with Sugar

put,

put into a Handkerchief, and it will appear finer, being dress'd the first side uppermost, to be serv'd up to Table.

Pastes of Currans.

Let your Currans be set over the Fire, to cause them to cast their Juice, and laid upon a Sieve, when cool'd Let them also be strain'd thro the same Sieve, and dried over the Fire, whilst an equal quantity of Sugar, that is to say, a Pound for every Pound of Fruit, is brought to its Crack'd Quality, which is to be incorporated with it, in the same manner, as for making Marmelade of Currans, explain'd Pag 78 Thus the Paste may be dress d, after having caus'd it to simper for a while, if you have a mind to dry it at the same time Otherwise, let this Marmelade be boil'd over again in other Crack'd or Feathered Sugar; observing, for the rest, what has been already deliver'd, upon the like Occasion, concerning Fruit-pastes, in general.

Rasberry-paste

The Body of this sort of Paste is usually made in the same manner, as for the Marmelade, that is to say, with Currans, and a few Handfuls of Rasberries, and the whole Work is finish d, as the former · Both these sorts are also to be strew'd with Sugar, as the Cherry-paste, as they are turning to be dried on the other side, and ought to be serv'd up to Table with the first side uppermost

Pastes of ripe Apricocks.

Apricock-paste is usually made, as the Marmelade of the same, specified Pag 78. or else the Apricocks may only be scalded at first, as the rest of the Fruits, without Sugar. If your Apricocks are not thoroughly ripe, they must be bruis'd, as much as is possible, and even pounded in a Mortar. Afterwards, the Sugar must be boil'd, till it become Crack'd, that is to say, a Pound for every Pound of Fruit, and temper'd with the Paste that has been well dried over the Fire. Then, having caus'd it to simper, dress it as the others, in order to be dried in the Stove. This Paste is not so grateful to the Palate, when kept for a considerable time; because it is apt to grow greasy, as that of green Apricocks.

A 2 4 *Plum-*

Plum-paste.

This Paste may be made of dried Marmelade of Plums, putting to it, some new Feathered Sugar, as it has been intima ted, in the beginning. Or else having prepar'd your Fruit, that is to say, strain'd and dried it, cause it to be incorporated with Crack'd Sugar. Afterwards, let all simper together, and let the Pastes be dress'd after the usual manner.

Pastes of Apples and Pears.

Scald these Fruits in Water, as the former, and when they are become soft, let them be drain'd, pass'd thro' a Sieve, and dried over the Fire, stirring them with a *Spatula*, both on the bottom and round about, lest they should burn. When the Paste slips off from the bottom and sides of the Pan, remove it from the Fire, and cause some Sugar to be greatly Feathered, or Crack'd, which must be well temper'd with it, allowing a Pound of Fruit, for the like quantity of Sugar. Afterwards, set your Paste again over the Fire, to simper, and dress it, as the others, with a Spoon, either upon Slates, or in Moulds, putting them into the Stove, at the same time, to be dried.

Pastes of roasted Apples and Pears

These sorts of Pastes may be made at all times, and more especially during the Winter-season. To that purpose, your Apples, or Pears being well roasted, take that Part of them which is reddish and most done, and strain it thro' a Sieve Then let as many Pounds of Sugar, as of Fruit, be brought to the crack'd degree of Boiling, and let the Work be finish'd, after the same manner, as for all other sorts of Pastes.

Peach-paste.

When the Peaches are somewhat ripe, they may be order'd, according to either of those Ways, express'd for ripe Apricocks, Pag 83. And as for the Paste of green Peaches, it is only requisite to follow the Directions given, for green Apricocks, Pag. 82.

Quin&c

Quince-paste.

Take the yelloweft and foundeft Quinces that can be procur'd, pare them, and cut out the Cores, if you fhall think fit,
or elfe let all be left; contenting your felf, only to cut the
Quinces into quarters Then, having caus'd fome Water to
boil over the Fire, throw in your Fruit, and let them be boil'd,
till they become very foft, in order to be drain'd upon a Hurdle
or Grate, and pafs'd thro' the Hair-fieve. Afterwards, the Pafte
muft be fet over the Fire again, to be dried, and temper'd with
Crack'd Sugar, to the quantity of fomewhat more than a
Pound, for every Pound of Fruit Laftly, you muft caufe your
Pafte, to fimper, for a while, and to be drefs'd, as the others.

Orange-paste.

This Pafte is ufually made as Orange-Marmelade, according
to the Method explain'd under that Article, Pag 79, and 80. or elfe
of the Marmelade it felf, as it has been already declar'd, in treating of the Fruit-paftes, in general, that is to fay, it muft be
incorporated with new Sugar, brought to its Feathered Quality, till it flips off from the bottom of the Pan. Then, having
caus'd it to fimper, drefs it after the ufual manner, to be dried
in the Stove Thus Orange-paftes may be prepar'd at all times,
provided there be a conftant Supply of the Marmelade; which
will keep very well for that purpofe, and for the making of
Conferves.

Lemmon-paste.

For this Article, recourfe may alfo be had to the Lemmon-
Marmelade, defcribed Pag 80. if you have none ready made
in the Repofitory: But if there be any left, you need only renew it, with Feathered Sugar, as in the preceding Article, and
having caus'd your Marmelade, or Pafte to fimper, a little while,
drefs it with a Spoon, upon the Slates, or in Moulds, fo as it
may conveniently be dried in the Stove.

Paftes

Pastes of Orange-flowers.

Take pure Marmelade of Orange flowers, or the other sort specified, Pag. 80, and 81 accordingly as Occasion may serve, and for the rest, follow the same Method that is us'd in ordering the former sorts of Paste. For want of Marmelade, take Orange flowers, which are to be prepar'd, as for the same Marmelade, and mingle them with any other Marmelade, that you shall judge to be most proper for that purpose, as in the following Article.

Violet-paste.

After having made Syrup of Violets, take the grofs Substance that is left, and mingle it with the same quantity of Pearled Sugar. So that whenever you are minded to dry the Paste, it will only be requisite to incorporate it, with as much Marmelade of Lemmons, or of Apples, as is needful, adding some Feathered Sugar, and causing all to be well intermix'd: Then let your Paste simper for some while, and dress it after the usual manner, to be dried in the Stove.

If you have no thick Substance of Violets, the Flowers may be us'd in their Season; which are to be pick'd and pounded in a Stone-mortar, in order to be mingled with either of the above-mention'd Marmelades, and as much Feathered Sugar, as is requisite; till the Paste slips off from the bottom and sides of the Pan: Then having caus'd all to simper, let it be dress'd and dried in the Stove as before. When these Violet-pastes are turn'd to be dried on the other side, they must be lightly strew'd with Sugar put into a Handkerchief, and by that Means a greater Lustre will be added to the Colour, on the first side, being that which is uppermost, when they are serv'd up to Table; as it has been already intimated, in treating of the Pastes, of Cherries, Rasberries and Currans.

Bell-grape-paste.

Having pick'd your Grapes off from the Bunches, throw them into hot Water, and let them boil till they break: Then let them be drain'd upon a Sieve or Cullander, and squeez'd hard, all at once, to separate the Grains and Skin. In the mean while, some

some green Apples are to be scalded, and the Pastes of both put into a Copper-pan, to be brought again to their Colour, over the Fire, and dried all together, continually stirring and turning them, till they begin to slip off from the sides of the Pan : Then let them be incorporated with an equal quantity of Feathered Sugar, and dress'd upon Slates with a Spoon, to be dried in the Stove, with a good Charcoal-fire As these Pastes are turn'd on the other side, strew them with Sugar as the former, and take care, that they be well harden'd.

Another Way of making Pastes of Bell-grapes.

Take good Bell-grapes, and having caus'd them to cast their Juice in a Copper-pan over the Fire, after the same manner, as Currans ; let them be drain'd upon a Sieve, and when cold, pass'd through the straining Sieve Then they are to be dried over the Fire, and continually stirr'd on all Sides, with the *Spatula*, whilst your Sugar is boil'd till it become Crack'd ; allowing a Pound, for every Pound of Fruit, in order to be incorporated with the Paste ; which ought to be dress'd upon Slates, as the others, and dried in the Stove. On the next Morning, or Evening, turn your Pastes, so as they may be dried in Sieves, on the other side, and shut them up in Boxes, with Paper, between every Row.

Pastes of Muscadine-grapes.

Pastes of Muscadine-grapes, are usually made in the same manner as these last, or else as those of Currans ; so that, it were altogether needless to insist on them, any longer in this Place.

C H A P. XXV.

Of the Jellies of Fruits.

ALthough it is a customary Practice, only to make Jellies of certain peculiar Fruits ; nevertheless they may be also prepar'd, with the most part of the others. To that purpose, measures may be taken, from those that have been before occasionally de-

defcrib'd, in treating of the Fruits, of which they are generally made, *viz* the Jellies of green Goosberries, white and red Currans, Bell grapes, &c But for the more clear underftanding of the whole Matter, it will be expedient, here to give a particular Account of thefe Jellies, beginning with that of Cherries :

Jelly of Cherries.

Take the beft fort of Cherries, that are very ripe, and extract their Juice by preffing them through a white Linnen cloth, or fomething elfe of the like nature ; whilft the fame Weight of Sugar, or fomewhat lefs, is boil'd till it be crack'd : Then pour in your Cherry-juice, after it has been ftrain'd to render more clear, and let all continue boiling , fo as the Scum may be carefully taken off, till the Syrup is brought again to a degree between Smooth and Pearled : At that very Inftant, the Jelly will be made, which may alfo be perceiv'd, when fome of it taken up in a Spoon, or Ladle, falls in thick Drops , or elfe, by putting fome of the Drops upon a Plate, from whence they'll rife up, when cold Afterwards, the Jelly may be pour'd into Pots or Glaffes, taking off the thin Scum that rifes on the top ; but thefe Veffels ought to be left three Days, without covering ; which muft be done at laft, with round pieces of Paper

The Juice extracted from Cherries, over the Fire, in order to make Paftes and Marmelades, may likewife ferve for this fort of Jelly ; if you have no mind to make ufe of it for *Ratafiaz* And in regard, that this Juice would be only of a fomewhat pale red Colour, it is expedient, to mingle it with a little of that of Currans, or elfe, the Colour may be heighten'd with fome prepar'd Cochineal ; although it may alfo be of Ufe, in its natural Condition, when red Colours, more, or lefs deep, are to be reprefented in a Pan-pie, or any other Device, of the like nature

Jellies of Goofeberries and Currans.

The particular Way of making a Jelly of green Gooleberries has been already explain'd, Pag 33. as alfo feveral Methods of preparing thofe of Currans, Pag. 34, 35.

Rasberry-jelly

Some mention has likewise been made of the manner of ordering this kind of Jelly, Pag 35 under the Article of *Curran-jelly, with a Tincture of Rasberries* To that purpose, it is requisite to provide four Pounds of Rasberrirs, with two of Currans, and five of Sugar, which being brought to its Crack'd Quality, the Fruits must be thrown in, and boil'd together, till the Scum ceases to rise, and the Syrup has attain'd to a degree of Boiling, between Smooth and Pearled. Then let all be pour'd into a Sieve set over a Copper-pan, and a very fine Jelly, will pass through, even without squeezing the Fruit, if you shall think fit At last, having given it another Boiling, take off the Scum, and dispose of it in Pots, or other Vessels, after the usual manner.

Jelly of Apples and other forts of Fruit.

Cut your Apples into pieces, and set them over the Fire, in a Copper-pan, with Water, to make a strong Decoction; causing them to boil, till they turn, as it were to Marmelade. Then having strain'd the Liquor through a Linnen cloth, or a fine Sieve, for every Quart of this Liquor, take three quarters of a Pound of crack'd Sugar, in which all must be lightly boil'd to a degree between Smooth and Pearled; carefully taking off the Scum. If it be requir'd to give the Jelly a red Colour, it must be cover'd, as it is boiling, at the same time, adding some red Wine, or prepared Cochineal But if you would have the Jelly left white, as that of Pippins, nothing is to be put therein, neither ought it to be cover'd at all

A Jelly may also be made of Pears, and other forts of Fruit, accordingly as it shall be judg'd expedient, by using the same Method.

Jelly of Bell-grapes.

Several Ways of preparing this Jelly, have been already explain'd at large, Pag. 48.

Quince-

Quince-jelly.

Quince-jelly is ufually order'd after the fame manner, as in the making of Marmelade of Quinces ; for which, recourfe may be had to the 49, and following Pages : or elfe, obferve what has been even now deliver'd, with refpect to the Jelly or Apples ; it being only requifite, to boil the Quinces a little longer, to get a good Decoction of them.

Other forts of Jellies.

Another kind of Jelly, or rather thick Confection, is fome times made in the Country, only with the Juice of Fruits, without Sugar ; Boiling and Scumming it till it comes to the Confiftence of a Jelly : But in regard that this Way is not extraordinary, nor conformable to the Rules of Art, it does not deferve any farther Confideration.

C H A P. XXVI.

Of Biskets.

BIskets are generally made in all Seafons, and conftitute part of the Entertainment throughout the whole Year. The beft fort of them, are thefe that follow, *viz.*

Almond-biskets.

Having provided a Pound of fweet Almonds, with a quarter of a Pound of bitter ones, let them be blanch'd and pounded in a Mortar ; tempering all from time to time, with the White of an Egg, to hinder them from turning to Oil : When they are well pounded, fo that no Clods, or Lumps are left ; take out the Pafte, and put it into one Scale of a Ballance, with the fame Weight of Powder-fugar into the other, as alfo fome Whites of Eggs : Then knead and mingle all well together in a Copper-pan, with the *Spatula*, or with your Hand, if it be neceffary, as when a greater quantity of it is to be made, proportionably augmenting
the

the Ingredients Afterwards, take up some of your Paste in a a Spoon, with which you are to scrape the Sides of the Pan, drawing it towards your Body, with the Edge downwards, so as only to get an entire Spoonful , which will be sufficient to make three or four of these Biskets of the breadth of a Shilling, or Copper Half-penny To that end, take part of this Paste, with the tip of your Finger, and having turn'd it upon the edges of the Spoon, to make it of a round Figure ; as it is spread along your Finger, let it fall upon a sheet of Paper, provided for that purpose, ordering the rest of the Paste, after the same manner.

To manage the Business with greater Neatness, some of this Paste may be taken up, with the blade of a Table knife, and without touching it with the Fingers, the Biskets may be dress'd with another Knife ; taking as much Paste, as is requisite for every one, from the first, on which it was spread When the sheet of Paper is fill'd with them, at the distance of about a Finger's breadth, one from another, set them into a Campain-oven, with Fire only at the top, at first, and as soon as the Biskets begin to rise, and are sufficiently brought to a Colour, let some Fire be likewise put underneath, to make an end of Baking them Afterwards, another sheet of Paper, that has been dress'd in the mean time, may be laid in the Oven, and so on, till the whole Mass of Paste is us'd These Biskets may serve for the garnishing of Dishes, to dress Pyramids upon *China*-dishes, and for other Uses.

Another Way of making Almond-biskets.

Take about a quarter of a Pound of bitter Almonds with the like quantity of sweet ones, and having scalded them in boiling Water, let them be blanch'd, without throwing them into fresh Water · Then let them be pounded in a Mortar, without one drop of any Liquor ; so that 'tis no great matter, whether they turn to Oil or not : In the mean while, having beaten up four or five Whites of Eggs at most with a Spoon, in an earthen Pan, put in it your Almond-paste, and temper it well with a Spoon. Afterwards, adding a Pound and two Ounces of Powder-sugar, and mingling all well together with the *Spatula*, let the Paste be dress'd upon white Paper, with two Knives; spreading it upon one, and shaping the Biskets with the other, of the thickness of the tip of your Finger. At last, they are to be set into the O-
ven,

ven, with a gentle Fire, in the beginning, but when they rife, it muft be made fomewhat quicker. As foon as they are bak'd, and have acquir'd a good Colour, they may be taken out of the Oven, but muft not be cut off from the Paper till they are cold, in order to be kept dry in the Stove.

Chocolate-biskets.

Scrape fome Chocolate upon the white of an Egg, but not too much, becaufe it is only requifite to give it the Tafte and Colour of the Chocolate   Then take Powder-fugar, and mingle it well with the reft of the Ingredients, till they become a pli able Pafte: Afterwards drefs your Biskets, upon fheets of Paper, in any Figure, that you fhall think fit, and fet them into the Oven, to be bak'd with a gentle Fire, as well on the top, as underneath.

Orange and Lemmon-biskets.

Thefe forts of Biskets are made after the fame manner, only inftead of Chocolate, fome grated Orange or Lemmon-peel is to be us d, with a little Marmelade, if there is any at hand   O ther Biskets of the like Nature may alfo be prepar'd with O- range-flowers, and thofe of Jeffamine, pounding them well, before they are intermix'd with the other Ingredients.

Another Way of making Orange-biskets.

Let fome old Orange-pafte, with fome dried Pulp of Oran- ges and Lemmons, be well pounded in a Mortar, and let the Whites of four Eggs be whipt, as it were, for the making of *Savoy*-biskets: Then flip in the four Yolks, which are alfo to be well whipt together, and add three good Handfuls of Powder-fugar, ftirring the whole Mafs with a Spoon · Afterwards throwing in a Handful of Flower, ftir all again, with the Marmelade, al- ready pounded in a Mortar, to the quantity of about a Pound, and let all be well beaten with the Spoon   In the mean time, certain Moulds being made of white Paper, an Inch thick, the Confection is to be laid on them, and fet into the Oven, with- out Icing ; but a quick Fire ought to be made, both on the top, and underneath. As foon as the Biskets are bak'd, they muft be turn'd upfide down, and the Paper is to be gently taken a-

way

way from the bottom, fo as they may be conveniently cut into fquare Pieces, as ftuff'd March pane, and fet by to cool Some time after, they may be ic'd on one fide, with Orange-flower-water, and on the other, if it be thought fit, with another Colour, and at laft the Ice muft be bak'd, with the Lid of the Campain-oven.

Savoy, *or French Biskets.*

Take three or four New-laid Eggs, or more, according to the quantity of Biskets that you would have made, and having provided a pair of Scales, put your Eggs into one of them, as alfo, fome bak'd Flower into the other ; fo as there may be an equal Weight of both   Thus for Example, If four Eggs were put in, one is to be taken out, and the three others left   In the mean while, fome Powder-fugar is to be provided of the fame Weight as the Eggs, the Whites of which are to be taken, to make the ftrongeft Snow that poffibly can be, by whipping them well with a Whisk· To this is to be added, at firft, fome candy d Lemmon peel, grated, or beaten as it were to Powder, and then the Flower that was weigh'd before.   All being thus mingled together, let the Sugar be put in, and after having beaten the whole Mafs again a little while, add the Yolks of the Eggs , fo as the Pafte may be well tempei d.   The Biskets may be made upon Paper, with a Spoon, of a round, or oval Figure, and neatly ic'd with Powder-fugar, after having wafh'd them over with the Whites of Eggs   Afterwards, you are to blow off the Sugar that lies upon the Paper, and caufe the Biskets to be bak'd in an Oven, that is not over-heated; giving them an agreeable Colour, on the top   When they are done enough, they muft be cut off from the Paper, with a very thin Knife, and may ferve to fet off Fruit, or for the garnifhing of Pies, or Tarts

Some do not allow fo many Whites of Eggs, and of fix that have been weigh'd, only take two, to make the rocky Snow ; but this is an indifferent Matter   The Lemmon-peel may likewife be difpenfed with , as alfo, the baking of the Flower, and yet the Biskets will prove good: However, for fix Eggs, it is requifite to ufe Sugar, to the weight of four.

Bb

Ano-

Another Way of making French Biskets.

Let the Whites and Yolks of eight Eggs be set by separately, and let the former be well whipt, till they rise up to a Snow Then let the Yolks of nine Eggs be slipt in, and let all be whipt again ; adding a Pound of Powder-sugar, and beating them well with the *Spatula* : Let three quarters of a Pound of Flower be also weigh'd out, and put to the Mass, continuing to beat it with the *Spatula* ; a little grated Lemmon-peel may likewise be added, if you please, to heighten the Relish In the mean while, certain Tin-moulds being provided, are to be wash'd over, a little, on the inside, with fresh Butter melted, or else the Moulds may be made with Cards, which must not be butter'd : But the Paper on which the Biskets are laid, must be rubb'd with the same Paste, to the end that the Moulds may stick to it If you have a mind to make small Biskets of this sort, they may be dress'd with a Spoon, upon white Paper, of the bigness of a Half-crown Piece, and ic d with Powder-sugar, which is to be strew'd upon them, and blown off a little, lest too much of it, should be left on the top. Afterwards, they are to be set into a Baker's Oven, moderately heated, and to that end, a tryal may be made with a single Bisket · But care ought to be taken, that they do not languish in the Oven, and as soon as they are drawn, the Moulds must be taken away, or the sheet of Paper, if the Biskets are small, which may be done, by slipping a Knife underneath, for if they were cold, they could not be any longer cut off, without breaking the Ice.

Lisbon-*biskets*.

Take three or four Eggs, according to the quantity of Biskets design'd to be made, and beat the Whites a little with the Yolks; adding as much Powder-sugar, as can well be taken up between your Fingers, at four or five times, with Lemmon-peel, and four or five Spoonfuls of bak'd Flower. When this Confection is well temper'd together, let it be turn'd upon a sheet of Paper strew'd with Sugar, and after having likewise strew'd the Paste on the top, with the same Sugar, let it be bak'd in an Oven, moderately heated. As soon as the Biskets are taken out, they must be cut all at once, with the Paper underneath, according to the Size and Figure, that you would
have

have them to be of, and then the Paper may be gently cut off, with a Pen-knife, for fear of breaking any part of them, which is soon done, because they ought to be very dry

Light Ic'd-biskets.

Having provided three quarters of a Pound of bitter Almonds, with one quarter of a Pound of sweet Ones, let them be scalded, blanch'd and pounded in a Mortar, as much as is possible; adding two Whites of Eggs, at several times. Then let all be insensibly mingled, with four Pounds of Powder-sugar, and well beat together, till the Paste becomes very pliable. Afterwards, this Paste must be squeez'd through a Syringe, one Roll after another, and the Biskets are to be made of it, cutting that which passes through, and is received upon a sheet of Paper, according to any length that you shall think fit; either into large, or small Pieces These Papers of Biskets are to be laid upon a Board, and the Oven-lid with Fire on the top, to give them a Colour, on that side. As soon as you perceive them to be done enough, and that they are considerably puff'd up, take away the Fire, and having gently slip'd them off from the Paper, cause them to be ic'd on that side, which lay undermost. This Ice is usually made, with the White of an Egg and Sugar, well temper'd and beaten together, till it turns almost to a kind of Pap Then it may be spread upon the Biskets with a Knife, and dried with a gentle Fire, till it is thoroughly coagulated. These sorts of Biskets may also be cover'd with an Ice, made of sweet Water, or some other Water and Sugar beaten and temper'd together, as the former.

Common Biskets.

Break six or eight Eggs, and having slipt the Whites and Yolks into an earthen Pan, or Bason; beat them well for some time, with the *Spatula* Then adding a Pound of Powder-sugar, with as much Flower, let all be well mingled together, and dress your Paste in Paper-cases, or Tin-moulds, in any Form or Figure, that you shall judge most expedient After- wards, let the Biskets be Ic'd, strewing them with fine Sugar, put into an Handkerchief, and set into an Oven moderately heated, till they rise, and come to a good Colour When they are sufficiently bak'd, take them up, with the point of a Knife,

B b 2 and

and make an end of drying them in the Stove, or ſome other Place, convenient for that purpoſe,

Biskets for Lent.

This ſort of Bisket is made with Gum-dragant, ſteept in the ſame manner as ſhall be hereafter explain'd for Paſtils, Pag. 104 Having cauſ'd the Gum-water to be well ſtirr'd about, add ſome Powder-ſugar, continuing to whip all together, as it is ſtrewing in, till the Liquor becomes as thick as Pap If you are minded to mix Marmelade, with this Paſte, as in making the *Biſcotins*; by that means it will be render'd ſo much the richer, and have a greater Conſiſtence, whereas, otherwiſe it is only a Compound of Sugar and Wind.   They may alſo be made, as the light Biskets above ſpecified ;   only retrenching the Whites of Eggs, in the place of which the Gum is to be ſubſtituted, and a ſomewhat leſs quantity of Almonds is to be uſd in preparing the Paſte   Theſe Biskets may be dreſs'd how you pleaſe, and bak'd as the former

Crackling-biskets.

The ſame ſort of Paſte is to be uſ'd, as for the *Savoy*-biskets, being brought to a due Conſiſtence, with four Eggs, and augmented with three or four Handfuls of Powder-ſugar :   Then having cauſ'd all to be well temper'd with a Spoon, let them be dreſs'd, as the Biskets of bitter Almonds, and bak'd in the Campain-oven; with more Fire on the top, than underneath. When they are taken out, the ſheet of Paper muſt be turn'd up ſide down, and laid under a wet Napkin, to the end that the Biskets may be clear'd from it , for if the Paper be not wet, it cannot poſſibly be done, by any other means   Afterwards, the Biskets are likewiſe to be laid upſide down upon other white Paper, and ſet into the Stove ; but they muſt not be dreſs'd on the Diſhes, before they are ready to be ſerv'd up to Table , becauſe they are too apt to give, and contract Moiſtneſs.

Biſcotins.

Take three Whites of Eggs, four Spoonfuls of Powder-ſugar, and one of any kind of Marmelade particularly, of Oranges, Lemmons, Apricocks, &c.   The reſt of the Confection is to be be made of fine Flower, which you are to knead all together, till the Paſte becomes very pliable, and then make your *Biſcotins* of different Figures, *viz* ſome round, others long, others in form of Love-knots, Ciphers, and other pretty Devices : They ought to be bak'd with a gentle Fire, and taken out of the Oven, as ſoon as you perceive them to have acquir'd a ſomewhat brown ruſſet Colour To clear them from the Paper, wet the ſheet on the back-ſide with Water, and the Buſineſs will be eaſily effected, but it muſt be done immediately after they are drawn

Another ſort of Biſcotin.

Having caus'd half a Pound of Sugar to boil in a little Copper-pan, or Skillet, till it become Feathered, remove it from the Fire, and throw in three quarters of a Pound of Flower, except one Handful, which is to be reſerv'd, to work it upon the Table ⋅ Then ſtir all about with the *Spatula,* and when the Paſte is well temper'd, take it out of the Pan, in order to be laid upon a very clean Table, or Dreſſer-board, ſtrew'd before with a little Sugar : The Paſte muſt alſo be ſtrew'd, both on the top, and underneath, with prepared Musk and Powder-ſugar, and continually work d, whilſt it is hot ⋅ At the ſame time, it muſt be roll'd out, and cut into Pieces, to make certain little Balls, of the thickneſs of a Man's Thumb ; which muſt be ſpeedily done, in regard that when the Paſte is cold, it will no longer take effect. Theſe Balls are to be bak'd in an Oven, without Paper, but afterwards ſome muſt be put underneath, when they are ready to be ſet into the Stove.

C h a p. XXVII.

Of March-panes.

MAarch-panes conſiſt of a ſort of Paſte made of Almonds and Sugar, and are in Uſe, as well as Biskets, during the whole Courſe of the Year ⋅ Only they may be diverſified in the ſeveral Seaſons, with different Marmelades, according to the variety of Fruits ; as it will more plainly appear, from the following Inſtructions. Bb 3 *Com-*

Common *March-panes*

The Almonds are to be firft fcalded in hot Water, and tofs'd into other cold Water, as they are done · Then being wip'd, and drain'd, they muft be pounded in a Marble-Mortar, and moiften'd from time to time, with the White of an Egg, to hinder them from turning to Oil In the mean while, let half as much clarified Sugar, as Pafte, boil, till it become Feathered, and let the Almonds be thrown in by Handfuls, or elfe the Sugar may be pour'd upon them, in another Veffel : Afterwards, let all be well incorporated together, with the *Spatula*, carefully ftirring the Pafte to the bottom, and round about, left it fhould ftick to the Pan, even tho' it were remov'd from the Fire You may know when this Pafte is done enough, by paffing the Back of your Hand over it, till nothing fticks thereto; at which inftant, it muft be laid upon Powder-fugar, and fet by to cool. To work it, you are to roll out feveral Pieces, of a convenient Thicknefs, out of which your March-panes muft be cut, with certain Moulds; gently flipping them off, with the tip of your Finger, upon Sheets of Paper, in order to be bak'd in the Oven, fo as the Fire may heat them at firft, only on one fide · Afterwards, the other fide is to be Ic'd over, and bak'd in like manner : Thus the March-panes are ufually made of a round, long, or oval Figure, curled or jagged, in the Shape of a Heart, &c The Pafte may alfo be roll'd out, or fqueez'd thro' a Syringe ; fo that the March-panes, will have as many particular Names, altho' they differ only in Shape, and in the manner of Icing them ; as it may hereafter, be more clearly obferv'd.

Another fort of *Pafte* for *March-panes.*

After having blanch'd, cool'd and drain'd your Almonds, as before, let them be pounded in a Mortar, and moiften'd with the White of an Egg, and a little Orange-flower-water beaten together. As foon as they are thoroughly pounded, fo that there does not remain the leaft Clod, or Lump, an equal quantity of Sugar muft be brought to its feather'd Quality · Then throwing in your Almonds, temper all together, with the *Spatula*, and fet the Pafte over the Fire again, to be dried ; continually ftirring it, till it becomes pliable, and flips off from the bottom

tom of the Pan · Afterwards, it muſt be laid in a Baſon, with Powder-ſugar underneath, and made up into a thick Roll, to be ſet by, for a little while, as the former ; in order to be ſhap'd and dreſs'd, in the ſame manner.

This laſt ſort of Paſte is more crackling and more grateful to the Palate than the former, and in that reſpect, it may be plainly diſtinguiſh'd from the common March panes.

Another ſort of March-pane.

The Almonds are to be pounded, as before, and moiſten d with the White of an Egg and Orange-flower-water, or ſome other ſort . The only difference is, that this Paſte muſt be drawn out, and dried in a Baſon, with Powder-ſugar, till it becomes very pliable, as it were ordinary Paſte ; ſo that after it has been ſet by, for ſome while, ſeveral Rolls may be made, of any thickneſs, which ſhall be judg'd expedient , out of which the March-panes are to be cut, and ſhap'd, according to Diſcretion.

Royal March-pane.

The Paſte of this March pane is the ſame with that of the preceeding, a Piece of which is to be roll'd out upon the Table, or Dreſſer, a Finger's breadth thick, and divided into as many Parts, as are requiſite to make ſeveral Wreaths, or Rings round about your Finger, cloſing the two ends, ſo as they may ſlip out, or be ſeparated again · Theſe Rings are to be dipt into the White of an Egg, with which a Spoonful of Marmelade of Apricocks has been intermix'd, and afterwards roll'd in Powder-ſugar : But you muſt not forget to blow upon them, as they are taking out, ſo that too much Sugar may not be left, and to lay them on Paper, in order to be bak'd in the Campain-oven, with Fire underneath, and on the top, becauſe at that Inſtant, they are ic'd on both ſides : Then a ſort of Puff will riſe in the middle, as it were in form of a Coronet, producing a very agreeable Effect ; to render which more certain, as the March-panes are dreſſing, you may put upon the void ſpace of theſe Rings, a little round Pellet of the ſome Paſte, or a ſmall grain of Fruit, ſuch as a Cherry, Rasberry, Piſtachoe, or any Thing of the like Nature.

Orange-

Orange-flower March-pane.

The Almonds being pounded and moiſten'd with the White of an Egg, are to be well temper'd with Feathered Sugar, adding a Spoonful of Orange flower-marmelade ; or you may content your ſelf only to mingle it with the Ice, with which they are cover'd, to be diverſified : For the reſt, the ſame Method is to be obſerv'd, as in preparing the common March-panes. Thus for Inſtance, Half a Pound of Sugar may be ſufficient for a Pound of Almond-paſte, and the Paſte muſt always be ſet by, for ſome time, before it is us'd For want of the Marmelade of Orange-flowers, ſprinkle your Almonds as they are blanch d, with a little Water of the ſame Flowers, and pound in a Mortar, ſome Orange-pulp that is preſerv'd Liquid, in order to be mix'd with the Almonds, or to conſtitute the Body of your Ice : But the Paſte ought to be dried at the Fire, by reaſon of the Orange-flower-water.

Lemmon March-pane.

Inſtead of what has been even now deliver'd in the laſt Article, theſe March-panes are to be diverſified with Lemmon-marmelade, or with the Pulp of preſerved Lemmons pounded in a Mortar : or elſe a little grated Lemmon peel may only be intermix'd, either with the pounded Almonds, before they are put into the Sugar, or with the Ice But this Peel ought to be grated very fine, and well beaten with the White of the Egg and the Sugar.

March-panes, with a Tincture of Raſberries, or other ſorts of Fruits.

During the Seaſon of Fruits, more eſpecially the red, your March-panes may be diverſified, ſeveral other Ways , by tempering ſome of them, with the Juice of Rasberries, and others with thoſe of Currans, Strawberries, Cherries, &c But obſerve by the way, That if thoſe Juices are us'd, for the ſoaking of your Almonds, when they are pounded with the White of an Egg, the Paſte ought to be well dried at the Fire, or elſe it muſt be done with Powder-ſugar, as in the third Article.

Iced

Iced March-panes.

When any sorts of March-pane, that is to say, the round, long, oval, or curled, are sufficiently bak'd and colour'd, on one side, they are to be gently cut off from the Paper, with a Knife, and ic'd on the other side, that lay undermost; according to either of the following Methods.

Having provided a sufficient quantity of sweet Water, either of Orange flowers, or some other sort, or else the above-mention'd Juices and Marmelades, according to the Quality, which you are minded to confer on your March-panes; intermix them by degrees with fine Powder-sugar, and temper all well together, till they come to the confistence of Pap: Then taking up some of this Ice, with a Knife, spread it neatly upon the March-panes, and set them again in order, upon Paper, with the O-ven-lid, and a little Fire on the top, to cause the Ice to coagulate. Afterwards, they may be lock'd up in Boxes, and kept for Use.

The other sort of Ice is made only with the White of an Egg and Powder-sugar, or mingled with some kind of Marmelade, compleating and using it, as the former. At another time, both these sorts of Ice may be prepar'd at once, to diversifie part of the March-panes; when different Figures are made of the same Paste, to the end that they may be more easily distinguished one from another

Stuff'd March-pane.

Having made the same sort of Paste as that of Royal March-pane, work it well upon a Table, or Dresser, with Powder-sugar, and roll out a Piece, as thin as is possible, strewing some Sugar underneath, to hinder the Paste from sticking to the Board: Then having divided it into two Parts, and cut it a little round about, spread any sort of Marmelade at pleasure, upon one of them, of the thickness of a Half-crown, and cover it with the other. Afterwards, you are to cut the Paste into great, or small Pieces, according to Discretion, and lay them in order upon White Paper, to be bak'd on one side, with the Oven-lid. As soon as they have taken Colour, set them by to cool, and ice them over on the other side, with the White of an Egg, beaten up with Powder-sugar, or else with Orange-flower-water, temper'd per'd in like manner with the ſame Sugar : Some time after, they are to be laid upon Paper again, and the baking of them finiſh'd upon the Table, with the Oven-lid, as before   Certain little Pies, or Tarts may alſo be made with the ſame Paſte ; to which purpoſe, taking a Piece as thick as a Walnut, ſhape it with your Thumb and Fore-finger, the tip of which may juſt enter into it, and work it very thin : Theſe little Pies are to be laid upon Paper, and gently bak'd in the Oven, with a little Fire, in the beginning, on the top, and underneath, till they come to a Colour ; and then fill'd with a preſerv'd Cherry, Rasberry, or Grape, or any kind of Marmelade · They may alſo be ic'd, if you pleaſe, and the Ice is to be bak'd with the Oven-lid ; but they muſt only be fill'd, as Occaſion requires.

C H A P. XXVIII.

Of Meringues and Macaroons.

THis ſmall Sugar-work is of great Uſe, and very eaſily prepar'd : It is alſo very convenient in an Office, in regard that it may be made in a trice, after the following Manner.

Meringues in Pairs.

Take three or four new-laid Eggs, according to the quantity of Meringues, that you would have made, and ſet a-part the Whites, to be whipt, till they make a rocky Snow   Then let a little grated Lemmon-peel be put into it, and three or four Spoonfuls of Powder-ſugar : A little Amber may alſo be added, and the whole Maſs muſt be whipt together, till it become very Liquid.   Afterwards, you may make your *Meringues* upon a Sheet of white Paper, with a Spoon, of a round or oval Figure, and of the thickneſs of a Walnut ; leaving ſome diſtance between every one of them : At the ſame time, they are to be ſtrew'd with fine Sugar put into a Handkerchief, and cover'd with the Oven-lid, with Fire on the top ; without removing them from the Table : Whereupon they'll immediately riſe and take Colour, leaving a void ſpace in the middle ;
which

which may be fill'd up, with a grain of preserv'd Fruit, according to the Season, such as a Rasberry, Cherry, Strawberry, &c. At last, every one of them is to be cover'd with another *Meringue*, enclosing the whole Substance, and these are call'd 'Twin-*Meringues.*

Dry Meringues.

Having caus'd the Whites of four new-laid Eggs to be whipt, as before, till they rise up to a Snow, let four Spoonfuls of very dry Powder-sugar, be put into it, and well temper'd with a Spoon : Then let all be set over a gentle Fire, to be dried a little at two several times, and add some Pistachoes, that are pounded and dried a little in the Stove. Afterwards, they are to be dress'd as the others, and bak'd in the Oven somewhat leisurely, with a little Fire underneath, and more on the top : When they are sufficiently done, and very dry, let them be taken out, and cut off with a Knife: Lastly, as soon as they are somewhat cold, let them be laid upon Paper, and set into the Stove to be kept dry

Pistachoe-Meringues.

Take a Handful, or two of Pistachoes, and blanch them in scalding Water · Afterwards, having whipt the Whites of Eggs, as for the other sorts of *Meringues*, and having beat them together with the Powder-sugar, put in the Pistachoes, well drain'd from the Water, and make the *Meringues*, with a Spoon, of what thickness you shall think fit, icing them over in the same manner If you have no mind to ice them, their natural Colour will be as white as Paper; but a Pistachoe must be allow'd for every one of the *Meringues* which will serve for the garnishing of Pies made of Crackling Crust, and also to Dress Pyramids upon the *China*-dishes, for the Desert.

Macaroons.

Macaroons are a particular Confection of sweet Almonds, Sugar, and the White of an Egg, and to make them it is requisite to provide a Pound of Almonds; which are to be scalded, blanch'd, and thrown into fair Water : Afterwards, they must be drain'd, wip'd and pounded in a Mortar; moistening ftening them at the fame time, with a little Orange-flower-water, or the White of an Egg, left they fhould turn to Oil Then taking the fame quantity of Powder-fugar, with three or four other Whites of Eggs, beat all well together, and drefs your Macaroons upon Paper, with a Spoon, in order to be bak'd with a gentle Fire : When they are half done, they may be ic'd over at Pleafure, as the March-panes , or they may be bak'd outright, without Icing, as the *Savoy*-biskets, or thofe of bitter Almonds, which they very much refemble in their Nature and Quality.

C H A P. XXIX.

Of Paftils.

PAftils are alfo a kind of Sugar-pafte, of which there are feveral forts, ufually drefs'd upon *China*-difhes, to fet off a Defert, or Banquet of Sweet-meats.

Cinnamon-paftils.

Let fome Gum-dragant be diffolv'd in Water, pour'd into a Pot, or earthen Pan ; that is to fay, one Ounce of it will be fufficient for four Pounds of Sugar At the end of two or three Days, when the Gum is well fteept and ftirr'd about with a Spoon, it muft be ftrain'd thro' a clean Linnen-cloth, to feparate all the Drofs from it Then this Gum-water being put into a Mortar, with one or two Whites of Eggs, all muft be well incorporated with fome Cinnamon beaten very fmall, and pafs'd thro' a fine Sieve. Afterwards, fome Powder-fugar muft likewife be fifted thro' a fine Sieve, and mingled with the reft, by little and little ; continuing to temper all together, till the Pafte become very pliable : At that Inftant, the Paftils may be made of a round, or long Figure, or of any Shape whatfoever , and if you have any Seals, or Ciphers at Hand, an Impreffion may be made with them, upon the Paftils ; which afterwards are to be dried in the Stove.

White-

White Pastils

The Gum is to be first steept in a little Water, with the Juice of three or four Lemmons, and the *Zests*, or Chips that were made of them At the end of two or three Days, when you perceive the Gum to be well dissolv'd, strain it thro' a clean Linnen-cloth, as before, and pour it into the Mortar, with double refin'd Powder-sugar, sifted thro' the Drum or fine Sieve : After having thrown in the first Handful of Sugar, let the whole Mass be well work'd and beaten, and add another Handful ; continuing to beat and temper your Compound on all sides, as it is augmenting with Sugar, till you have a very white and pliable Paste ; with which the Pastils are to be made, according to the former Method, and dried in the Stove.

Orange-flower Pastils.

These sorts of Pastils are usually prepar'd after the same manner, only some Leaves of Orange-flowers, and Water of the same, are to be intermix'd with the Lemmon-juice, in which the Gum is steept.

Apricock-pastils.

Instead of Gum-dragant take Gum-*Arabick*, which is dissolv'd a great deal sooner, and having caus'd it to be steept and strain'd thro' a Linnen-cloth, pour it into a Mortar, with Syrup of Apricocks Then let all be well temper'd together, and augmented with Sugar, at several times, till the Paste becomes pliable, in order to make round Pastils, which are dried in the Stove, to be made white, if you shall think fit, in the wide Pan, after the same manner as Sugar-plums

Violet-pastils, and other forts

The same sort of Gum-*Arabick* is to be used for these Pastils ; because they are usually made white in the Sugar-plum Pan, as well as the following Clove-pastils To give them the Colour and Smell of Violets ; some Indigo and Orrice is to be steept in Water, and mingled with the Gum, when it is dissolv'd and pour'd into the Mortar Afterwards, you are to add some fine

Pow-

Powder-fugar, continuing to work and temper the whole Mafs, till it turns to a pliable Pafte   Then round Paftils may be made of it ; or if defign'd for fine Sugar plums, they may be fhap'd in form of Hearts, Diamonds, Clubbs and Spades by the means of a Tin-mould, in which thefe Figures are exprefs'd, and at laft thefe Paftils are to be made white, after they have been thoroughly dried in the Stove

Clove-paftils.

Having caus'd your Cloves to be well pounded and fifted thro' the Drum, or fine Sieve, mingle them in the Mortar, with the fteept Gum-*Arabick* ; adding as much Sugar as is requifite to make a pliable Pafte : Then roll out a flip of this Pafte, to be cut into little Pieces, in the fhape of Cloves, which are to be made white in the Sugar-plum Pan : Otherwife, gray Paftils may be made of them, as thofe of Cinnamon.

C H A P. XXX.

Of the Caramel Sugar-work, and Candy'd Comfits.

THefe two forts of Sugar-works are very curious, and may be made upon feveral Occafions for the embellifhing of a Defert, according to the following Inftructions

Candy'd Cinnamon.

Cut your Cinnamon in form of fmall larding flips of Bacon, as alfo of the fame bignefs, and put them into thin Sugar, over the Fire, fo as they may boil only in a little Syrup : Then removing the Pan, let them imbibe the Sugar, during five or fix Hours, and let them lye a draining upon a Hurdle, or Grate in the Stove. As foon as they are half dry, they muft be gently taken off, and laid upon a Sieve in the fame Stove, to make an end of drying them. Afterwards, they are to be fet in order in Tin-moulds, upon little Grates made for that purpofe, and let into the Moulds ; fo as three Rows may be plac'd one above another, feparated with thofe little Grates ; but a piece
of

of Lead, or ſomewhat elſe of the like nature muſt be laid on the uppermoſt Grate, to keep all cloſe ſtopt In the mean while, having caus'd a ſufficient quantity of Sugar to boil till it is Blown, pour it into your Mould, ſo as ſome of it may lie upon the laſt Grate, and paſs thro' ſeveral parts of the Mould, which is to be ſet into the Stove the next Evening, with a good cover'd Fire, and to continue therein all Night · In the Morning, obſerve, whether the Cinnamon be well coagulated, and make a little Hole, at one Corner of the Mould, ſo as the Sugar may be drain'd thro' it : Then ſet the Mould again into the Stove, upſide down, with a Plate underneath, and when it is ſufficiently drain'd, take out your Cinnamon ſticks, which muſt be gently looſen'd, by little and little, and laid upon a Sieve, to be throughly dried in the Stove

Candy'd Fennel.

Take Fennel run up to Seed, as ſoon as it comes from the Flower, and having caus'd it to be well dried on a Board, cut it into halves, or quarters, according to the thickneſs of the Stalk : Then let it be ſcalded and put into thin Sugar, ordering it, for the reſt of the Work, in the ſame manner as the Cinnamon. The ſame thing may be done in the candying of pickt Cherries, and old Paſte, particularly thoſe of Quinces, either red or white, and of roaſted Pears, as alſo Orange or Lemmon-chips, Bell-grapes, *Biſcotins,* and Paſtils · But it is requiſite, that all be well dried before, in the Stove, to ſerve as a proper Garniture for all ſorts of Fruit.

Sugar-candy.

The preceding Methods are only an Imitation of that of preparing Sugar-candy, the Virtue of which is ſo well known, in the Curing of Defluxions and other Indiſpoſitions of the Breaſt : For it is made in like manner, by cauſing Sugar to boil to the Degree, call'd, *Blown,* and puting it into an earthen Pot, wherein certain ſmall Sticks are laid in order, round about which, the Sugar coagulates, when ſet into the Stove, with a Fire, as before. Some Confectioners, after having taken away the firſt Cruſt, ſet the reſt again into the Stove, till another is form'd, and ſo proceed, till the whole Work is finiſh'd ; more eſpecially if the Sugar be boil d over again, to cauſe it to return to its

Blown

Blown Quality : Others, having laid these little Sticks in Order, side-wise, cross-wise, or upright, pour in the Sugar, and leave all for the space of fifteen Days, in the Stove, or some other warm Place : Afterwards, having pour'd in hot Water, at several times, they leave them again, for a whole Day, and breaking the Pot, the next Morning, find the Sugar-candy round about the Sticks ; of which there are two sorts, *viz*. White and Red. The former being the best, is usually prepar'd with Sugar brought from the *Canaries*, and the other, with that of St *Thomas*'s Island

To make the Caramel *Sugar-work*.

One of the chief Uses of the Sugar-work, call'd, *Caramel*, is to make a kind of Cap or Net, to cover a Service of Cheese-curds. To that purpose, the Sugar must be brought to the *Caramel*, or last Degree of Boiling, whilst a Plate, or *China*-dish is provided of a convenient size , upon which, several sorts of small preserv'd Fruits are to be set in order, at a certain distance, one from another ; such as Cherries, Rasberries, Apricocks, green Almonds, Orange and Lemmon-slips, or other Things of the like Nature , artificially intermixing their different Colours, to render all more pleasant to the Sight, by the means of that agreeable Variety   The Fruits being thus disposed of, on the bottom and sides of the *China*-dish, a Pearling-pot is to be us'd, or else a Tin-mould in Form of a Funnel ; but the Hole of it ought to be very small , otherwise, a kind of Pin, or Stopple must be put into it, which may be slipt up and down, to cause the Sugar to run thicker, or finer, accordingly as it shall be judg'd most expedient . Then pour the *Caramel*-sugar into this Mould, and sprinkle your Fruits ; turning it about, from one to another, till you have fill'd up the whole Compass of the *China*-dish, or Plate.   As the Sugar thickens, and is dried in an instant, sticking to the Fruits, as it falls, a kind of curious Filigreen, or Net-work will be form'd, very proper, for the covering and adorning of the *China*-dishes, which will pleasantly deceive the sight of the Guests that have a mind to take up some of the Fruit, with a Fork. Besides that the broken Sugar falling among the Cheese-curds and Sweet-meats, will cause the whole Mess to be eaten together, with a great deal of satisfaction.

Thus

Thus Pyramids of raw Fruit, particularly, of Cherries, Strawberries, Plums, &c may be diversified, and when they are dress'd, some *Caramel*-sugar is to be pour'd upon them, in like manner, beginning at the bottom, and continuing to turn it about to the uppermost Point By which means the Fruit will be entirely hid, so as some part of their Colour may only be discern'd, making a very fine shew, under this Sugar-work.

CHAP. XXXI.

Of Mosses and Sultanes.

Mousselines or Mosses were in great repute, some Years ago, and may still, be us'd to very good purpose, as well as another sort of Sugar-work, call'd, *Sultanes* They are also convenient to fill up a large Desert ; for want of Fruits preserved dry, or other kinds of Sweet-meats.

Moss of several Colours.

To make white Moss, let some Gum-dragant be steept in fair Water, with Lemmon-juice, and afterwards strain'd thro a Linnen-cloth : Then take as little of it as you please, to work up a white Paste, with double refin'd Sugar pouder'd and pass'd thro' a Sieve, tempering and beating all well together, in a Mortar, till the Paste become pliable

For red Moss, let some of the same sort of Gum be put into the Mortar, with prepar'd Cochineal, to give it a red Colour. Afterwards, add Sugar, as before, causing all to be well mingled, and work d together, till your Paste be made no less pliable

At another time, let the Gum be intermix'd with Indigo and Orris, if you are minded to have it of a Blew, or Violetcolour . Then being put into a Mortar, with fine Powder-sugar, all must be thoroughly temper'd together, to make a Paste of the same nature as the others

A yellow Paste may likewise be made with Gum-booge or with Saffron, and a green Paste, with the Juice of Beat-leaves, which must be scalded a little over the Fire to take away their Crudity   C c   If

If you have a mind to make marbled Mofs of all thefe Paftes, take a piece of every one of them, and lay them one after another, upon a Sieve, fo that as they are fqueez'd thro' with a Spoon, certain little Rocks are form'd, which will be marbled, and of thofe different Colours

If it be requifite, to make fome of every fort of Pafte a-part, and of the fame Colour, they muft be feparately ftrain'd, in like manner, and thefe different Rocks are to be drefs'd in form of Pyramids upon *China*-difhes, for the Defert   They are dried in a very fhort fpace of time, without putting them into the Stove, or ufing any other means for that purpofe.

Sultanes.

Take the Whites and Yolks of four Eggs, with an equal Weight of Powder-fugar, and as much fine Flower, as will counterpoife the Weight of two Eggs: Let all be well temper'd together, and if you would have a grain of Musk added, it muft be pounded with a little other Sugar, and mingled with the reft : Afterwards, the *Sultanes* are to be drefs'd with a Spoon upon Papers, and ftrew'd on the top, with fine Sugar But a convenient diftance muft be left between every one of them ; becaufe they are apt to fpread very wide, and then they may be fet into the Oven, with Fire on the top and underneath As foon as they are fufficiently bak'd, and well colour'd, they are to be clear'd from the Papers; wetting them gently on the back-fide, and bringing them to the Fire, by which means they may be eafily flipt off   Laftly, the *Sultanes* are to be roll'd up in form of Wafers, fo as the Ice may remain on the out-fide, and drefs'd upright upon *China* difhes or Plates ; or elfe they may ferve for the garnifhing of fome Pie, or other fort of Ser vice

C H A P. XXXII.

Of certain natural and artificial Flowers.

BEfides Orange-flowers, the particular Way of preferving which, has been already explain'd, Pag. 52. Some other
forts

ſorts may alſo be prepar'd, for Curioſity, which will produce a very agreeable Effect: Indeed, thoſe Confectioners, who follow their Trade, have no regard to theſe little Knacks, becauſe they are unwilling to beſtow their time and pains about them, but they may be made in an Office, where the Officers ſometimes have more leiſure, and may lay hold of an opportunity to ſhew their utmoſt Skill

Tuberoſa-flowers.

Take Flowers that are not blown, and lay them a ſoaking in Water and Salt, as the Orange-flowers, to take away a certain Bitterneſs that is natural to them: At the end of two Days, they are to be ſcalded in Water, over the Fire, with the Juice of a Lemmon, then drain'd and thrown into clarified Sugar made luke-warm. To that purpoſe, a flat Copper-pan ought to be provided, or an earthen Pan of the like Form, to keep them from being ſqueez'd On the next Day, let the Sugar boil, till it become ſomewhat Smooth, and pour it upon your Flowers: On the third Day, having caus'd the Sugar to be thoroughly brought to its ſmooth Quality, or between ſmooth and Pearled, turn it in like manner upon the Flowers, and ſet them by to cool · Then let them be drain'd upon Hurdles, or Grates, and dried upon Sieves, ſtrew'd with Sugar, in order to be ſet into the Stove

Another Way of preſerving Tuberoſa-flowers.

After having order'd the Flowers, as before, or even without uſing that Method, let them be put into the Copper, or earthen Pan, whilſt ſome Sugar is boil'd till it become very much Pearl'd, or Blown Afterwards, let this Sugar be pour'd upon the Flowers, ſo as they may be ſufficiently ſoak'd therein, and let all be left in the Stove, till the next Day · Then they are to be drain'd upon Hurdles, or Sieves, and thoroughly dried. Orange-flowers may alſo be prepar'd, after the ſame manner, altho' that which has been elſewere deſcrib'd, is more certain, when they are to be kept for a conſiderable time.

Violet-flowers and other ſorts.

Take the fineſt double Violet-buds, with part of their Stalks,

and

and put them into a flat earthen, or Copper-pan, as before
Then having caus'd ſome boil'd Sugar to be Blown, pour it upon the Flowers, ſo as they may be well ſoak'd in it, and finiſh
the whole Work, according to the Method, laid down in the
laſt Article

The Flowers of Spaniſh Broom, may alſo be preſerv'd after
the ſame manner, and many other ſorts, at pleaſure   Some of
them may likewiſe be ic'd over, with Powder-ſugar, after they
have been dipt into the White of an Egg and Orange-flower
Water, in order to be dried at the Fire   In drying theſe Flowers, they may be dreſs'd in Bunches upon ſmall Twigs diſpoſd
of to that purpoſe, and they may be put to the ſame Uſe, as the
Artificial Flowers hereafter ſpecified ; or elſe they may ſerve
ſingle, for the garniſhing of ſome other Diſh

Counterfeit, or Artificial Flowers.

It is requiſite at firſt to make Paſtes of divers Colours, according to the Inſtructions already given in the Article of *Maſ-
ſes* ; that is to ſay, with Gum dragant thoroughly ſteept, and
mingled with Powder-ſugar, which is to be well temper'd and
beaten in the Mortar, till the Paſte become pliable   For the
Red, ſome prepared Cochineel may be added , for the Blew,
Indigo and Orris, for the Yellow Gum-booge ; and for the
Green, Beet-juice, which ought to be firſt ſtew'd over the Fire
in a Pan or Silver-diſh   The Paſtes being thus order'd and
roll'd out into very thin Pieces, may be ſhap'd in the Form of
ſeveral ſorts of Flowers, as Tulips, Wind-flowers, Roſes, &c
by the means of certain Tin-moulds ; or elſe they may be cut
out, with the point of a Knife, according to Paper-models   Then
the Flowers muſt be finiſh'd all at once, and dried upon Egg-
ſhells turn'd upſide-down, or otherwiſe   As for the leſſer ſort,
particularly the Wind-flowers, they may be ſtuck upon Thim-
bles, or ſomething elſe, of the like nature, that may facilitate
the forming of their Shape   In the mean while, different ſort
of Leaves are to be cut out of the green Paſte, to which you
may likewiſe give ſeveral Figures, to be intermix'd among
your Flowers, the Stalks of which are to be made with ſmall
Slips of Lemmon-peel   For the Wind-flower, a Raſberry preſerv'd dry, is to be us'd, after it has been dipt into Indigo and
Orris, becauſe the top or Bud of thoſe Flowers, repreſented by
this Fruit, is generally of that Colour. For Tulips, ſome ſmall
point

points of Lemmon-flips may be put in the middle; for Rofes, a little Bud of Lemmon or Orange-chips; and fo for the other kinds of Flowers: In all thefe Particulars, their natural Figure and Colour may be very well imitated, with a little Precaution, and by that Means you may have the Satisfaction, of pleafantly impofing upon the Credulity of fome Perfons, when they fee fuch variety of Flowers in the midft of Winter. The tops of the Pyramids of dryed Fruit, may be garnifh'd with thefe artificial Flowers, or elfe a feparate Nofegay may be made of them for the middle of your Defert, or they may be laid in order in a Basket, or kind of Cup, prepar'd with fine Paftry-work of crackling Cruft, neatly cut and diied for that purpofe. If they are tied up in a Bunch, a Foot or Stock may be made of March-pane, roll'd out and wreathed after the fame manner, as Nofegays are ufually bound with Wire, or Thread; and the Branches of this Stock are to fupport on the top, a kind of winding Wreath, neatly fhap'd or cut, into which your Leaves and Flowers are to be put, artificially intermixing them, according to their various Colours: So that for the bringing of the whole Bufinefs to perfection, 'twill be requifite to beftow fome time, with a particular Application of Mind.

All thefe forts of Works may alfo be made with the Pafte that is proper for *Bifcotins,* and which has been already defcrib'd, Pag 96 and 97.

Of Fennel.

Forafmuch as Fennel, or Anis may have a place among the above-fpecified Confections, it will not be improper, here to fubjoyn the manner of ordering them to the beft Advantage; befides the Ufe that may be made of the Stalks alone, for the dreffing of Flowers that are preferved dry; more efpecially thofe of Spanifh *Jeffamin.*

Fennel may be ferv'd up to Table iced, after it has been foak'd in Orange-flower Water and the White of an Egg, and then roll'd in Powder-fugar, caufing it to be dried in the Sun, or at the Fire, upon Paper It it be judg'd expedient to give it divers Colours, an Ice may be made with Pomegranate-juice, or Cochencal, and the White of an Egg beaten together, for the red Colour, or with Indigo and Orrice-powder, for Blew, and fo of the reft.

As for the Anis, it is to be fteept in like manner, and dried n the Stove, upon Sieves or Grates. It may also be cover'd, as thick as you please, with that Ice, by soaking it several times in the same.

Moreover, when any Oranges, or Lemmons are preserv'd dry, the Fennel may be thrown into the Sugar, as soon as it is made white on the sides of the Pan; or else it may be candy'd, according to the Method elsewhere explain'd under the Article of *Candy'd Confections.*

C H A P. XXXIII.

Of Pies made of Crackling-crust and Puff-paste.

THis Article having so near a Relation to the Art of prese-ving Sweet-meats, ought not to be omitted here, and in-deed, it is not sufficient to know how to make these sorts of Paste, but 'tis also requisite to be well vers'd in the Method of ordering and disposing them for a Desert, and upon all other Occasions Now it cannot be denied, that Pan pies hold a considerable rank among these Particulars, more especially those made of Crackling-crust, which are at present, very of ten prepar'd, even for the most curious Palates, and serv d up, to the most sumptuous Tables, both at Court and elsewhere

Paste for Crackling-crust.

Having provided about two Handfuls of Almonds, which are sufficient for one Pan-pye, let them be scalded, blanch'd, and thrown into fresh Water · Then they are to be wip'd, and pounded in a Mortar, moistening them from time to time, with a little White of an Egg and Orange flower Water, beaten to gether, to prevent them from turning to Oil 'Tis very mate-rial, that they be well pounded, and they may also be squeez'd through a Sieve, to take away all the Clods, or Lumps The Almond-paste being thus prepar'd, must be spread on a Bason, or Dish, and dried with Powder-sugar, as an ordinary sort of Paste, till it become very pliable Afterwards, having set it by for some time, you are to roll out a Piece for the under-crust, to be dried in the Oven upon the Pie-pan; whilst other small
Pa-

Paftry-works are making, with what was par'd off, fuch as *Petits Choux,* Ciphers, Knots and other Devices, that may ferve for the garnifhing of your Pie.

Cracrling-crust made after another manner.

After the Almonds have been thoroughly pounded and moi-ften'd, as before, let as much Sugar as Pafte, at leaft, be put into a Copper-pan, and boil'd till it become Feathered . Then throwing in your Almonds , let all be well temper'd and mingled together with the *Spatula,* and having fet them over the Fire again, keep continually ftirring the whole Mafs, till your Pafte flips of from the bottom and fides of the Pan. Afterwards, it muft be laid in a Difh, ftrew'd with Pow-der-fugar on the top, and fet by, for a while, as the former, in or-der to make a Pye of it, after the fame manner.

In preparing the Pafte conformably to either of thefe Methods, the Pie will certainly become crackling and delicious to the high-eft Degree · But if you are minded to avoid the trouble, and perhaps the charge of Almonds, very good Pies may alfo be made according to the following Inftructions

Another Way.

Take one, or two Whites of Eggs, with three or four Spoon-fuls of fine Sugar, and as much Flower, if you would only make one Pan-pye · The Sugar being firft temper'd with the Whites of the Eggs, and then the Flower, knead all together, till your Pafte become pliable, and roll out a very thin Piece ; ftrewing it with fine Sugar Afterwards, having put it into the Pie-pan, let the Sides be neatly pinch'd, at certain Intervals, and prickt with the point of a Knife, to hinder them from puff-ing In the mean while, the remaining part of the Pafte is to be roll'd out into Slips of the thicknefs of a Lace, to compleat the infide of the Pie; which may be made in form of a Sun, Star, *Malta*-crofs, Flower-de luce, Coat of Arms, or the like. At laft, it muft be gently bak'd in the Oven, and when ready to be brought to Table, the void Spaces are to be fill'd up, with feveral forts of Marmelades, or Jellies, according to the Co-lours, that fhall be judg'd moft expedient. The fame thing ought alfo to be obferv'd, with refpect to Pies made of the preceding Paftes. To the latter, may be added a little Orange-

flower

flower Water, or ſome other ſweet Water, and if it be requiſite to prepare a greater quantity of either ſort of Paſte, another Piece, of an equal thinneſs, may be roll'd out for the Lid, which muſt be cut round, and dried in the Oven, upon a Piepan, or Plate, in order to cover the Pie, after it has been ic'd over, if you have no mind to leave it in its natural Colour.

Wafers.

Let as much Flower, as you pleaſe, be mingled, with new Cream in the Evening; taking care that it do not ſour On the next Day, when they are well temper'd and clear'd from the Lumps, add a ſomewhat greater quantity of Powder-ſugar than that of the Flower, and intermix all with a Spoon Then pour in more Cream, with a little Orange-flower Water, till the whole Meſs becomes almoſt as thin as Milk, and ſtirr all well together In the mean while, the Wafer-iron is to be heated, and rubb'd on both ſides, from time to time, with freſh Butter, put into one corner of a Napkin Then let your prepared Cream, or Batter be turn'd upon the Iron, but it muſt not exceed a Spoonful and half for every Wafer; which will be render'd ſo much the more delicious, if the Iron be preſs'd a little. Afterwards, the Wafer-iron is to be laid upon the Furnace, ſo that when the Wafer is bak'd on one ſide, it may be turn'd on the other: To know whether the Wafer be done enough, let your Iron be gently open'd a little and obſerve whether it be come to a good Colour At that very inſtant, take off your Wafer from the Iron, with a Knife; rolling it a little round the ſame Laſtly, let the Wafers be ſpread hot upon a Wooden Roller, made for that purpoſe, to give them their due Shape, and ſet them into the Stove, as they are finiſh'd, to the end that they may be kept very dry.

Rock-cream.

Let a Quart of ſweet Cream, more or leſs, according to the quantity that you would have made, be put into an earthen Pan, with Powder-ſugar, according to Diſcretion, and as much Culverized Gum-dragant: as you can take up between two Fingers. Then having cauſ'd all to be well whipt together, it will riſe, as high as you ſhall think fit, and continue two Days in the ſame Condition · A little Orange-flower Water may alſo be added as the Cream is Whipping.

Boil'd

Boil'd Cream.

Having boil'd a Quart of Milk, with what quantity of Sugar you please, when it begins to rise, slip in six Yolks of Eggs well beaten, and a little fresh Butter Then keep continually stirring all together, till your Cream is brought to a due Consistence, and dress it in *China*-dishes, or Cups.

Puff-paste.

Let some Paste be made after the usual manner, with Flower, Water, Salt, and if you please, the yolk of an Egg : As soon as it is well kneaded, and made very pliable , roll it out upon the Dresser-board, of a convenient length and thickness Then cover it with as much good Butter, and having turn'd one of the ends upon the other, so as all the Butter may be enclos'd on the inside, roll it again, continuing to do the same thing five or six times Two Pounds and half of good fresh Butter, ought to be allow'd for every three Pounds of Flower.

This sort of Paste is proper for other Pan-pies that are brought to Table without a Desert, in which it is not customary to serve up any thing that is prepar'd with Butter However, *Feuillantins* and *Mazarines*, which are certain small Tarts of the breadth of the Palm of a Man's Hand, may be made of it, being usually fill'd with Sweet-meats, to garnish some other Pie of a larger size, set among the Intermesses; but if these little Tarts are design'd for the Desert, they may be made of Crackling-crust, as before

---

C h a p. XXXIV.

Of Chesnuts and Mulberries ; with some particular Observations upon several other sorts of Fruit.

IT remains only to give some Account of Chesnuts and Mulberries, in regard that no notice has been taken of them among the other sorts of Fruit, and we shall afterwards add certain New and particular Remarks upon the Way of preserving
some

ſome of them ; ſo that it is preſum'd, That nothing will then be
wanting that relates to the whole Art and Myſtery of Confectioners.

To preſerve Cheſnuts.

Having choſen the beſt ſort of large Cheſnuts, let them be
ſcalded in Water, and neatly peel'd with a little Knife, proper
for that purpoſe, paring off the two Skins, and taking care that
they do not break : Afterwards, ſome clarified Sugar made luke-
warm being pour'd upon them, in a Copper-pan, they are to be
left for a while, in order to have ten, or twelve Boilings the
ſame Day : But it is not requiſite, to ſoak them entirely in the
Sugar, or to give them a cover'd Boiling, becauſe by that means
they would be all broken into pieces   On the next Day, boil
your Sugar till it be greatly Feathered, and almoſt ready to be
blown, and ſlip in the Cheſnuts: This ſtrong Boiling of the Sugar, cauſes them abſolutely to caſt their Juice, and then it returns to its Pearled Quality, which is the uſual Degree for Sweet-
meats: The Cheſnuts ought not to be ſet over the Fire any longer, left they ſhould grow Black ; but to dry them, they are to
be drain'd from their Syrup, and turn'd into Feathered Sugar .
Then having caus'd the Boiling to be cover'd, take them off from
the Fire, and ſet them by for ſome time · As ſoon as they are
cool'd a little, let the Sugar be made white by rubbing it with
the Ladle, or Skimmer againſt one of the Sides of the Pan, and
put your Cheſnuts into it, with a Spoon and Fork, as dextrouſly
as is poſſible, for fear of breaking them   Afterwards, being
dreſs'd upon Hurdles, or Grates, in the ſame manner as Lemmons, they will be ſoon dried, and finely Ic'd over.

If you have any other Sweet-meats to be dried at the ſame
time, ſuch as Oranges, or Lemmons, it is expedient to begin
with them ; more eſpecially the latter, which ought to be very
White , becauſe the Cheſnuts extremely blacken the Sugar ; ſo
that it is no longer fit for any other Uſe, but only to ſerve for
Compotes.

Of Mulberries, as well dry as liquid.

For the former, take ſuch Mulberries as are not too ripe, but
rather ſomewhat greeniſh and tart   In the mean while, having
caus'd ſugar to be Blown, throw in your Mulberries, and give
them

them a cover'd Boiling Then remove the Pan from the Fire, take off the Scum, and leave all in the Stove till the next Day: And it ought to be obferv'd, that as much Sugar is requifite as Fruit, and that it may be alfo melted with the Juice of Mulberries to clarifie it. As foon as they are taken out of the Stove, and cool d, let them be drain'd from their Syrup, and drefs'd upon Slates, in order to be dry'd in the Stove, ftrew'd with Sugar, as the other forts of Fruit, laftly they muft be turn'd again upon Sieves, and when thoroughly dry, lock'd up in Boxes to be ufed as occafion requires.

For liquid Mulberries, let the Sugar be boil'd till it be a little Pearled, allowing three Pounds of it, for four Pounds of Fruit, and let them have a light cover'd Boiling in the fame Sugar ; gently ftirring the Pan by means of the Handles · Then take it off from the Fire, and having fet it by, till the next Day, drain off the Syrup, in order to be brought to its Pearled Quality Afterwards flip in your Fruit, adding a little more Pearled Sugar, if it be needful, and difpofe of them in Pots, as foon as they are fufficiently cool d.

Mulberries may alfo be preferv'd wet after the following manner : Take five Pounds of Fruit, with three Pounds of Sugar boil d till it become Feathered , into which you are to flip them, giving them at the fame time, twelve, or fifteen Boilings: Then they are to be augmented, all at once, with two, or three other Pounds of Sugar, likewife Feathered, and brought to Perfection, without removing them from the Fire, only caufing the Syrop to return to its Pearled Quality

Additional Obfervations upon green Figs.

Befides the Inftructions elfewhere given, Pag 44. for the preferving of green Figgs, it may be obferv d here, That before they are fcalded, the cutting of them is fometimes difpenfed with, only pricking them along their whole length, from one end to the other · Then fet them over the Fire in a Copperpan, with Water, and give them ten, or, twelve Boilings : Afterwards, being cool'd in the fame Liquor, and turn'd into frefh Water ; they are to be brought to the Fire again, with a Glafs of Verjuice, and boil'd, till they become very green and foft. At that inftant removing them from the Fire, let them be cool'd, drain'd and put into earthen Pans. In the mean while, fome clarified Sugar, that is to fay two Ladles fullof it for one of Water, is to be heated, and pour'd upon the Figgs, so as they may be well foak'd therein. On the next Day, drain off the Syrup, give it two, or three Boilings, and turn it upon your Fruit: Some time after, the whole Work may be finished, almost in the same manner as is exprefs'd Pag 45 by caufing the Syrup to be boiled one Day, a little fmooth, at another time very Smooth, then to a degree between Smooth and Pearled, and at laft, entirely Pearled And the Figgs muft be fet over the Fire, from one Day to another, alternately, only to fimper, and at the other times, it will be fufficient only to pour the Sugar upon them: However the laft time, your Fruit ought to have feven, or eight cover'd Boilings, and then being fet by for a little while in their Syrup, they may be either immediately dried, or laid up in Pots, till a more convenient Opportunity, fhall offer itfelf for that purpofe.

Additional Remarks upon Bell-grapes.

It has been already obferv'd Pag 48 That pared Bell-grapes are ufually preferv'd after the fame manner, as thofe that are left in their natural Condition • But it ought to be underftood only with refpect to the Sugar; becaufe they are not to be fcalded, in water as the latter, nor foak'd to bring them again to their Colour, as being riper, otherwife the Skin would not be fo eafily par'd off If it be perceiv'd, that the Pearled Boiling is not ftrong enough, the firft time that fuch juicy Fruits are put into Sugar, it may be boil'd till it become greatly Feathered, allowing the fame quantity of it, as of the Grapes; which ought to have four, or five Boilings, at once, before the Pan is remov'd from the Fire: For the reft, the whole Work may be finifh'd, altogether according to the Directions before laid down, for unpared Bell-grapes; unlefs, inftead of leaving them to fimper a little, every time that they are fet over the Fire, after having brought the Sugar, to the neceffary Degree of Boiling; you have a mind to give them feveral Boilings together, as at the firft.

For Paftes made of Bell-grapes, as they are fcalding over the Fire, in their own Liquor, according to the Inftructions given in the fecond Article of *Bell-grape-paftes*, Pag 86 remember to take off the Scum as foon as it boils, and when your Pafte lies a drying at the Fire, after having fqueez'd it through the Sieve, add, if you pleafe, a little Powder-fugar: Neither muft

you

you forget, to cause the same Paste to simper for a while, when incorporated with the Blown Sugar, before it is dress'd upon the Slates , it being more especially requisite to observe this particular Circumstance, in the preparing of all sorts of Pastes.

Additional Observations upon Quinces.

Forasmuch as the Method of preserving Quinces explain'd Pag. 50. may seem somewhat tedious, we shall now try another that is easier, and of greater dispatch, being also at least, of equal efficacy and certainty

Having caus'd your Quinces to be cut into pieces, clear'd from the Cores and par'd, let all boil together in a sufficient quantity of Water; and when they are become very soft, remove the Pan from the Fire   Then taking up the Pieces that are to be preserv'd, with the Skimmer, put them into fresh Water, to cool ; set the rest over the Fire again, and give them twenty other Boilings : Afterwards, this Decoction being strain'd thro' the Straining-bag, or thro' a doubled Napkin, take two Ladles full of it, with one of clarified Sugar, proportionably to the quantity of your Fruit, and turn all into a Copper-pan, with the Quinces , in order to boil over a gentle Fire : Let some Sugar be also added ; accordingly as the first Syrup consumes away, without pouring in any more Decoction, and let the whole Mess be well boiled, till the Syrup becomes Pearled : Then let it be cool'd, and dress your Quinces in Boxes, Pots, or Glasses; pouring the Syrup upon them, which will be very fine, and of a lively red Colour, if the Pan were cover'd in the Boiling.

Additional Remarks upon Oranges.

When mention was made of *China*-oranges, Pag 54 it ought only to be understood of the large and sweet ones, as it may be easily discern'd   The lesser Sort of *China*-oranges are not to be clear'd from their Juice, but being lightly Zested, or par'd, to take away the Yellow, they must only be prick'd, with a Knife, making a little slit on the top, and thrown into fair Water: Then they are to be scalded and boil'd in fresh water, till they slip off from the Pan, adding a Handful of pounded Allum, in order to have twenty other Boilings, which Method may also be observ'd in the preparing of other sorts of Oranges   Afterwards, they must be cool'd, and put into clarified Sugar, newly

ly

ly pafs'd thro' the ftraining-bag, with a very little Water , becaufe a great deal of Juice will be extracted from them ⋅ For
that very reafon, it is requifite to boil them at the fame time,
till the Sugar be fomewhat fmooth; which neverthelefs will be
altogether undone, the next Day   Then let it be brought again
to its fmooth Quality, augmenting it with other Sugar, and having flipt in the Oranges give them fifteen, or twenty Boilings.
On the Day following, let them be drain'd again, whilft the Syrup is made Pearled; in which they are to have ten, or twelve
cover'd Boilings : A little while after, they are to be cool'd and
drain'd, and difpofed of in Pots or Glaffes, and the Syrup being boil'd till it become greatly Pearled, muft be pour'd upon
them in the ufual manner   But you muft not forget to augment
it with as much Sugar as is needful, to the end that the Fruit may
be fufficiently foak'd therein.   The particular way of drying
thefe Oranges, is the fame with that which is proper for other
Fruits of the like nature, and it has already been defcrib'd at
large, more efpecially, in the Article of Lemmons

Barley-Sugar.

Having caus'd Barley to be well boil'd in Water, ftrain it
thro' the Hair-fieve, and let this Decoction be put into clarified
Sugar, brought to the *Caramel*, or laft Degree of Boiling: Then
remove the Pan from the Fire, till the Boiling fettles, and pour
your Barley-fugar upon a Marble-ftone rubb'd with Oil of O-
lives, taking care to hinder it from running down   If the Mar-
ble be wanting, a Silver-difh, or one of fome other fort of Metal, may be us'd, for the fame purpofe ⋅ So that as the Sugar
cools, and begins to grow hard, it muft be cut into pieces, and
roll'd out of what length you pleafe, in order to be kept for Ufe

C H A P. XXXV.

Of the Accidents that may happen to Sweet-meats, and of proper Means for the remedying of them.

IT may be perhaps be affirm'd, That all forts of Sweet-meats,
well made according to Art, are not apt to decay, or to be
spoil'd,

spoil'd, and that this Defect proceeds from the Unskilfulness of those Persons who are employ'd in the preparing of them ; nevertheless it may so happen sometimes, notwithstanding the utmost Precautions that have been taken to prevent such Inconveniences. So that altho' we have laid down the most certain Methods for the due Preserving of every Particular, yet it is expedient to shew the bad Accidents that may befal them, and the manner of applying proper Remedies :

The most usual Inconvenience is, that wet Sweet-meats are subject to sour, and puff, which proceeds from the moistness of the Fruit, which not having sufficiently cast their natural Juice, or the Liquor they imbib'd, as they were Scalding and Cooling, cause the Sugar to give, in process of time; so that the Sweet-meats grow mouldy, and throw out a kind of Scum. This ill Accident is soon perceived in frequently visiting the Store-house, or Repository, and it ought to be immediately remedied, whilst an Opportunity offers itself; otherwise, by neglecting a Matter, which at first might be easily reduc'd to good order, you'll run the hazard of rendering it desperate, and of utterly spoiling your Sweet-meats   To prevent this Disaster, it is requisite to put them into a Copper-pan, over the Fire ; causing the Sugar, or Syrup to give a little, with a cup full of Water · Then let all boil together, taking of the Scum, that rises on the top, and having brought them again to the Pearled Boiling, remove the Pan, and put your Fruit into Pots, or Glasses as at the first, by which means they'll be thoroughly free'd from their sourness, and in a condition to keep to the end, provided they be not laid up in too moist a Place Otherwise, the Syrup alone may be set over the Fire, at first, with a little Water, and after having scumm'd it, as before, the Fruit may be slipt in ; which are to boil till the Syrup has attain'd to the Pearled Degree, and then they are to be disposed of in the usual manner.   Thus the sourness may be taken away from all sorts of Fruits preserv'd liquid, particularly Walnuts, Plums, Orange and Lemmon-slips &c.

The Inconvenience incident to preserv'd Fruits, is, that they sometimes candy. but this is not properly a Defect, as being only occasion'd by giving the Syrup too strong a Boiling ; so that there are grounds to fear, least such an Accident should do your Sweet-meats any Injury, on the contrary, you are assur'd, that they will keep very well, and that the Sugar was good   To repair this slight Damage, you need only put all that part which is candied into a Pan, with a little Water, and when it is brought

to

again to the Pearled Quality, mingle it with the rest, or else let all have a few Boilings together When the sweet-meats are only candy'd on the Surface, such as Jellies, this Candy may be taken off, by passing hot Water over them, which will easily disperse the Candy and render the Sweet-meats as fine, as they were in the Beginning These Jellies of Gooseberries, Currans, or other sorts of Fruit, being stale, may also be renew'd, by setting them over the Fire, in a Copper-pan, with a little Water, to dilute and cause them to give · So that as soon as they return to their former Degree of Boiling, which is Pearled, or between Smooth and Pearled, they are to be pour'd, into a Sieve set over an earthen Pan, and afterwards put again into the Pots or Glasses

There are certain Fruits which are apt to grow greasy, more especially green and ripe Apricocks, and in that Condition, they cannot be well dried The proper Remedy is, to boil them in new Pearled Sugar, after they have been drain'd from their for mer Syrup If the same Cost were bestow'd upon all other sorts of Fruits, they might be much more easily dried, and would be come finer, than when the Confectioner, or Officer contents himself according to the usual Method, only to drain them from the Sugar with which they were preserv'd, and afterwards to dress them upon Slates, or little Boards, in order to be dried in the Stove strew'd with Sugar.

Dry Sweet-meats, that are kept for a considerable time, ought to be laid up in a Place free from all manner of Moisture, that is to say near the Stove, or else in some Closet into which a lit tle Fire ought constantly to be put, from time to time, during the Winter-season: and in regard, that Fruits preserv d dry, are apt to lose their Ice, when kept for too long a time; it is expedient to dry them Occasion requires, by which means they will also be secur'd from another Accident, that is to say, from being shrivell'd and wrinkled, altho' both may be remedied, by causing those Fruits to be boil'd again over the Fire, in the like Syrup, or other new Sugar, in order to be dried again, after they have been boil'd in it to the Pearl'd Degree, and set by to cool.

C H A P.

C H A P. XXXVI.

The Way of Ordering and Setting-out a Defert, or other Regalio of the like nature, to the best advantage, with fome Models of fuch Entertainments.

AFter having treated of every Thing that may give Satisfaction to the niceft Palates, the preparing of which is the peculiar Province of Confectioners, Butlers and other Officers; it is expedient to conclude the whole Work, with the Method of ferving up all thofe refpective Meffes, in due Order, either for a Defert, or fome other Entertainment of the like nature

To that purpofe, it ought to be obferv'd, That a Banquet of Fruits, as well Raw, as Preferved, with its Appurtenances, may be drefs'd either upon a Level or in a Basket This laft Way is only us'd in preparing Entertainments for certain Fraternities, or particular Societies; where as many little Baskets are ferv'd up at firft to Table, as there are Guefts · Thefe Baskets are ufually adorn'd with fmall Ribbands, and Taffety-covers, according to the allotted Expences, and fill'd up with all forts of Sweet-meats, Biskets, March-panes, Orange and Lemmon-faggots, dried Fruits, &c fo as the moft delicious Comfits may lye on the top At laft, after all have been fet in good Order, and contributed much to the Decoration of the feveral Courfes, every individual Perfon fhuts up and takes away his Basket, to treat his Family and Friends at home, contenting himfelf only to eat the liquid Sweet-meats, fuch as Compotes and Marmelades, or elfe the raw Fruits, which were provided, to ferve for the Out-works.

A Banquet of Sweet-meats is faid to be drefs'd upon a Level, when difpofed of upon *China*-difhes, and Machines made of Wood, or Ofier-twigs, having a great Board in the middle, in form of a Square, or Hexagon, that is to fay, with fix Panes in length, or of any other Figure · This Board is encompafs'd with divers other Works of different Shapes, *viz* That of a Club at Cards, round, oval, or otherwife, and feveral *China*-difhes are fet upon thefe Boards, by the means of certain fmall wooden Leggs, or Cups; fo as the Oval may contain

D d two,

two, and the Clubs three ; whilst the Oval serve for Compotes, and the Middle-board for a large Pyramid of Fruit, with *China*-dishes round about, fix'd, as before   Or else it may be fill'd up altogether with *China*-dishes , that in the middle being rais'd higher than the others ; upon which several small Pyramids are to be erected, of an exact Proportion ; so that the same sorts of Comfits, and the same Colours may appear on every side, at the opposite Angles   Lastly, a Row or Border of raw Fruits may be made round about the Dishes, upon every Board to garnish the top, and the whole Desert is to be set out with Flowers, Greens, and other Ornaments, according to the Season.

For the more clear Illustration of this Method, it will not be improper here to produce some Examples, or Models of such Deserts, or Banquets of Sweet-meats, according to which, Measures may easily be taken, for the dressing of those of a greater, or lesser Size.

The Model of a Desert, for an Oval Table of twelve Coverings.

pag 126

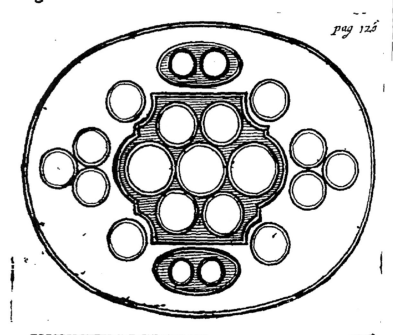

The Explication

The Board in the middle is usually made of Osier-twigs, in form of a Basket, and may be gilt, silver'd over, or painted like fine earthen Ware, with this convenience, that they may be clean'd by Washing There is also a thin Board, that lyes almost at the Entrance, over-against the Border, to serve for a Ground-plot for the Sweet-meats which are to be dress'd upon it, the Ledge of the Osier basket, or Board being indented; so that besides the Ornament, to which it contributes, it serves also to keep in the Fruit, with which a Border may be made round about the *China*-dishes Seven of these Dishes are express'd in the above-specified Model, and the Order of them may be clearly discern'd, but that in the middle ought to be a little larger, and rais'd somewhat higher than the rest For want of *China*-dishes, certain Tin-moulds of the same shape may be substituted in their room, the Quality of which is not so easily discover'd, in regard, that before any Thing is dress'd upon them, the bottom ought always to be cover'd with Leaves, or Paper These round Moulds may also be fasten'd upon the Leggs, and by that means the Desert will become more solid.

Those Persons who have no mind to make use of Wicker-boards according to the Model even now describ'd, may cause some to be made, of the same Form, or otherwise, that consist only of a wooden Bottom, supported by little Knobs, or other sorts of Feet, with a Ledge round about, to keep in the Fruit, as before, and this Ledge may be gilt, or done over with Silver. The same Thing may be observ'd, with respect to the other Boards which are added to the greater, as so many Out-works, and upon these wooden Bottoms the several Leggs are to be fix'd, for the *China*-dishes, in which the Sweet-meats are laid in order

As for a common Desert prepar'd for few Persons, the Confectioner or Officer may content himself, only to make use of the middle Board, without the Out-works, and in disposing those Out-works otherwise, may find Means to diversifie the Service at another time, or for other Tables, as it appears from the following Model

The Model of a Desert, or Banquet of Sweat-meats, for a round Table.

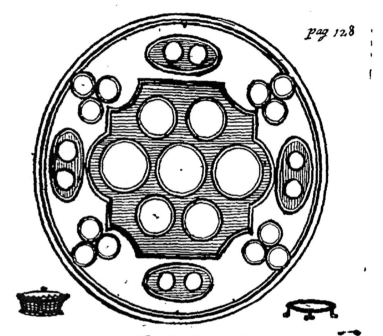

pag 128

The Explication.

This Desert contains two Oval Out-works more than the former, and the round ones are absolutely retrench'd : In this case, the Compotes may be set upon the Clubs, and certain small Pyramids of Biskets, March-panes, or other Comfits may be rais'd upon the Sides that remain empty and naked If it be perceiv'd, that the Figure is not sufficiently round, by reason that the Machine in the middle is not so broad, as it is long, the Round Out-works may be introduc'd again, or else two Ovals with their Ends plac'd inwards; garnishing the whole Desert, as it may be observ'd, with real *China*-dishes, or Tin-moulds representing their Figure, upon which the Fruits and Sweet-meats are to be dress'd in small Pyramids · Neither are there express'd in this Model above seven of these Dishes for the middle Board, altho' for the most part, a greater number is admitted, when it is requisite to provide a somewhat larger Desert.

A

A square Machine set in the middle of such a Table, will render the Figure more round, placing the Oval and Club-Out-works in the same situation: But forasmuch as in such a square Piece, the *China*-dishes leave a void Space, at the four Corners, they may be fill'd up with as many *China*-cups, into which other fine Fruits are to be put, or only some of the same, and the same thing may be done with the other Intervals; garnishing the rest with lesser sorts of Fruit, the thickness of which does not exceed the height of the *China*-dishes: And in a simple Desert, for four Persons, these four Corners may be taken up with little Cups of iced Waters, or other Liquors, according to the Season.

One of the two separate Figures that appear at the Bottom of the Model, or Scheme above delineated, denotes the Form of the above-mention'd Wicker-baskets, either round, or oval, and the other, the simple wooden Machines, with Feet, which may supply the Place of the others, as it has been already intimated. The Clubs, and the Board in the middle are also of the same Construction, and in the little Basket is to be seen the thin Board that lyes on the top at the Entrance, upon which the *China*-dishes are usually rais'd · This Board ought to be cover'd with marbled, or painted Paper, and always set out with Leaves and Flowers, or other Ornaments, according to the Season, more especially in the void Spaces, and Intervals, caus'd by the Indentings on the top of this Wicker-machine. And indeed, very convenient Boards are made for little Tables, where the several Pieces of the like nature, with their whole Contexture is form'd, are all fasten'd together; so that the Desert may be readily serv'd up to Table, all at once, without any manner of trouble, or impediment, and without running the hazard of confounding or spoiling the Sweet-meats, provided a little Care be taken in the ordering of the Machines

For greater Tables, other Machines of proportionable Dimensions, may be prepar'd at Pleasure, and upon any emergent Occasion, when all these Instruments are wanting, a Desert may nevertheless be very neatly disposed of upon the ordinary Table-furniture, after having taken a particular account of the Size and Number of the Dishes, Basons and Plates, which are necessary for that purpose; so that as many *China*-dishes, or Cups may be set in order upon them, as shall be judg'd requisite, to contain the Sweet-meats and Fruits, accordingly as an Opportunity may serve, or the Diversity of Seasons may require

Upon the whole Matter, it were to be wish'd, that exact Models were produc'd of all the sorts of Materials, with which Deserts might be prepared for different Tables: But considering, that these Circumstances depend upon the Abilities and Inclinations of particular Persons, and the Conveniencies of Houses, such Models would be of no great use, when the Managers are not in a condition to act conformably to those Measures. A certain Officer, for example, thinks fit to serve up *Switzerland*-cneese, cut into Quarters, or Slices, whilst another makes use of Parmesan, or Cheese-curds, during the Festival of *Easter*, with a *Caramel*-embellishment Another in like manner, judges it expedient only to present a Service of iced Cherries, whilst others are employ'd in preparing a Banquet of more costly and delicious Sweet-meats Therefore it is sufficient, that we have already given some Account of the several sorts of Comfits and Fruits, which are proper to be serv'd up to Table, in every Month throughout the whole Year So that recourse may be had, as Occasion serves, to the Rules before laid down in this Treatise; and as for those Persons, who are desirous to be farther instructed in the Method of Dressing an entire Desert, or Banquet of Sweet-meats, to the best advantage, they need only cast an Eye upon the following Model, neatly engrav'd upon a Copper-plate, wherein Endeavours have been us'd, to represent as exact and intelligible a Draught of it, as possibly could be done with no small a Compass

In this Figure, the middle Board is a Hexagon, consisting of six Angles, or Corners, and the Out-works are of the same nature as those express'd in the first Model The Club-figures, at the two Ends, are for iced Waters, the Round ones adjoyning, for *Compotes*, and the Oval on both Sides, serve each to hold a Couple of Club-dishes, for two small Pyramids Thus the Quantity of those contain'd in the principal Machine may be very well distinguish'd, and supposing, this Desert were provided for the Month of *July*, you may easily find out, of what Materials it ought to consist, by turning back to Page 12. of this Treatise, in which is contain'd a Description of all sorts of Sweet-meats and raw Fruits, that are proper for that Season The same thing may be done at any other time, accordingly as Occasion shall require

N E W

NEW INSTRUCTIONS FOR LIQUORS;

SHEWING

How to Prepare feveral Sorts of WATERS and DRINKS that are proper for every Seafon of the Year.

CHAP. I.

Of the iced Waters of Flowers.

THat nothing may feem to be wanting for the compleating of this Work, it is only requifite here to add a few plain Directions relating to certain Liquors and Syrups ufually prepar'd by Confectioners, which are of two forts, *viz* fome cooling to be us'd in the Spring and Summer, and others ftrong for Autumn and Winter, more efpecially proper to revive and cheer the Spirits during that rigorous Seafon, fome of which are very particular and remarkable

Violet-water

Having provided two good Handfuls of Violets for every two Quarts of Liquor, let them be pick'd and put into Water

Dd 4   with

with a quarter or half a Pound of Sugar When all have been well infused from Morning till Night, at leaft, for five or fix Hours, ftrain the Liquor thro' a Linnen-cloth, or only thro' a Sieve, and fet it by to be iced, according to the Method for all forts of Waters in general, hereafter explain'd in the laft Article of this Chapter

Another Way.

Whenever you have not leifure enough to let the Ingredients infufe, as before, the pick'd Violets may be thrown into a convenient quantity of Water, with the Sugar, and foak'd as long as it is poffible . Then pour off the Liquor out of one Pot into another, as it were beaten Water, till by this continual agitation, it has acquir'd the fmell of Violets, which may be farther improv'd with Orrice-powder Laftly, ftrain your Liquor, and fet it by to cool.

Orange-flower Water

Take only the Leaves of a Handful of Orange-flowers, without the Yellow and Green, thofe being fufficient to give the Smell and Tincture Let thefe Flowers be infufed in a Quart of Water, with a quarter of a Pound of Sugar, in order to be ftrain'd, cool'd and iced, as occafion requires Otherwife, if you would make a quick difpatch, beat up your Water, with the Flowers and Sugar, by pouring them feveral times out of one Veffel into another, and finifh the Work after the fame manner as in preparing Violet water

Jonquil-water

Let a good Handful of thefe Flowers be well pick'd and infus'd in Water, with Sugar, from Morning to Noon, or from Noon till Night; and one Hour before the Liquor is ferv'd up let it be cool'd and iced, after having ftrain'd it thro' a Sieve, or a Linnen-cloth The Work may alfo be more fpeedily done, by beating up the Water, with the Flowers and Sugar, after they have been fteept, as long as the time will admit Then ftrain off the Liquor and pour it into the Ciftern to be iced

Musk.

Musk-rose Water.

Take, as before, only the Leaves of your Rofes, and let them infufe in two Quarts of Water, with a quarter of a Pound of Sugar, otherwife beat and pour them out of one Ewer into another: Then ftraining all fet them by to cool, and it will prove a very delicious Liquor

Pink-water.

Having pick'd the Leaves, throwing away the White and the Green, let them be foak'd in the Morning, or during the Afternoon, with a quarter of a Pound of Sugar, in two Quarts of Water, in order to be ftrain'd and iced: Otherwife pour off the Liquor out of one Pot into another, till it has imbib'd the Scent of the Pinks, after they have been fteept therein for a quarter of an Hour. Laftly, ftrain it thro' a Sieve, or a clean Napkin, and fet it by to cool

Tuberofa-*flower Water.*

The Leaves of thefe Flowers are to be taken likewife, without the Yellow and the Stalks, and infus'd from the Evening till the next Morning, or for the fpace of half a Day; with a fufficient quantity of Sugar. Otherwife, if it be requifite to prepare it fooner, the Liquor may be beat up, as before, by pouring it out of one Pot into another, till it be well impregnated with the *Tuberofa*-flowers Then it muft be ftrain'd thro' a Sieve, or a Linnen-cloth, and well iced.

Jeffamin-water

Take two Handfuls of *Jeffamin*-flowers, and let them infufe in one or two Quarts of Water, with a good quarter of a Pound of Sugar · For a quicker difpatch, the Liquor may be beat up, ftrain'd and fet by to cool

Thus fuch Waters as thefe may be eafily made after the fame manner, of all kinds of Flowers that have a fweet and pleafant Smell.

How

How to ice all ſorts of Waters and Liquors.

For that purpoſe, a kind of Ciſtern in form of a Box is to be provided, which may be of any convenient ſize, but ſet out on the inſide with Tin-moulds, into which the Liquors are to be put. Theſe Moulds or other Veſſels being fix'd in order on this Ciſtern, and cover'd with their reſpective Lids, the remaining void Spaces are to be fill'd up with broken Pieces of Ice, as alſo with ſeveral Handfuls of Salt ſtrew'd up and down every-where and laid over the Moulds, by which means, the Liquors will effectually congeal. A Hole ought alſo to be made in the Ciſtern, about the middle of its height, to give paſſage to the Water, into which the Ice diſſolves by degrees, leſt it ſhould over-flow the Moulds · Then care muſt be taken from time to time, to break the Ice, that is firſt made on the Sur face, and to put Salt again quite round about the Moulds, to cauſe the reſt to freez Laſtly, when the Liquors are ready to be ſerv'd up to Table, the *China*-diſhes and other Cups, are to be fill'd with theſe little Pieces of Ice.

C H A P. II.

Of the iced Waters of Fruits, &c.

Cherry-water.

HAving made choice of Cherries that are very ripe, let them be clear'd from their Stones and Stalks, bruis'd, and ſteep in Water; allowing a Quart for every two Handfuls of Fruit, with a quarter of a Pound of Sugar. If they are not ſet by to infuſe for ſome Hours, the Water muſt be beat up, by pouring it ſeveral times out of one Pot into another, then it may be ſtrain'd, and iced in the Ciſtern.

Strawberry-water.

After the Strawberries have been well pick'd and bruis'd, let the Juice be mingled with ſuch a quantity of Water and Sugar, as may be sufficient to make a pleasant Liquor. Then let all be clarified and strain'd, squeezing out the gross Substance strongly, to give the Water a red Colour. If you have no mind to ice this Liquor it must be made clear, by passing it thro' the Straining-bag, or thro' a Napkin folded into three or four Doubles.

Rasberry-water.

This Water is made after the same manner as the former; the proper Tincture and Smell may also be given to both sorts, without the Colour, by making use of white Strawberries or Rasberries.

Curran-water.

Let the ripest Currans be bruis'd, squeez'd and infus'd in Water, with Sugar for five or six Hours, then strain the Liquor thro' a Sieve, if you would have it iced: Otherwise if it be design'd for a cooling Drink, you need only clarifie it, by passing it thro' the Straining-bag

Apricock-water.

Let very ripe Apricocks, that have been pared, ston'd, and cut into Pieces, be put into Water that has boil'd for some time; adding a quarter of a Pound of Sugar to every Quart of Water: After the Fruit has infus'd for some time, the Work may be finish'd according to the preceeding Method, by often beating and pouring the Liquor out of one Vessel into another: Then it may be strain'd or made clear, in order to be iced, or cool'd

Peach-water

Is prepar'd after the same manner as that of Apricocks; but 'tis observable, That all these sorts of Liquors, made of Fruits, that have no great smell, may be perfum'd with Amber or Musk, at discretion.

Orange-

Orange-water.

Squeez out the Juice of three or four *Sevil*-Oranges, into two Quarts of Water, and steep the Pulp and Zests in the same Water, during some Hours, with a good Piece of Sugar This Liquor for a quicker dispatch, may be beat up by pouring it often out of one Pot into another ; and then it may be strain'd thro a Bag or Sieve, in order to be cool'd or iced : The Juice of a Lemmon added, will give it a more agreeable tartness.

Lemmon-water.

Having in like manner squeez'd out the Juice of three or four Lemmons into two Quarts of Water, let the Pulp and Zests be soak'd therein, with a quarter of a Pound of Sugar, during some Hours: Then strain the Liquor, as before and let it by, to be iced or cool'd.

Orangeade.

To make this Liquor, a greater quantity of Oranges is require than for the common Orange-water, that is to say, six Oranges and two Lemmons, for every Quart of Water The Juice of their is to be squeez'd out, and the Zests left to steep for some time, or else the Water must be beat up by pouring it out of one Pot into another Then pressing the Oranges, the Liquor may be strain'd and set by to cool

Limonnade.

A very good sort of Limonnade may be prepar'd, by allowing three Lemmons to a Quart of Water, with a quarter of a Pound of Sugar, and these Ingredients may be proportionably augmented, according to the Quantity designed After having squeez'd out the Juice of your Fruit into the Water, leave the Pulp and Zest to infuse for a considerable time, then press the Lemmon Pulp and Peel, strain the Liquor, and set it by to cool Several sorts of sweet-smelling Flowers may be added to this Limonnade, to heighten its Scent and Flavour, which may also be done with Amber or Musk, beaten before in a Mortar, with a little Sugar, or Sugar-candy, and afterwards put into the Liquor.   *Ano-*

Another sort of Limonnade.

Let two Quarts of Wine, one Pint of Water, with the Juice and Zests of two Lemmons, be put into an earthen Pan, adding nine or ten Ounces of Sugar, more or less, according to your own inclination and the Quality of the Wine: Afterwards having left these Ingredients to infuse about half an Hour, pour the Liquor thro' the Straining-bag, and dispose of it in Bottles.

Another sort.

Having provided *Cedres,* Citrons, or large Lemmons, take all that part which contains the Juice, and separate them from the Kernels; cutting them into Quarters, or otherwise · In the mean while, let some Sugar be boil'd up to its Blown Quality, that is to say, a Pound for every douzen of Citrons, or Lemmons, and when it has attain'd to that Degree, throw in the Juice; leaving all to boil together, till it return to the Pearled Degree · Then pour the Syrup thro' a Sieve set over an earthen Pan, and keep it in Glass-bottles for use: This Liquor is very delicious and cooling, when a small quantity of it is mingled with Water beaten and pour'd several times out of one Vessel into another, that it may be well diluted.

A *Limonnade* may also be made even with the Leaves of the Citron-tree; which are very odoriferous and full of a pleasant and cooling Juice; but it can only be put in practice in Countries, where such Trees are more common than in these Climates. Lastly, a kind of Liquor may be prepar'd without any Citrons or Lemmons, which nevertheless has the taste of *Limonnade*; by the means of a few drops of Spirit of Salt, being no less useful and wholesome, for the Virtues of this Spirit are very particular and well known; upon which account, it is sometimes used instead of Verjuice in Sauces and Ragoos

White Water, or Virginal Water.

Take as much Milk as may be sufficient to whiten the quantity of Water you would have prepar'd, and to give it a tincture or relish; adding a quarter of a Pound of Sugar to every Quart, and squeezing in the Juice of a Lemmon, which will

much

much promote the pleaſantneſs of its taſte : Then pour it thro'
a Sieve as other Liquors of the like nature, to clear it from the
droſs of the Sugar ; but if you do not deſign to ice it, only let
it paſs thro' the Straining-bag.

Chocolate-water.

This Water, as well as the former, may be us'd in the Winter, and at any time when the above-mentioned Flowers and
Fruits are wanting. It is prepar'd only by grating ſome Chocolate into Water, accordingly as the quantity requires, and adding a good quarter of a Pound of Sugar to every Quart Afterwards, all being well ſteept and infus'd for ſome time, the
Liquor muſt be ſtrain'd in order to be iced or cool'd.

Roſade

Is a pleaſant Liquor made of pounded Almonds, with Milk
and clarified Sugar ; but it will not keep long ; becauſe it is
ſoon apt to grow ſo greaſie and unctuous, that it afterwards
becomes very diſagreeable to the Palate, and conſequently fit
only to be thrown away.

C h a p. III.

Of Liquors that are proper for the Winter-Seaſon.

SOme of the Liquors above-deſcribed, as Orangeade, Limon
nade, Roſade, Chocolate-water, Milk-water, &c may
alſo be uſed in the Winter ; but thoſe that more properly belong to this Quarter, which may likewiſe reciprocally take place
in the other Seaſons, are the particular Waters of Cinnamon,
Coriander, Anis, and Juniper, ſeveral ſorts of Hippocras, Ratafiaz, &c

Cinnamon-water.

Take the beſt Cinnamon well beaten, and infuſe it for the
ſpace of three Days in a Veſſel of double Glaſs, with Roſe
water, or common Water, a Pint of White-wine, and Sugar
pro-

proportionably to the quantity To that purpose, the Veſſel muſt be ſet upon hot Embers, or in a warm Place, and well cover'd; then the Liquor may be ſtrain'd and kept for uſe.

Another Way of Preparing it.

Upon any urgent occaſion, ſome beaten Cinnamon may be taken, that is to ſay half an Ounce for every Quart of Water, and boil'd together with Sugar, till it be half conſum'd : Then ſtrain your Liquor and it will be very pleaſant.

The Water may alſo be boil'd alone, and when it is taken off from the Fire, the beaten Cinnamon is to be thrown in, with a quarter of a Pound of Sugar, as ſoon as the Liquor is cold, it muſt be ſtrain'd as before.

Another more ſimple Water may be made only by cauſing the Cinnamon to be ſteept in it at Night till the next Morning, or from Morning to the Evening of the ſame Day· Then it muſt be ſtrain'd and ſet by to cool after the ſame manner as the above-mentioned Liquors.

Coriander-ſeed Water.

Let a Handful of Coriander-ſeed taken out of its Husk or Cod, be put into a Quart of Water, with a quarter of a Pound of Sugar, leaving all to ſoak, till the Water taſtes ſtrong of the Seeds, and the Sugar is diſſolved· Afterwards, having beat up the Liquor, by pouring it out of one Pot into another, let it be ſtrain'd and cool'd, or iced, accordingly as occaſion ſerves.

Anis-ſeed Water

Take a Handful of Anis-ſeed well cleanſed, and infuſe it in a Quart of Water, with a quarter of a Pound of Sugar: As ſoon as the Water is ſufficiently impregnated, ſtrain it off, and if you think fit, add a little Brandy, to enrich it, when it is not deſign'd to be cool'd or iced.

In the Summer, a ſort of Anis-water may be made, by cauſing the Leaves only of that Plant, eſpecially the tops of them, to be ſteept for a conſiderable time The ſame thing may be done with another ſort of Herb call'd *Burnet*, ſo that theſe two Liquors may well be added to the others that have been before deſcribed and appropriated to the Summer-Seaſon.

Cleve-

Clove-water.

This Water is not made of Cloves alone, becaufe its Scent would be too ftrong and offenfive to the Brain; therefore fome Cinnamon is ufually intermixt, and eight or ten Cloves may be fufficient for a Quart of Water, with a good Piece of Sugar After all has been infus'd for fome time over hot Embers, or in a warm place, the Liquor may be ftrain'd, and it will prove very pleafant.

Juniper-water

Is prepar'd by infufing a Handful of Juniper-berries in two Quarts of Water, with fome Sticks of Cinnamon and Sugar Then the Work may be finifh'd as before; unlefs you have a mind to add a little Brandy, to render the Liquor more pleafant and efficacious.

Kernel-water.

Having pour'd two Quarts of good Brandy into an earthen Pitcher, put in two Ounces of the Kernels of Cherries well pounded, or elfe an Ounce and a half of Apricock-kernels like-wife well pounded, with the Skin; as alfo, almoft a quarter of a Dram of Cinnamon, two Cloves, as much Coriander-feed as may be taken up between two Fingers, nine or ten Ounces of Sugar, and about two Glaffes of boil'd Water, after it is be-come cold: Then the Pitcher muft be well ftopt and all the In gred.ents left to infufe for the fpace of two or three Days Af terwards pour your Liquor thro' the Straining-bag, till it be clear and put it into Bottles, which muft be kept clofe ftopt.

CHAP. IV.

Of Hippocras and fome other Liquors.

THefe Liquors are generally prepar'd for Entertainments du-ring the Winter-feafon, among them the different forts of Hippocras are more efpecially remarkable, *viz.* *Whit*

White Hippocras.

Take two Quarts of good White-wine, with a Pound of Sugar, an Ounce of Cinnamon, a little Mace, two Grains of whole black Pepper and a Lemmon cut into three quarters: Let all infuse together for some time ; and afterwards pass thro' a Straining-bag, which is to be hung up in a convenient place, with a Vessel underneath to receive the Liquor, and kept open by the means of two little Sticks · The Liquor must be strain'd thus three or four times ; but if you perceive upon such Occasions, that it does not pass freely, pour in half a Glass or a whole Glass of Milk, and that will soon produce the desired effect. The smell of Musk or Amber may be given to this Hippocras, by using a Grain of either pounded with Sugar, and wrapt up in Cotton, which may be fasten'd to the end of the Bag through which the Liquor is strained.

Pale Hippocras.

Let half a Pound of Loaf-Sugar broken into small Lumps, with half a Lemmon, three or four Cloves, a little Cinnamon, three or four Grains of white Pepper and Coriander-seed, and a few Almonds cut into pieces, be infus'd for an Hour or half an Hour in a Quart of pale Wine · Then having caus'd all to be stirr'd about and well mingled together let the Liquor pass thro' the Straining-bag, as before

Red Hippocras.

Having pour'd two Quarts of good red Wine into an earthen Pan, take half a Dram of Cinnamon ; a Grain and a half, or two Grains of white Pepper, a little long Pepper, half a Leaf of Mace ; and about a Spoonful of Coriander-seed, all beaten separately, 'tis also requisite to provide a Pound or a Pound and a quarter of Sugar only bruised in a Mortar and six sweet Almonds likewise bruised, with half a Glass of good Brandy Let all these Ingredients be steept in your Wine, for the space of an Hour, taking care that the Vessel into which they are put, be well cover'd and stopt , and let it be stirr'd a little with a Spoon, from time to time, to cause the Sugar to dissolve Then strain the Liquor according to the usual method,

and

and if you please, give it a sweet smell, but the first Liquor that distills from the Straining-bag, must be put into it again two or three several times, till it become very clear Afterwards, set a Bottle with a Funnel underneath, and when it is full, keep it close stopt

Hippocras made more speedily.

Take any sort of Wine that you shall think fit, with the requisite quantity of Loaf-Sugar broken into pieces, adding some beaten Cinnamon, a few Grains of Coriander-seed, three or four Grains of Pepper, and a piece of Lemmon, the Juice of which is to be squeez'd in Otherwise instead of all these Ingredients, only use a little Cinnamon-essence, if you have any at hand, and having strain'd your Hippocras through the Bag with a little Milk, it will very well answer your expectation.

Hippocras without Wine

Let half a Pound of fine Sugar and a little Cinnamon, with the other Ingredients above-specify'd, be put into one or two Quarts of Water, and let all infuse from Morning to Noon, or from Noon till Night, the Vessel being well covered : Then let the Liquor pass thro' the Straining-bag five or six times, and give it the smell of Musk, or Amber, at discretion.

Besides this variety of Hippocras, several Dishes of burnt Wine and burnt Brandy are also serv'd up at Entertainments, the particular manner of preparing which is every where so well known that it needs no description

A delicious sort of Wine.

Put two Lemmons cut into slices, and two Pippins cut in like manner, into a Dish, with half a Pound of Powder-Sugar, a Quart of good *Burgundy*-Wine, six Cloves, a little beaten Cinnamon and Orange flower Water, let all be well cover'd and infus'd for three or four Hours: Then strain it thro' the Bag, and give it a tincture of Amber or Musk, as either is most agreeable to your Palate

C H A P

C H A P.   V.

Several sorts of Ratafiaz.

THis Liquor is at prefent very much in vogue, and may be made of Cherries, Apricocks and Mufcadine-grapes, according to the following Inftructions

Ratafiaz *of Cherries.*

Let your Cherries be bruifed together with their Kernels, and put into an earthen Jarr, or into a wooden Barrel, but a Cask that has held Brandy, is more efpecially proper for that purpofe: To twenty Pounds of thefe Cherries add three Pounds of Rasberries likewife bruiled, with five Pounds of Sugar, three Penny-worth of Cinnamon, a Handful of white Pepper in grain, a few Nutmegs, twenty Cloves, and ten Quarts of good Brandy. Leave the Veffel unftopt during ten or twelve Days, then ftop it up, and let it continue untouched for the fpace of two Months: Thus a greater quantity may be made, by mingling the Ingredients proportionably, and the whole may be enrich'd with fome Drops of Effences and fweet Scents. When the *Ratafiaz* is fit for drinking, the Barrel muft be pierc'd above the Lees, as the Wine-casks are, but if it be kept in an earthen Jarr, it muft be ftrain'd thro' the Bag, and put into other Veffels carefully ftopt up, to be us'd as occafion ferves.

Another Way of making Cherry-Ratafiaz

Having provided ten Pounds of Cherries, let them be bruifed and put into earthen Pitchers with two Quarts of Brandy; then let the Veffels be well ftopt, and fet by for five or fix Days, at the end of which, the Cherries muft be prefs'd in a Linnen-cloth to get out all their Juice In the mean while, let five Pounds of large Currans be boil'd with three Pounds of Sugar, and prefs'd as the Cherries; fo as both forts of Juices may be mingled together, allowing for every Quart of that Liquor, a Quart of Brandy, and a quarter of a Pound of Sugar. Then add the Kernels of your bruifed Cherries, with half a Pound of Coriander-feed, a little Mace, Cloves, Cinnamon and long Pep-

E e 2   per,

per, all pounded together, and fill your Pitchers or other Veffels with the Liquor, leaving it to infuse for the fpace of fix Weeks: Afterwards it muft be pafs'd thro' the Straining-bag, and put again, with the Kernels of Apricock-ftones or Cherry-ftones, into the Pitchers, which are to be kept clofe ftopt, and the *Ratafiaz* may be drawn off clear, upon all occafions.

To give the *Ratafiaz* a tincture of Rasberries, or Strawberries, fome of it may be prepar'd feparately, with Brandy, Sugar and Cinnamon; or elfe the Juice of thefe Fruits may be infus'd at any convenient opportunity in part of the *Ratafiaz*. Orange-flowers may alfo be preferv'd, which will give it a very pleafant fmell, and to improve its colour, the Juice of Mulberries may be us'd mingled with Brandy, and clarified by ftraining it thro' the Bag. Thofe that are prepar'd with Strawberries and Rasberries may alfo be order'd after the fame manner; and a great variety may be produc'd even out of one fort of *Ratafiaz*. Mulberries likewife ferve to bring it to a good confiftence, and make a very fweet Liquor, when infus'd with the other above-mentioned Ingredients.

White Ratafiaz.

Take a Gallon of Water, a Pound of Sugar, an Ounce of Cinnamon, with Cloves, white Pepper and Ginger tied up in a Rag; as alfo fome Nutmeg and Mace, and put thefe Ingredients into a Copper pan fet over the Fire: To clarifie the Sugar, throw in the White of an Egg, clear it well from the Scum, and let all boil together, till at leaft one third part be confum'd; if you perceive that the Liquor has not fufficiently acquir'd the tafte of the Ingredients. Then take it off from the Fire, adding a Quart of Brandy, and let it pafs thro' the Straining-bag, or only thro' a fine Sieve, you may alfo give it a fragrant fmell, with the Juice of white Strawberries or Rasberries, provided feparately in a Pot, as upon other occafions, or elfe it may be done with Orange-flowers. If for want of the red forts of *Ratafiaz*, above-defcribed, you are minded to give this the fame tincture, it may be coloured by the means of Mulberry-juice; or elfe with thick *Orleans*-Wine, or fome other of the like nature; or laftly, with prepared Cocheneal.

Moreover it is expedient for the making of the like white *Ratafiaz*, to keep in a Pot, the Kernels of Cherries and Apricock

cock

cocks fteept in Brandy, which will ferve to enrich it by putting in a little at difcretion.

Apricock-Rataffaz

May be prepar'd two feveral Ways, *viz.* by caufing the Apricocks cut into pieces to infufe in Brandy for a Day or two; at the end of which Term the Liquor muft be ftrain'd thro'. the Bag and impregnated with the ufual Ingredients. Other-wife, the Apricocks may be boil'd in White-wine, and by that means more eafily made clear, adding to every Quart of fuch Liquor, a Quart of Brandy, and a quarter of a Pound of Su-gar, with Cinnamon, Cloves, Mace, and the Apricock-kernels: After all have been well fteept during eight or ten Days, the Liquor muft be ftrain'd again, and put into Bottles or earthen Pitchers, to be kept for ufe.

Mufcadel-Ratafiaz.

Having made choice of the beft Mufcadel-grapes, that are very ripe, let them be well prefs'd; allowing for every Quart of their Juice a Quart of Brandy and a quarter of a Pound of Sugar: Then this Liquor muft be pour'd into earthen Pitchers, with Cinnamon, Cloves, Mace, and a few Grains of Pepper, and left to infufe for the fpace of two or three Days; after-wards let the *Ratafiaz* be clarified by paffing thro' the Strain-ing-bag, and conveniently put into Bottles; adding a Grain of Musk, if it be not fufficiently perfum'd.

C H A P. VI.

Of the Syrups of Flowers.

WE are now come to an Article, that has a nearer relation to the Confectionary Art, than the preceding; altho' fome of the Syrups contain'd therein, are more commonly pre-par'd by Apothecaries, &c.

Syrup of Violets.

Take a Pound of pick'd Violets, and beat them in a Mortar, with half a Glass of Water, to moisten them a little; whilst four Pounds of Sugar are brought to the Pearled Quality: Then taking the Pan off from the Fire, as soon as the Boiling sinks, throw in your Violets and let all be well stirr'd together: Afterwards you are to press them thro' a fine Linnen-cloth, so as the Syrup may be receiv'd into an earthen Pan, and put into Bottles, when cold

The gross Substance that remains may likewise be slipp'd into two Pounds of Pearled Sugar, after the Boiling is settled: Then let all be well mingled together, and pour'd into a Pot; to be us'd in the making of Pastes and Conserve of Violets, according to the Instructions elsewhere laid down. The best Violets for this purpose, are such as are of a dark Purple-colour, not pale, and of a very sweet scent; they ought to be gather'd in the Morning, when no Rain has fallen, and before the Sun has impair'd their Virtue

Another Way.

Syrup of Violets may also be made by an Infusion of the Flowers, according to the following Method · Having caus'd fifteen Quarts of hot Water to be pour'd upon six Pounds of these Flowers, let all soak during eight Hours in an earthen glazed Pot, that has a straight Mouth, which must be close stopt, so as the Virtue and Smell may not exhale: Then the Liquor being heated again, and squeez'd out, add the like quantity of fresh Flowers, which are to be left to infuse in the same manner for eight Hours, and to be strongly press'd again Afterwards Sugar may be put in, as it shall be hereafter shewn in the Article of *Clove-gilliflowers*, or this Infusion may be kept, according to the common practice of Apothecaries.

Syrup of Roses

This Syrup may be well prepai'd after the two manners but now explain'd for that of Violets, or else according to the following particular Way. Take entire Roses, put them into a Pot, as before, and pour in as much warm Water, then cover
the

the Pot, and let all infuse for eight Hours on hot Embers: Afterwards, set them in a Copper-Pan or in the same Pot over a clear Fire, till the Liquor be ready to boil, and squeez it thro' a new Linnen-cloth Lastly, pour this strained Liquor, on the same quantity of other fresh Roses, let them infuse again, and continue to do so for nine Days, changing the Roses every time. This Infusion may be kept a whole Year, without being spoil'd in Glass-Viols, provided they be well stopp'd with Cotton and double Paper, to the end that its Smell and Virtue may be preserv'd

Syrup of Violets may be made after the same manner; but the Infusion will not keep so well

Syrup of Clove-gilliflowers.

Having provided the best sort of Clove-gilliflowers of a lively red colour, weigh out three Pounds of those that are well pick'd, and put them into an earthen Vessel with a straight Mouth, varnish'd on the inside · Then pour in nine Quarts of Spring-water boiling hot, and dip the Flowers in the Water, with a wooden Spatula: Let the Pot be well cover'd, and set over hot Embers for the space of an Hour; at the expiration of which the Infusion must have a little Boiling, in order to be strain'd and squeez'd, it must also be heated again, and pour'd hot on three Pounds of fresh Flowers put into the same Vessel: This Liquor is to be mingled with six Pounds of good Sugar boil'd till it become Pearled, and clarify'd with the White of an Egg: Afterwards, the whole Mess must be pour'd into a Sieve set over an earthen Pan, or else strain'd thro' a fine Linnencloth.

This Syrup is of admirable efficacy against any Infection of the Air and malignant Feavers, and is a great Restorative for Weakness of Body, more especially strengthening the Heart and Brain, when taken alone in a Spoon, or in ordinary Drink.

C H A P.

CHAP. VII.

Of the Syrups of Fruits, &c.

THe remaining forts of Syrups are no lefs advantagious than the former, and of fingular ufe in private Families.

Syrup of Mulberries.

After having caus'd two Pounds of good Sugar to be boil'd till it has acquir'd its Blown quality, let a Pound of Mulberries be thrown in, and give them eight or ten Boilings: Then pour all into a Sieve-fet over an earthen Pan, and put the Syrup into Bottles, to be kept as long as you fhall think fit and us'd as occafion ferves.

It may alfo be made by preffing the Mulberries to get their Juice, which is to be put into a Pan with a Pound of Sugar, and the whole boil'd till it become Pearled   This Syrup is well known to be a Soveraign Remedy for Diftempers of the Throat and other Indifpofitions of the like nature.

Syrup of Cherries.

Let two Quarts of the Juice of Cherries be firft pafs'd thro' the Straining-bag, to cleanfe it, (which is alfo requifite to be done in all other cafes) and then put to a Pound and a half of Sugar: Afterwards having brought the Syrup to the Pearled Degree of Boiling, as before, let it be fet by, and put into Vials, when cold ; to be mingled with beaten Water, in order to make a cooling Drink, upon any emergent occafion.

Otherwife (according to the firft Method for the ordering of Syrup of Mulberries) you need only to bruife the Cherries and throw them into Sugar that has attain'd to its Blown Quality, fo that after ten or twelve Boilings, all may be pour'd into a Sieve, fet over fome Veffel, to receive the Syrup

Moreover having caus'd the Cherries to caft their Juice by preffing them in a Copper-Pan over the Fire, this Juice likewife may be put into Blown Sugar, and left to boil till it becomes Pearled.

Syrup of *Currans* and other forts of cooling *Fruit*.

Having provided Curran-juice clarify'd by paffing it thro'
the Straining-bag, let as much Sugar be made almoft Crack'd :
Then mingle both together, and you'll perceive, that the Syrup has attain'd to the neceffary degree of Boiling   This Syrup
may alfo be prepar'd after the fame manner, as that of Mulberries already explain'd, as well as Syrup of Pomegranates, and
others of the like nature that are proper for cooling.

Syrup of *Apricocks*.

Forafmuch as this Syrup is apt to grow greafie, it ought only
to be made for prefent ufe, according to one of the two following Methods.   Let very ripe Apricocks be cut into pieces and
thrown into Blown Sugar, with the Kernels bruifed, fo as they
may have eight or ten Boilings between Smooth and Pearled :
Then pour all thro' a Sieve, and let the Syrup that runs thro'
be put into proper Veffels, allowing a Pound of Sugar for every half Pound of Fruit.   The other Way is as follows, Having
par'd and flit your Apricocks in the middle, fet them in order
upon little Sticks laid a-crofs an earthen Pan, and put Powder-
Sugar on every Bed or Row; making ufe of the above-mentioned Quantity,   thus they are to be left in a cool place, till
the next Day.   Afterwards flip the Apricocks into a little hot
Water, and turn all out upon a Linnen-cloth to drain without
preffing the Fruit, fo that this Juice together with that which
the Apricocks have already let fall into the Pan, will ferve to
make the Syrup, by caufing them to boil, with the ufual Precautions, to the Pearled Degree.

Syrup of *Quinces*.

This Syrup may be made with the Pulp of Quinces grated
or cut into fmall flices, and fqueez'd in a Linnen-cloth, to get
their Juice, which is to be clear'd by leaving it to fettle in the
Sun, or before the Fire   In the mean while, having caus'd a
Pound of Sugar to be brought to its Blown Quality, let it be
mingled with four Ounces of this Juice, but if the Sugar fhould
by that means be too much deprefs'd, it may have a few Boilings afrefh, till it returns to the Pearled Degree; and the Syrup,
when cold, may be put into Bottles.

F f   *Syrup*

Syrup of Bell-grapes, and others.

Syrup of Bell-grapes is made with their Juice clarified after the same manner as that of Quinces, and four Ounces of it are likewise sufficient for a Pound of Sugar, which must attain to its Blown degree of Boiling, before the Juice is incorporated with it. If the Grapes are more ripe, a Syrup may be made of them, according to the Method before laid down for Mulberries

Syrup of Lemmons may also be prepar'd conformably to these Instructions.

Syrup of Sugar.

Pour Spirit of Wine upon Sugar-candy to the height of a Finger's breadth, and set all over the Fire, till it comes to the Confistence of a Syrup; which may be us'd to very good purpose in promoting the Cure of Distempers of the Lungs and Coughs.

The Juices of all sorts of Fruits.

To get the Juice of Cherries, Currans, Mulberries, Rasberberries, Strawberries, &c you only wrap them up in a new Linnen-cloth, and cause them to be well prefs'd: The Juice of Oranges, Lemmons, Pomegranates, Quinces and other Fruit of the like nature is usually extracted by cutting them first into pieces or round slices, and then squeezing or pressing them, as before Afterwards, take care to clarifie these Juices by putting them into Bottles to settle in the Sun for several Days, and when the gross Substance sinks to the bottom, pour off the Liquor by degrees, in order to be pafs'd thro' the Straining-bag. Then the Juices may be us'd for Syrups, or kept in Bottles, covering their Surface with Oil of Olives, which as occasion serves is to be gently taken away with Cotton Lastly, In the Winter-season these Juices are to be preserv'd in a warm Place to prevent them from freezing, and by this means, they'll be always ready at hand for present use.

F I N I S.

Lightning Source UK Ltd.
Milton Keynes UK
UKOW020727201111

182387UK00005B/6/P